Atlas of Orthopedic Oncology Volume 2

Ajay Puri
Wan Faisham Nu’man Bin Wan Ismail
Editors

Atlas of Orthopedic Oncology Volume 2

An Anatomical Guide to Resection of Extremity Bone Tumours & Tips and Tricks of Biological Bone Reconstruction

Springer

Editors
Ajay Puri
Department of Surgical Oncology
Tata Memorial Centre
Mumbai, Maharashtra, India

Wan Faisham Nu'man Bin Wan Ismail
Prince Court Medical Centre
Universiti Sains Malaysia
Kuala Lumpur, Kuala Lumpur, Malaysia

ISBN 978-981-95-8961-6 ISBN 978-981-95-8962-3 (eBook)
https://doi.org/10.1007/978-981-95-8962-3

This Springer imprint is published by the registered company Springer Nature Singapore Pte Ltd.
The registered company address is: 152 Beach Road, #21-01/04 Gateway East, Singapore 189721, Singapore

Foreword

Having had the opportunity to witness the factors over the past five decades that were important in achieving our current levels of success in musculoskeletal oncology, one clinical factor that is clear is the one that was emphasized by Bill Enneking: while surgeons have little control over the development of metastatic disease, it is the responsibility of surgeons to achieve adequate clear margins, to minimize the chance of local recurrence with the subsequent adverse consequences. This two-volume book is a great asset for surgeons of all levels of training and experience to achieve the resection goals, promoting precision surgery and confidence in resections. Following this anatomical approach advocated by the authors allows the surgeon to avoid important adjacent structures, and maximize functional recovery!

The Case Atlas format highlights the tremendous volume of experience and expertise of Professor Faisham and colleagues, providing comprehensive step-by-step surgical planning and resection tips; the high-definition photographs with clear anatomical structures enhance further understanding of the resection principles! The volume on bone tumours likewise provides well-illustrated, clear steps to the resection and offers a variety of reconstructions ranging from simple effective techniques, to more sophisticated techniques, depending on the circumstances!

All of our tumour patients will benefit from the knowledge imparted. In this two-volume case formatted book!

Emeritus Professor Orthopaedic Surgery
Mayo Clinic, Rochester, MN, USA

Franklin H. Sim

Introduction

In cancer treatment, surgical procedures play a crucial role in removing tumours, preventing their spread and restoring function and aesthetics. Collaborative approach for sarcoma entails close cooperation between surgical, medical and radiation oncologists, pathologists and radiologists, with surgical oncologists playing a crucial role. This collaboration ensures comprehensive and tailored care for each patient. Understanding sarcoma behaviour, the surgical anatomy, compartmentalization concept and margin are important to achieve oncological margin and improve local control and the survival of patients with sarcoma. Preoperative planning with advance radiology, including CT scan, MRI and PET scan, is important for surgical execution for good margin as well as minimized contamination.

The purpose of this atlas is to illustrate radiological evaluations and detailed surgical techniques with anatomical correlation for each procedure. Each anatomical procedure of bone and soft tissue sarcoma is written in detail from simple resection to complex procedures, such as limb salvage with advance microsurgical and flap technique.

Each chapter starts with a simple and important introduction, anatomical description of the surgical structures of limb salvage surgery, anatomical compartmentalization concept for sarcoma growth and relevant structures to achieve surgical oncological margin. Important vital structures related to specific area of sarcoma have been highlighted to achieve optimum functional outcome and, most importantly, to avoid surgical complication to the vital structures. This atlas will facilitate readers in understanding the anatomic correlation of important structures in specific regions for surgical planning for sarcoma resection. Potential sarcoma infiltration, compartmentalization concept and anatomical barrier of sarcoma have been described in a concise manner for better understanding. Potential areas of infiltration and contamination by sarcoma for evaluation and surgical planning have also been highlighted.

Preoperative radiological assessment and the importance of sarcoma extension and surgical margin, which plays a crucial role in achieving local control, have been explained. This atlas also provides concise critical points used during most limb salvage surgeries combined with labelled preoperative MRI as well as step-by-step live surgery photographs. Each topic will highlight the radiological evaluation, including an MRI, as part of the assessment prior surgery. Relevant structures related to sarcoma involvement, specific areas of involvement and important neurovascular structures, which are critical for major decision, are also discussed. The assessment includes a series of important labelled combine images of MRIs for a better understanding of this crucial part of sarcoma management. The assessment includes combine axial, sagittal, or coronal with labelling for better understanding of each level evaluation of sarcoma. Serial MRI images for evaluation of vital structures are also included.

The main part of this atlas is the step-by-step surgical procedures with high-quality labelled surgical photos for all the anatomical region of sarcoma management. The procedures start with general surgical access and each anatomical layer of surgical procedures for sarcoma resection. Vital structures, including the major vessels and nerves, and other relevant important structures have been labelled for a better understanding of its correlation with the main sarcoma prior resection. This atlas has been designed to describe simple to complicated procedures, including different surgical approaches, and modifications for sarcoma resection. Options of bone and joint reconstruction have been described in detail and advanced techniques of microsurgeries and flaps are also included. Surgical procedures have been presented in a clear and easily comprehensible manner using both important anatomical and surgical landmarks. Attractive labels and arrows are inserted alongside the figures. The cases illustrated comprise the main surgical approach of each anatomical site with a view to share the surgical principles to achieve oncological margin and optimum function in complex heterogenicity of sarcoma in general.

This book aims to share armamentarium of my surgical procedures to all orthopaedic oncology surgeons who dedicate their lifelong journey to salvage limb for patients with sarcoma. It will also be a valuable reference and excellent guidebook for junior surgeons and trainees' in orthopaedic surgical oncology specialty.

Contents

Bone Tumour Resection and Reconstruction: Lower Limb

Proximal Femur Resection and Replacement 3
Wan Faisham Nu'man Bin Wan Ismail

Extra-Articular Proximal Femur Resection 23
Wan Faisham Nu'man Bin Wan Ismail

Total Femur Resection and Replacement 39
Wan Faisham Nu'man Bin Wan Ismail

Distal Femur Resection and Reconstruction 53
Wan Faisham Nu'man Bin Wan Ismail

Proximal Tibial Resection and Reconstruction 91
Wan Faisham Nu'man Bin Wan Ismail, Muhamad Naseh Sajadi Budi, Muhammad Phetrus Johan, Istan Irmansyah Irsan, Vivek Ajit Singh, Azura Mansor, and Nor Faissal Yasin

Distal Tibia Resection and Reconstruction 125
Wan Faisham Nu'man Bin Wan Ismail, Arman Zaharil Mat Saad, Wan Azman Wan Sulaiman, Zulmi Wan, and Ahmad Sukari Halim

Distal Tibia Resection and Endoprosthesis Reconstruction 143
Vivek Ajit Singh

Fibula Resection 159
Wan Faisham Nu'man Bin Wan Ismail

Foot Tumour 175
Wan Faisham Nu'man Bin Wan Ismail

Intercalary Resection and Reconstruction 203
Wan Faisham Nu'man Bin Wan Ismail, Ferdiansyah Mahyudin, Mohammad Hardian Basuki, Istan Irmansyah Irsan, Achmad Fauzi Kamal, Vivek Ajit Singh, Azura Mansor, Nor Faissal Yasin, and Ajay Puri

Bone Tumour Resection and Reconstruction: Upper Limb

Scapulectomy 223
Wan Faisham Nu'man Bin Wan Ismail

Resection Proximal Humerus and Shoulder Girdle 253
Wan Faisham Nu'man Bin Wan Ismail

Total Humerus Resection and Replacement 277
Wan Faisham Nu'man Bin Wan Ismail

Distal Humerus Resection 285
Wan Faisham Nu'man Bin Wan Ismail

Radial Neck-to-Humerus Trochlea Transposition 293
Ajay Puri, Rudra Pratap Singh, and Ashwin Prajapati

Distal Radius Resection 303
Wan Faisham Nu'man Bin Wan Ismail and Ajay Puri

Editors and Contributors

About the Editors

Ajay Puri currently serves as the Chief of Orthopaedic Oncology and Professor and Head of Surgical Oncology at the Tata Memorial Centre. He has held esteemed positions including founder President of the Indian Musculoskeletal Oncology Society, Past President of the Asia Pacific Musculoskeletal Tumor Society, and past Chairman of the Indian Orthopaedic Association (Oncology). He is a member of the Global Steering Committee of the International Sarcoma Kindred Study (ISKS), the largest multi-institutional international trial aimed at understanding the genetic background of sarcomas. He has pioneered the development of a low-cost indigenous megaprosthesis, extensively used in India and other Asian and African nations. Additionally, he has popularized novel methods of biological reconstruction after oncologic resection. He serves on the editorial board of the *Journal of Bone & Joint Surgery* (formerly JBJS [Br]), *Bone & Joint-360*, *Bone & Joint Open*, and *Sarcoma*. He has published numerous papers and book chapters, establishing himself as a leading authority in Orthopaedic Oncology.

Wan Faisham Nu'man Bin Wan Ismail is an orthopaedic oncology surgeon at Prince Court Medical Center, a prestigious oncology centre in Malaysia. He previously served as a professor and consultant surgeon at Universiti Sains Malaysia and is renowned as one of the pioneers of limb salvage surgery for orthopaedic cancer. Throughout his career, he has been involved in numerous clinical research endeavours and multidisciplinary collaborations in oncology. For his significant contributions to the field, he has been honoured with five distinguished awards and appointed as the International Advisor to the Asian Pacific Musculoskeletal Oncology Society. He has authored over 100 research papers in medical journals and 4 textbooks related to his expertise. Currently, he is a leading figure in oncology applicable to sarcomas in Malaysia and is recognized as an orthopaedic oncology expert within ASEAN and the Asia Pacific region. He is actively involved in training both national and international orthopaedic oncology fellows. His research interests primarily focus on survival and functional outcomes following surgery for orthopaedic cancer. Internationally, his surgical method utilizing allograft and vascularized tissue has been recognized as a trademark in the field.

Contributors

Mohammad Hardian Basuki Orthopaedic and Traumatology Department, Faculty of Medicine of Universitas Airlangga/Dr. Soetomo General Academic Hospital, Surabaya, Indonesia

Muhamad Naseh Sajadi Budi Department Orthopaedic and Traumatology, Hasan Sadikin General Hospital, Padjadjaran University, Bandung, Indonesia

Ahmad Sukari Halim Reconstructive Sciences Department, School of Medical Sciences, Universiti Sains Malaysia, Kubang Kerian, Kelantan, Malaysia

Istan Irmansyah Irsan Department of Orthopaedic Surgery, Saiful Anwar Hospital, Brawijaya University, Malang, Indonesia

Wan Faisham Nu'man Bin Wan Ismail Prince Court Medical Center, Kuala Lumpur, Malaysia

Orthopaedic Oncology Reconstructive Unit, Universiti Sains Malaysia, Kubang Kerian, Kelantan, Malaysia

Muhammad Phetrus Johan Department Orthopaedics and Traumatology, Faculty of Medicine, Hasanuddin University, Makassar, Indonesia

Achmad Fauzi Kamal Department of Orthopaedic and Traumatology, Faculty of Medicine, Universitas Indonesia/Dr. Cipto Mangunkusumo General Hospital, Jakarta, Indonesia

Ferdiansyah Mahyudin Orthopaedic and Traumatology Department, Faculty of Medicine of Universitas Airlangga/Dr. Soetomo General Academic Hospital, Surabaya, Indonesia

Azura Mansor Department of Orthopaedic Surgery, Faculty of Medicine, University Malaya, Kuala Lumpur, Malaysia

Ashwin Prajapati Department of Surgical Oncology, Tata Memorial Centre, Mumbai, India

Ajay Puri Department of Surgical Oncology, Tata Memorial Centre, Mumbai, India

Arman Zaharil Mat Saad Plastic Reconstructive & Microsurgery, MSU Medical Centre, Management and Science University of Malaysia, Shah Alam, Selangor, Malaysia

Rudra Pratap Singh Department of Surgical Oncology, Tata Memorial Centre, Mumbai, India

Vivek Ajit Singh Department of Orthopaedic Surgery, Faculty of Medicine, University Malaya, Kuala Lumpur, Malaysia

Wan Azman Wan Sulaiman Reconstructive Sciences Department, School of Medical Sciences, Universiti Sains Malaysia, Kubang Kerian, Kelantan, Malaysia

Zulmi Wan Prince Court Medical Center, Kuala Lumpur, Malaysia

Nor Faissal Yasin Department of Orthopaedic Surgery, Faculty of Medicine, University Malaya, Kuala Lumpur, Malaysia

Bone Tumour Resection and Reconstruction: Lower Limb

Proximal Femur Resection and Replacement

Wan Faisham Nu'man Bin Wan Ismail

Introduction

The proximal femur is a common site for sarcoma and metastatic bone disease. Resection and reconstruction of proximal femur tumour has been shown to achieve good functional outcome and long-term survival using prosthesis. Gait impairment still remains an issue owing to poor abductor 'gluteus medius' tendon insertion and incorporation to the prosthesis.

Surgical Anatomy

Anatomical boundaries and tumour extension are important to improve oncological clearance and minimize the risk of local recurrence. Anatomical boundaries of the proximal femur:

- The anterior compartment—the vastus lateralis and quadriceps femoris muscle
- Medially, the adductor brevis and magnus and illiopsoas tendon insertion
- Posterior, the gluteus maximus attachment and short rotator
- For proximal lesions, the gluteus medius attachment and hip capsule

W. F. N. B. W. Ismail (✉)
Prince Court Medical Center, Kuala Lumpur, Malaysia

Orthopaedic Oncology Reconstructive Unit, Universiti Sains Malaysia, Kubang Kerian, Kelantan, Malaysia

A. Puri, W. F. N. B. W. Ismail (eds.), *Atlas of Orthopedic Oncology Volume 2*,
https://doi.org/10.1007/978-981-95-8962-3_1

Most of the proximal femoral resection is performed through an intra-articular approach. The retained labrum and part of the hip capsule is used to anchor the head of the femur to improve stability.

Three important structures can be displaced from their normal anatomical by a proximal femur tumour:

- The sciatic nerve, which leaves the pelvis via the greater sciatic foramen, is inferior to the piriformis muscle and progresses down to the posterior compartment and can be displaced or involved in tumour with posterior extension. Mobilization and protection of the sciatic nerve are major steps in posterior approach for proximal femur resection.
- The femoral artery can be displaced and is sometimes situated over the margin in anterior extension of the tumour. The femoral vessels lies on the psoas, which separates it from the hip joint, pectineus and adductor longus and is at risk during resection. An anterior approach and mobilization of the femoral vessels are important steps for achieving margins control and to minimize injury.
- The profunda femoral artery, which passes between the adductor longus and magnus and enters the medial fascial compartment of the thigh, can be displaced medially by extension of the tumour and has to be secured during resection.

Assessment

A large proximal femur tumour will displace the sciatic nerve and femoral vessels. Hence, MRI evaluation of these structures is important. Anatomical boundaries around the proximal femur are an important part of the assessment to achieve a wide surgical margin:

- Distal marrow extension for femoral osteotomy
- Hip joint capsule and intra-articular involvement
- Gluteus medius and all the short rotator and iliopsoas tendon attachments
- Group of muscles that envelope the proximal femur for direct infiltration

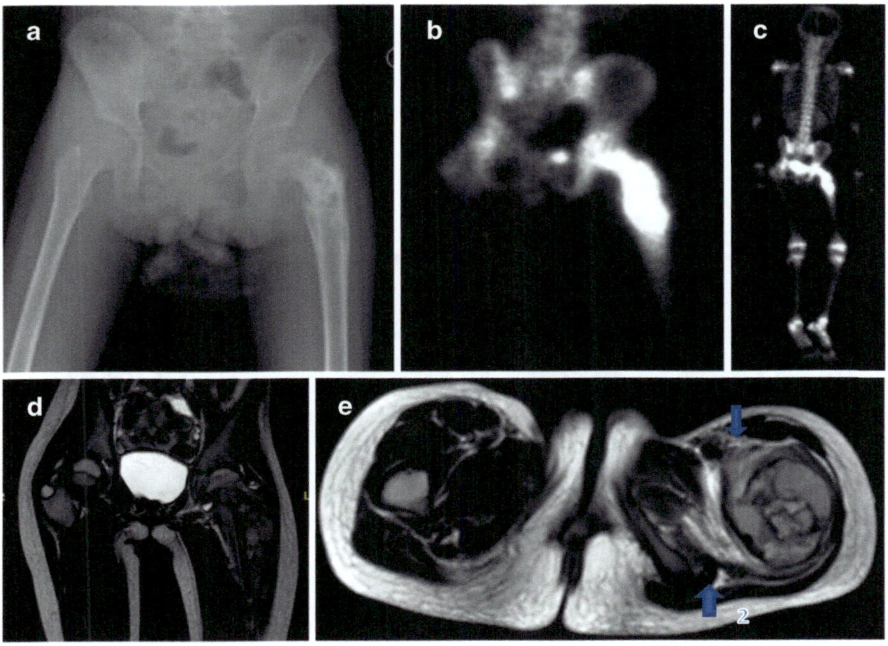

1. Femoral vessels
2. Sciatic nerve

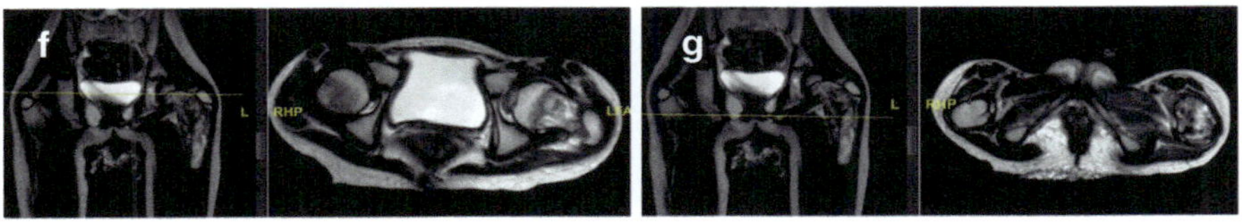

A 6-year-old girl with localized Ewing's sarcoma responded well to chemotherapy. The tumour was confined to intraosseous extent and had not infiltrated the surrounding muscle. The hip joint was spared (Fig. 1a–g).

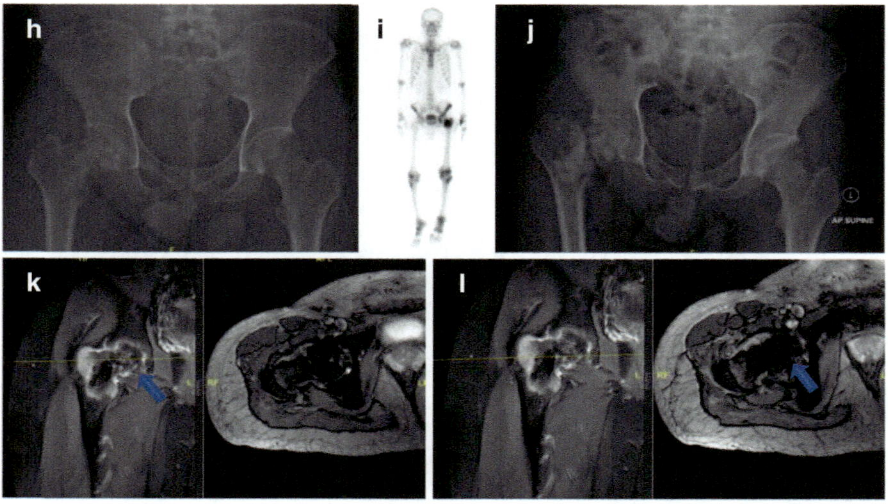

- Hip joint contamination

A 20-year-old man with osteosarcoma proximal femur with pathological fracture neck of the femur. MRI showed localized tumour with intra-articular contamination that required extra-articular resection for clear margin (Fig. 1h–l).

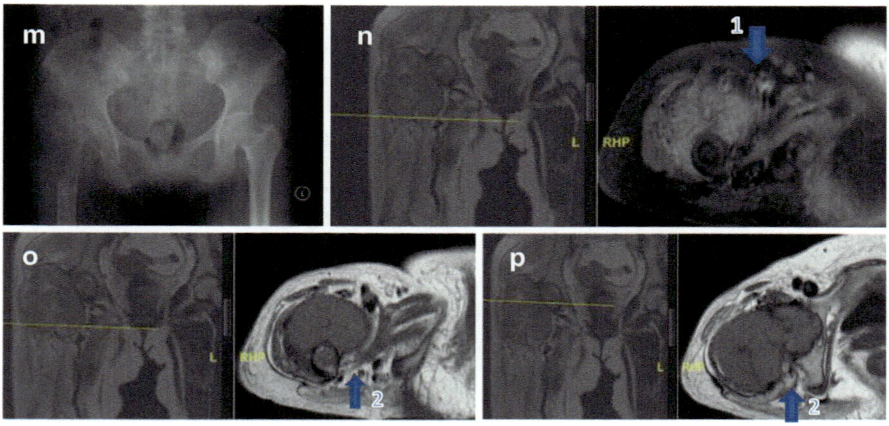

1. Femoral vessels
2. Sciatic nerve

Thyroid metastases with extraosseous extension and pathological fracture. The anteromedial mass displaced the femoral artery; however, the sciatic nerve was spared (Fig. 1m–p).

Surgical Steps

Lateral Approach-Wide Resection of the Proximal Femur

The incision is centred over the greater trochanter and posteriorly directed to PSIS along the gluteus maximus fibres. The gluteus maximus attachment is detached from the posterior femur, and all the external rotator and sciatic nerves are exposed. The first femoral perforator within the gluteus muscle insertion is ligated and can sometimes cause excessive bleeding. The circumflex femoral artery at the inferior border of the quadratus femoris also must be ligated before the entire short rotators and capsule are sectioned to expose the hip joint (Fig. 2a–c).

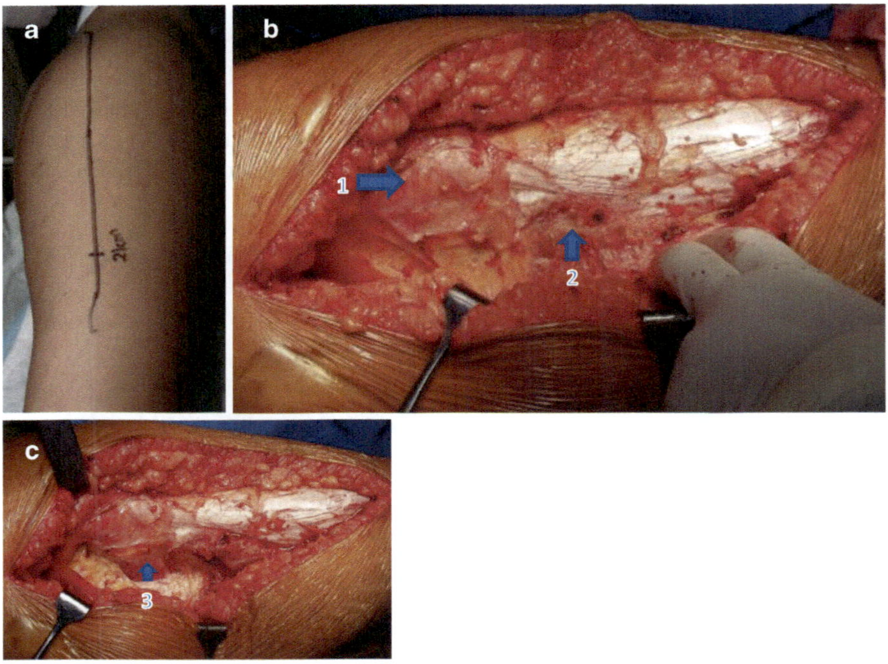

1. Greater trochanter
2. Gluteus maximus insertion
3. Short rotators and quadratus femoris

The vastus lateralis muscle is elevated from the femur origin ‘vastus ridge’ leaving in a cuff of muscle around the femur, including the superior margin of the vastus intermedius. This can act as an oncological barrier for resection. Remnant of the vastus lateralis can be used as coverage for the lateral part of a prosthesis. However, when the tumour involves the lateral part, the entire superior part of vastus lateralis must be removed (Fig. 2d).

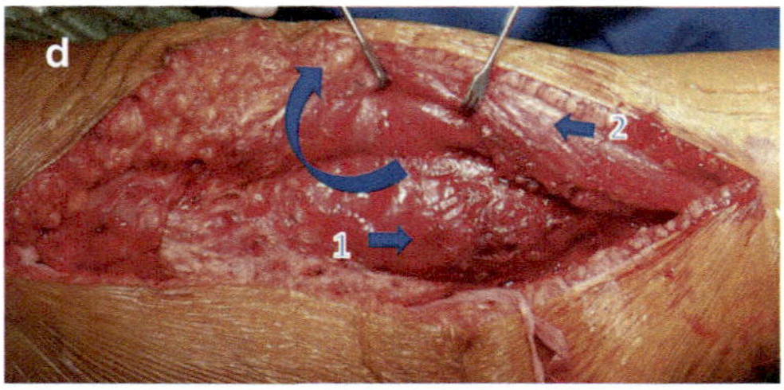

1. Vastus intermedius
2. Vastus lateralis elevate through plane from posterior border

The greater trochanter can be osteotomized if it does not compromised the oncological margin. The entire posterior and anterior capsule can be exposed and cut to deliver the entire head of the femur. The inferior capsule and lesser trochanter are visualized posteriorly by lateral subluxation of the hip in flexion and internal rotation. Preservation of the capsule and short rotators is important for reconstruction and purse-string suture around the neck of the prosthesis to prevent dislocation (Fig. 2e, f).

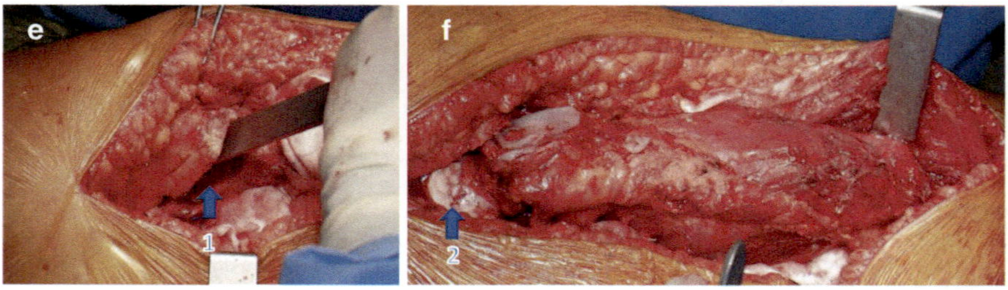

1. Trochanteric osteotomy
2. Femoral head

The femoral head is dislocated, and the medial border of the adductor compartment is visualized for evaluation and resection of respecting the oncological margin. Care must be taken to identify the profunda femoral artery and clear it from the resection margin (Fig. 2g, h).

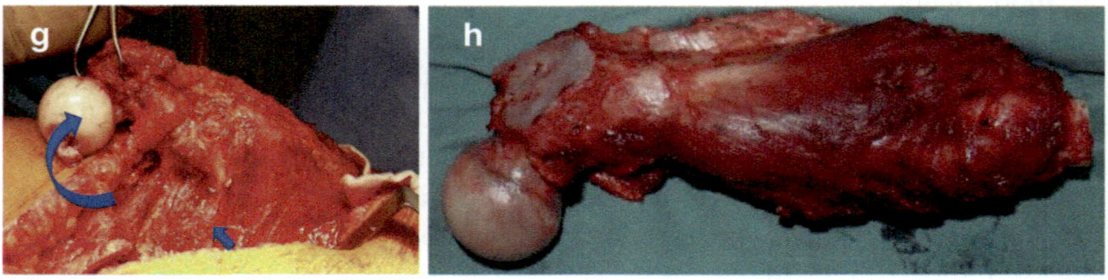

- Adductor muscle group attachment at the medial border of femur

Options for Proximal Femur Reconstruction

- Modular endoprosthesis replacement
- Allograft prosthesis composites

Modern modular endoprosthesis allows for accurate segment length reconstruction. The proximal femoral component has multiple holes for soft tissue reconstruction and is porous coated to improve surface for bony integration and attachment. The prosthesis bone junction is also covered with porous coating for better integration with formation of an extracortical bone bridge interface. Position and rotation of the proximal femur replacement is crucial to achieve correct anteversion of the hip and can be done by positioning the knee and leg in 90/90 prior to final insertion (Fig. 3a–f).

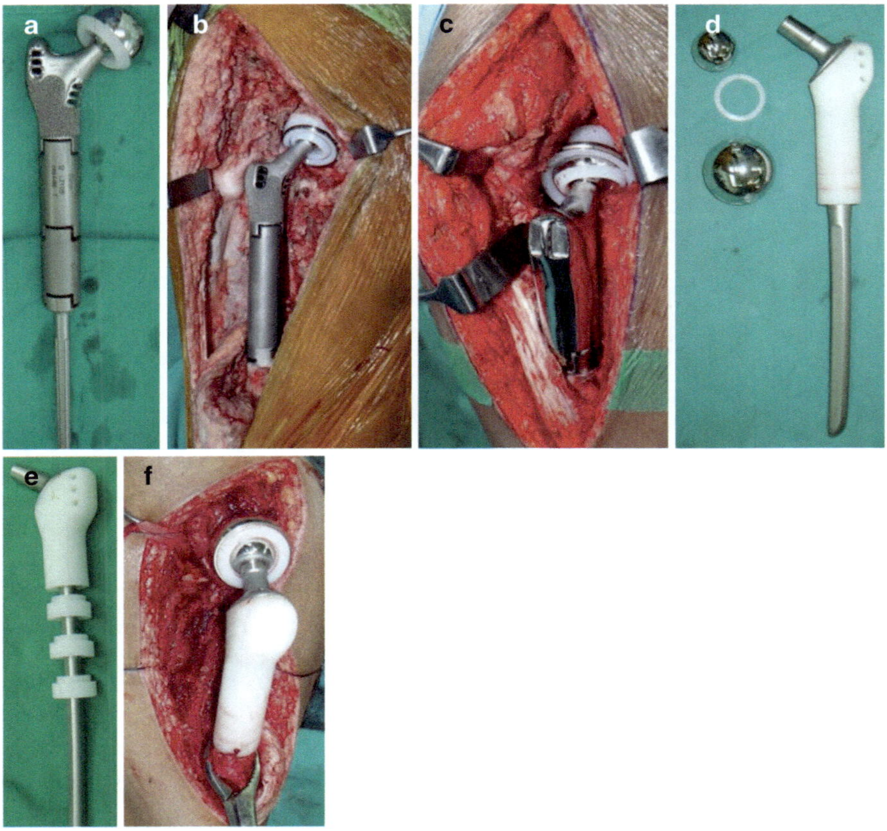

An allograft is another option for proximal femur replacement. Segment loss reconstruction is built by a cemented allograft. In cases of metastases, we cement the entire allograft and stem to the distal femur for immediate stability and ambulation. Advantages of an allograft are that it provides remnant of the abductor tendon for gluteus medius reconstruction and minimizes abductor lurge. An allograft is also used for the revision of proximal femur loosening as biological reconstruction. Combination with a vascularized fibula graft can improve the entire construct (Fig. 3g–k).

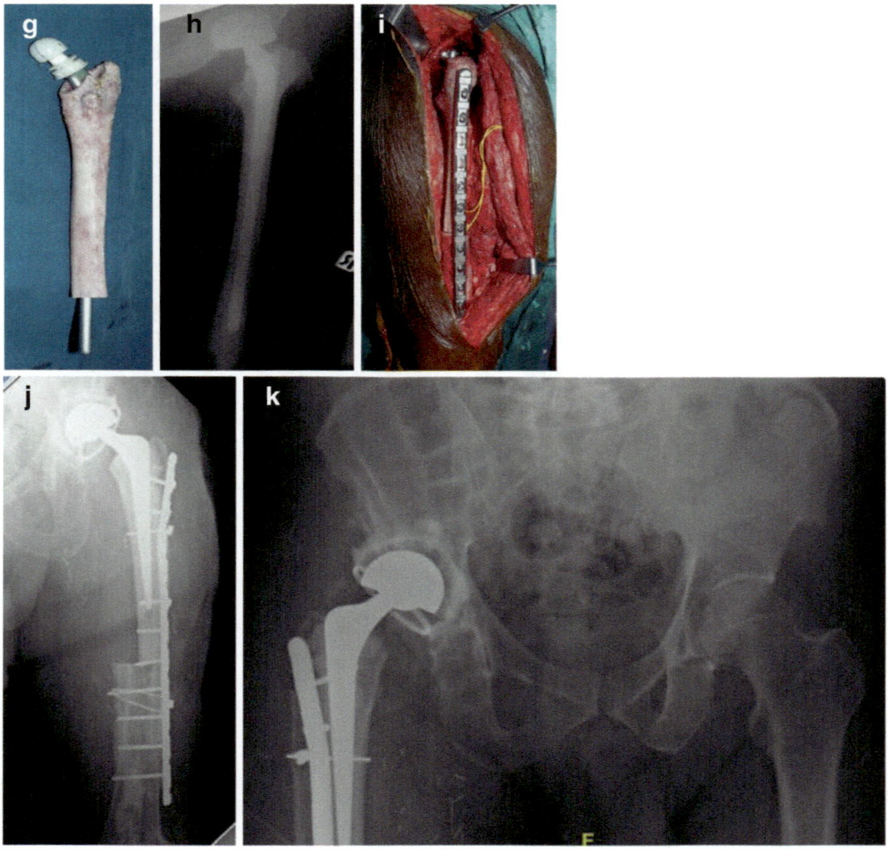

Reconstruction of the gluteus medius is important to maintain hip joint function. However, in majority of the cases, the abductor function is weak, and reconstruction is suboptimal.

Hip joint stability can be achieved by various methods:

- Purse-string the hip capsule (Fig. 3l–n)
- Dacron graft or trevira tube
- Constrained acetabulum cup

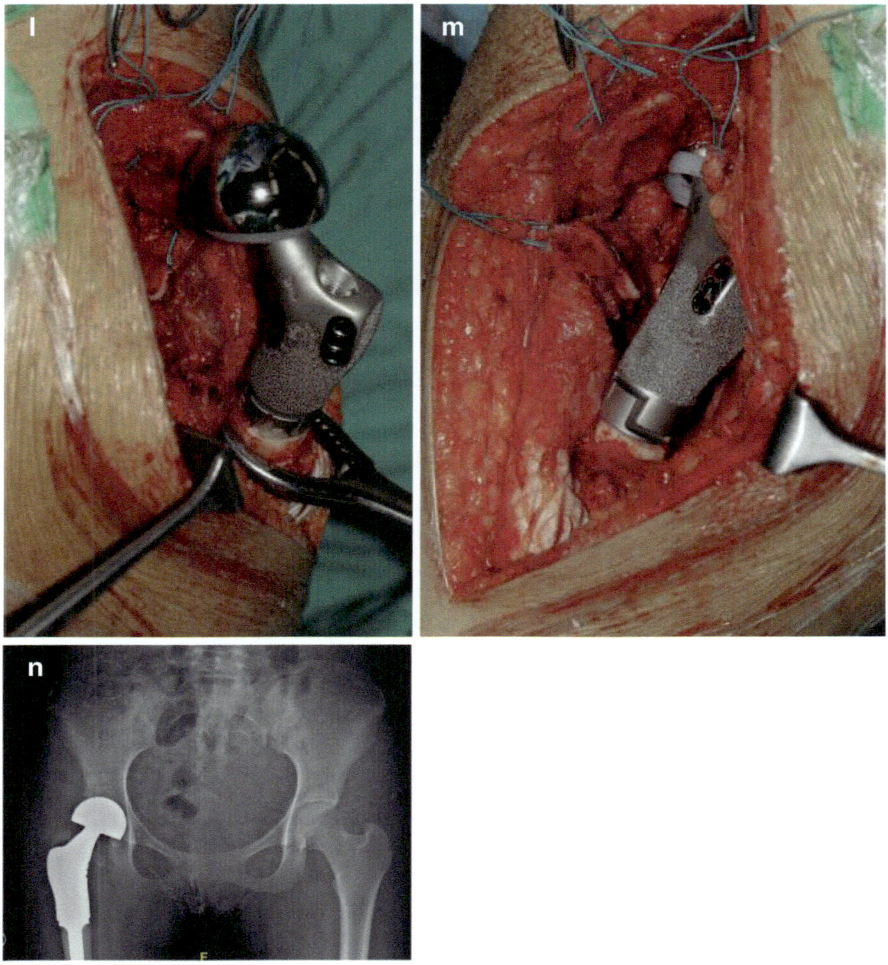

Inadequate capsule for purse-string sutures can be augmented with a dacron graft or trevia tube to improve hip joint stability (Fig. 3o–q).

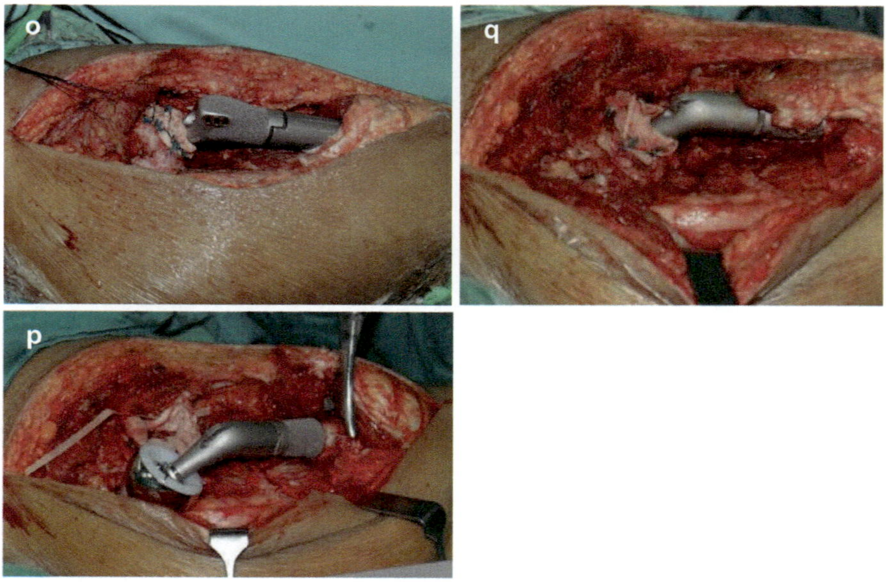

Capsular reinforcement purse-string technique can be used to improve stability during total hip replacement (Fig. 3r–t).

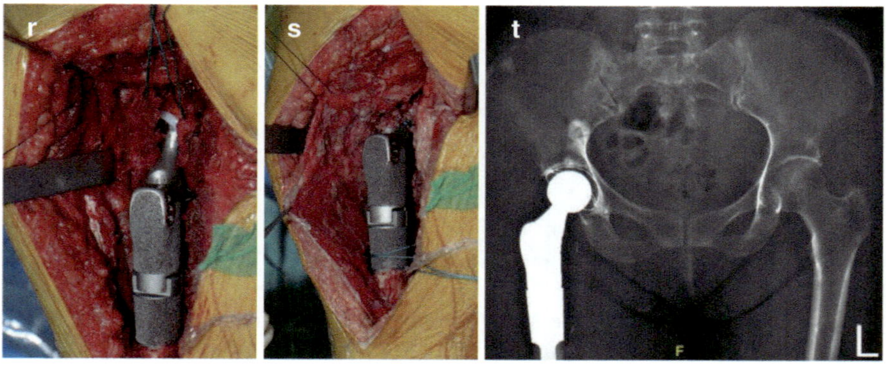

Constrained acetabulum cup is an option when the hip capsule and acetabulum labrum have to be removed for oncological clearance (Fig. 3u, v).

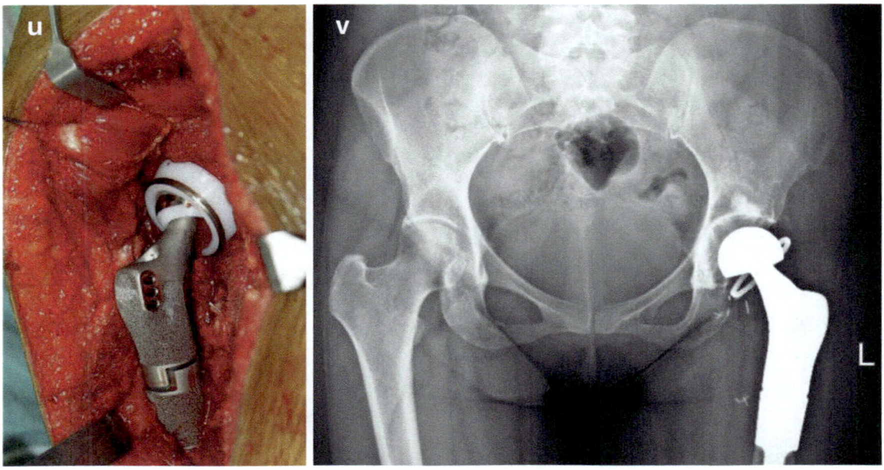

In children, unipolar replacement (sizes 28, 32 and 36) is an option for a smaller femoral head (Fig. 3w–y).

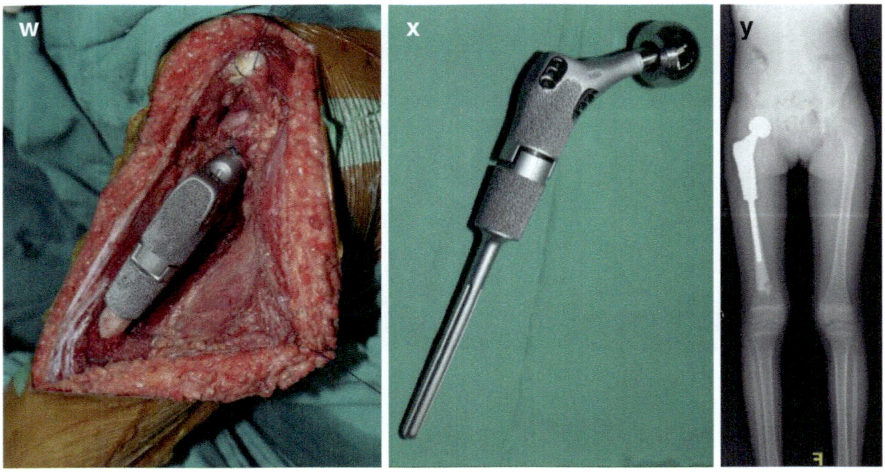

Anterior Approach-Wide Resection of the Proximal Femur

Sarcoma with extensive anterior soft tissue extension requires exploration of the femoral artery and nerve (Fig. 4a–d). Motor unit to the rectus femoris must be maintained for knee extension function. This approach with superior extension is also suitable for extraarticular resection of the hip joint.

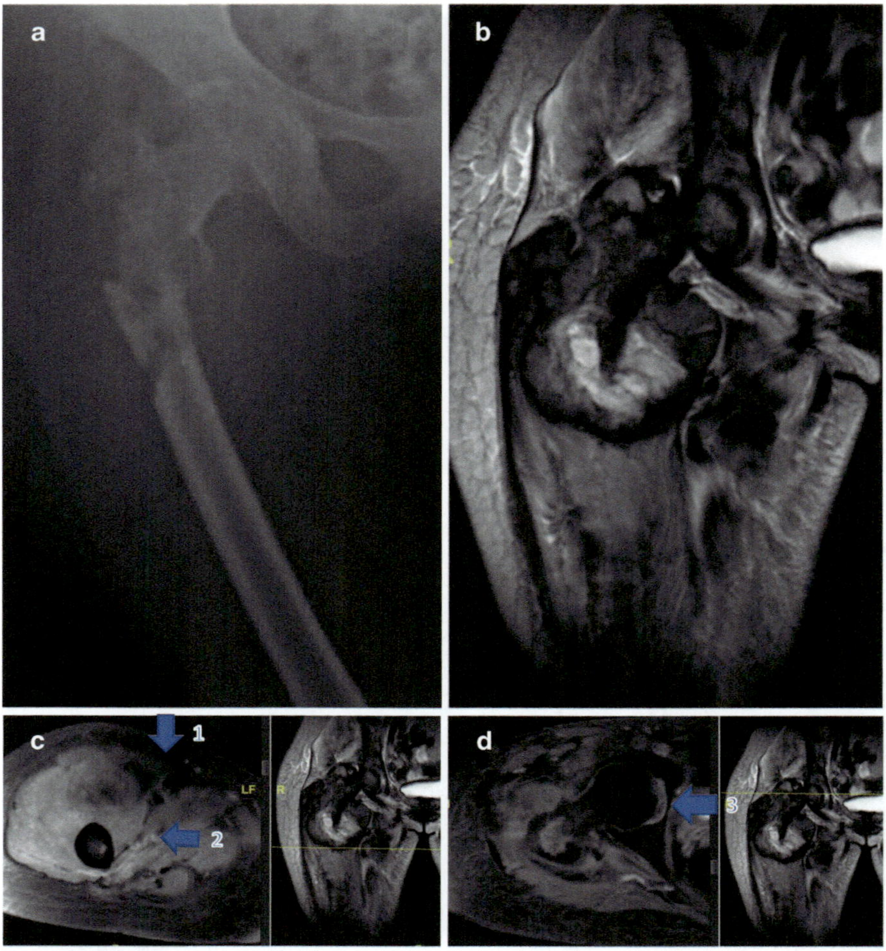
a
b
c
1
2
LF
R
d
3

1. Femoral artery
2. Profunda femoral vessels and adductor muscle infiltration
3. Hip joint free of tumour infiltration

Surgical Steps

- Exploration of the femoral vessels and nerve with motor unit to the sartorius, vastus lateralis and rectus femoris muscle. The proximal part of the vastus intermedius and vastus lateralis are usually included as the surgical margin (Fig. 4g, h).
- The iliopsoas tendon can be identified below the femoral vessels and resected as the surgical margin.
- Posterior approach by reflecting the entire gluteus maximus and exploration of the sciatic nerve. Part of the gluteus maximus attached to the proximal femur is resected as part of the oncological margin.
- Elevation of the entire tumour after dislocation of the hip joint. The adductor compartment is evaluated for surgical margins and resection. The profunda femoral artery is usually ligated and included in the resection margin (Fig. 4i, j).
- The final reconstruction needs a stable hip joint using a constrained cup. Hip function is compromised due to extensive tissue resection. However, with good motor unit for knee extensor, the patient can ambulate with the help of a walking stick (Fig. 4k, l).

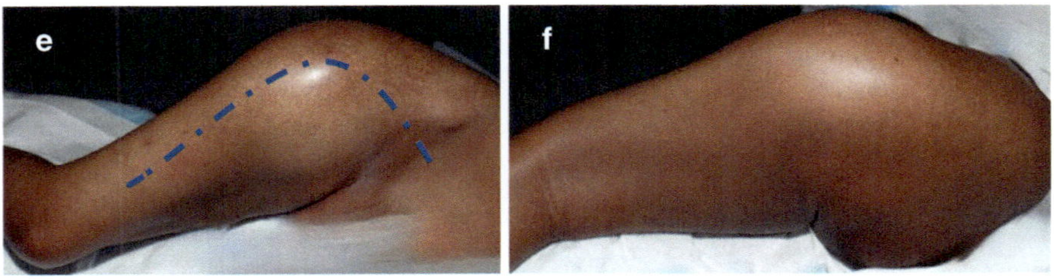

- Line of incision (Fig. 4e, f)

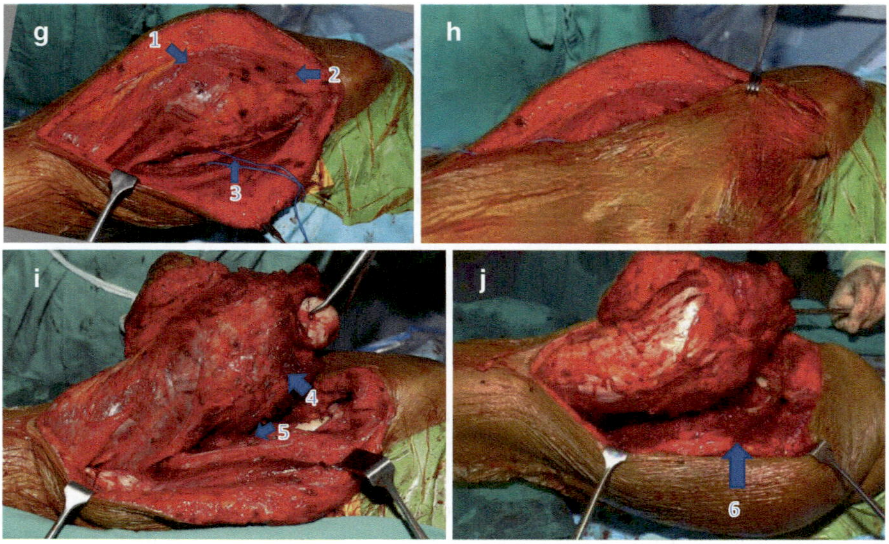

1. Greater trochanter
2. Gluteus medius
3. Femoral vessels
4. Lesser trochanter and remnant iliopsoas
5. Profunda femoral artery
6. Sciatic nerve

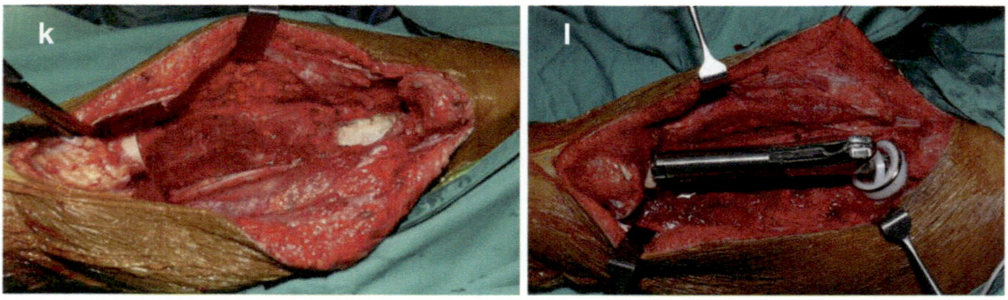

Sarcoma with Extensive Circumferential Soft Tissue Extension

Sarcoma with massive circumferential soft tissue extension of the femur requires exploration of the sciatic nerve and femoral neurovascular structures. Soft tissue extension includes the proximal vastus lateralis, intermedius and all the rotators (Fig. 4a–d). The adductor brevis and magnus must be resected as a wide margin surgery (Fig. 4e–i). Soft tissue reconstruction and closure is possible with mobilization of the tensor fascia latae, gluteus maximus and remnant of the gluteus medius (Fig. 4j–l).

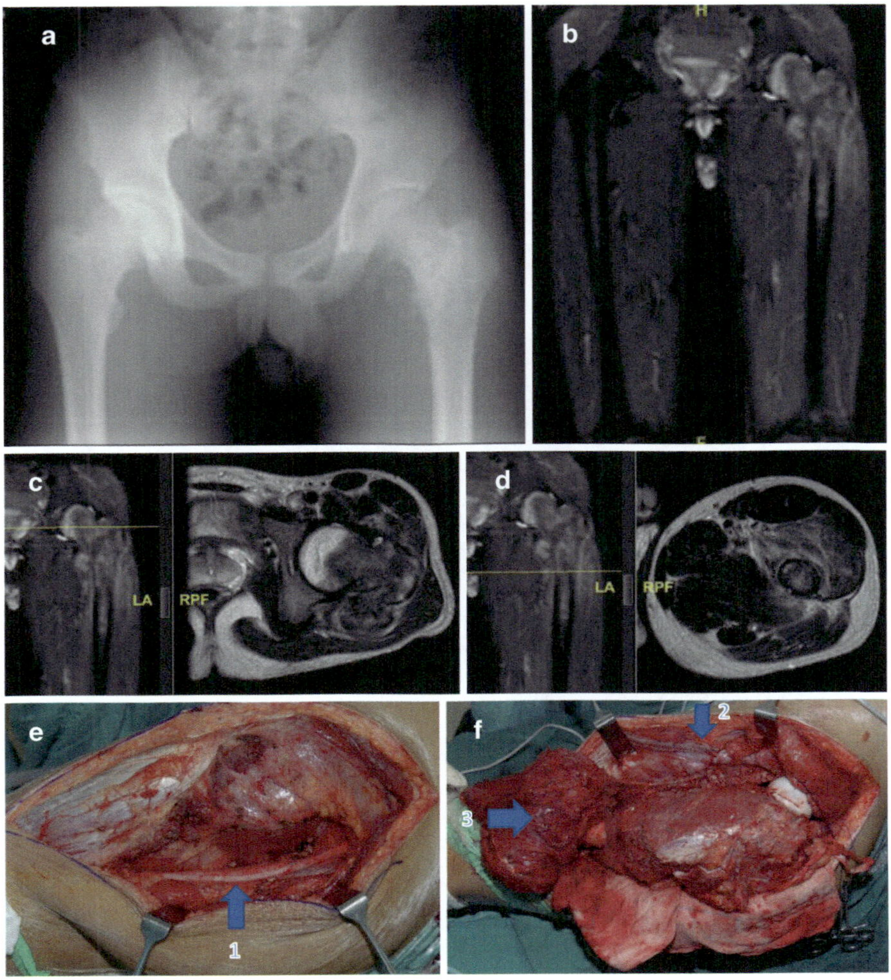

1. Sciatic nerve
2. Femoral vessels
3. Vastus lateralis

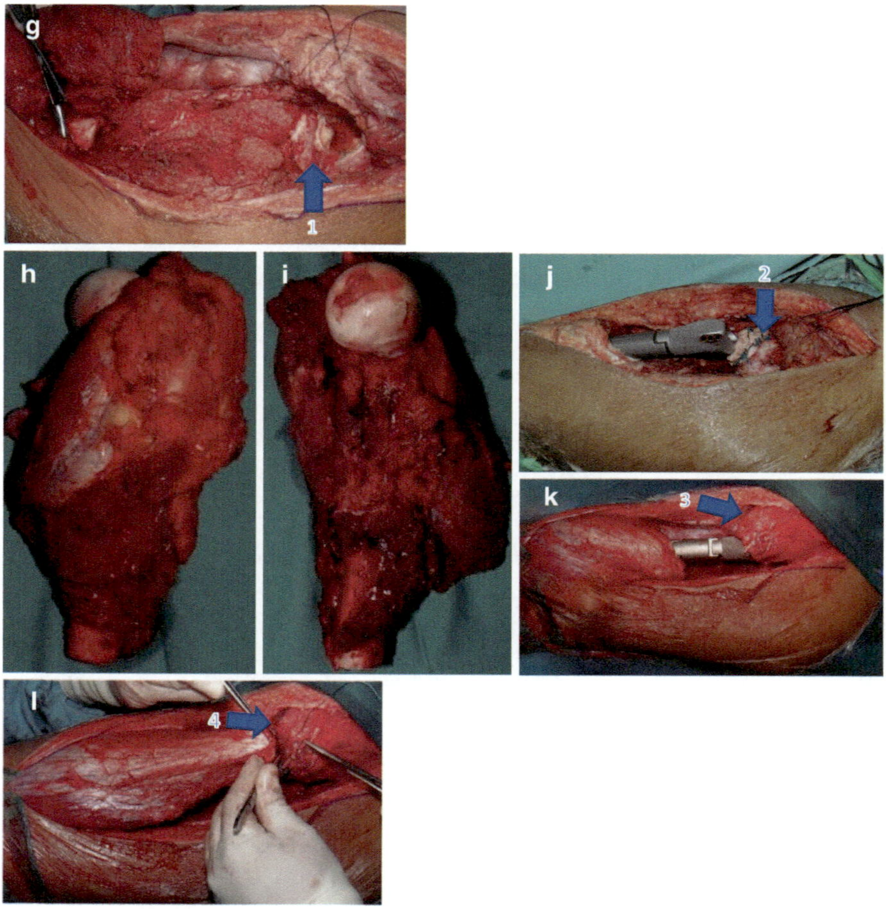

1. Minimal capsule remnant for reconstruction
2. PTFE graft for hip stability
3. Gluteus medius 'abductor' reattachment to prosthesis trochanter
4. Soft tissue reconstruction

Sarcoma with Capsular and Acetabular Labrum Extension

Proximal sarcoma with superior extension to the capsule requires acetabulum labrum and rim resection for an adequate oncological margin (Fig. 5a–k). Reconstruction of the hip joint is by a constrained cup to achieve stability due to loss of soft tissue and rim for reconstruction (Fig. 5l–n). Trendelenburg gait is expected due to poor abductor tendon attachment to the endoprosthesis.

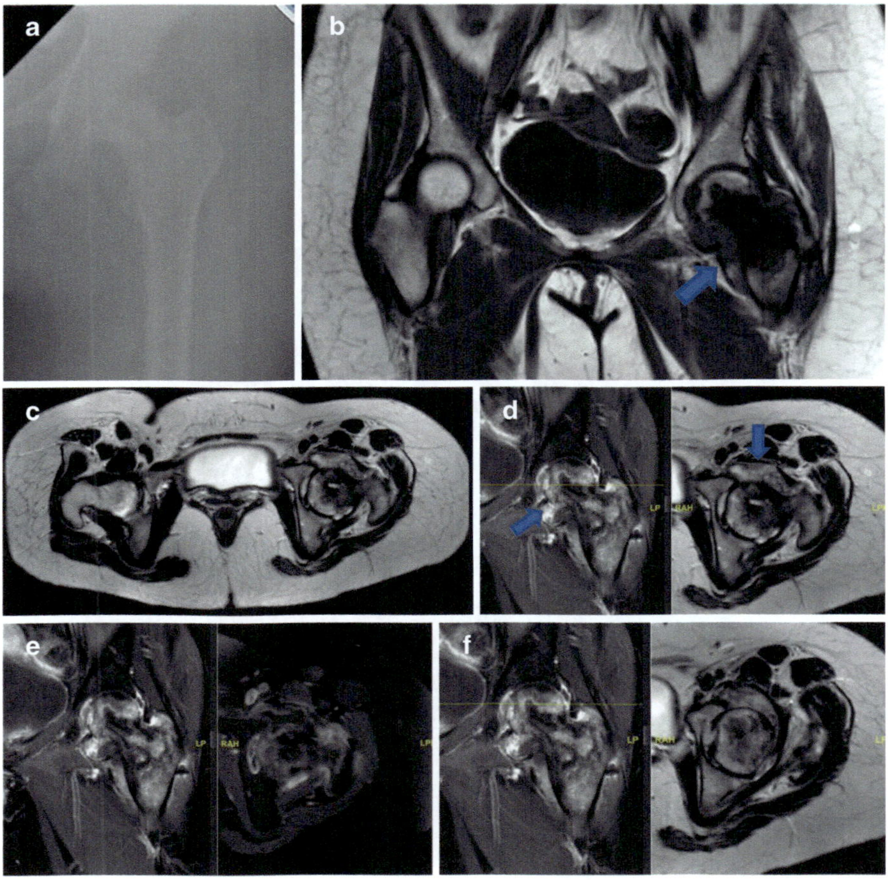

- Hip capsule infiltrated by proximal femur sarcoma
- Part of the anterior acetabulum ring was removed to achieve the margin.

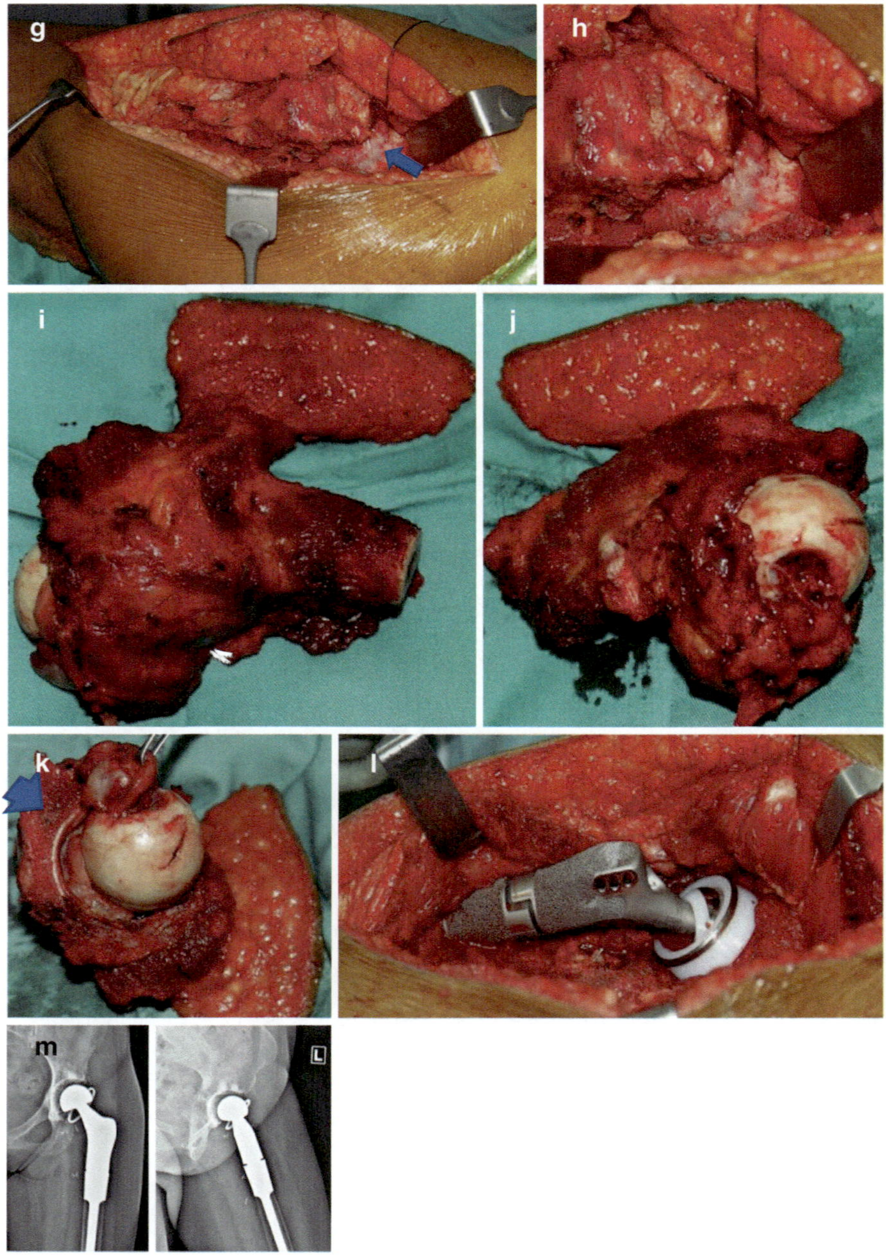

'Gluteus Medius—Vastus Lateralis Continuity'

Gluteus medius and trochanter reconstruction is important for hip stability and abduction function to minimize Trendelenburg gait. However, due to poor tendon or bone implant interface incorporation, late migration and poor tendon reattachment are commonly occur. We designed a technique to preserve continuity of the gluteus medius and vastus lateralis similar to the 'surgical hip dislocation' technique. It allows abductor vastus continuity during resection procedures, particularly for marginal resection margin, in metastases and benign aggressive tumours. The tension and forces of the abductors are maintained without the risk of superior migration and avulsion and thus provide better hip function.

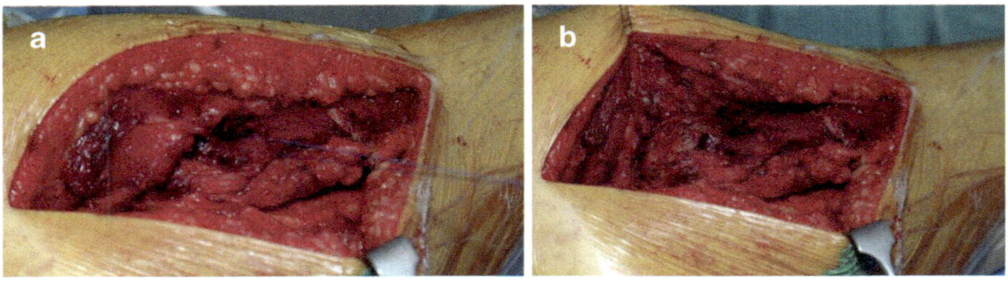

The gluteus medius is detached from the trochanter in intra-osseous proximal femur metastases in continuity with vastus lateralis tendon origin (Fig. 6a, b).

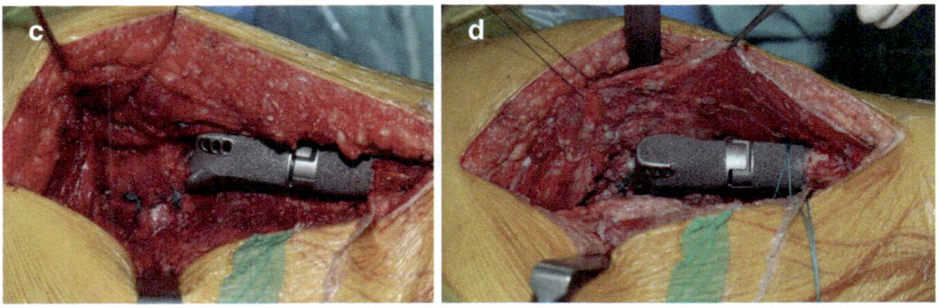

The gluteus medius and vastus lateralis continuity is maintained to minimize abductor forces for trochanteric reconstruction (Fig. 6c, d).

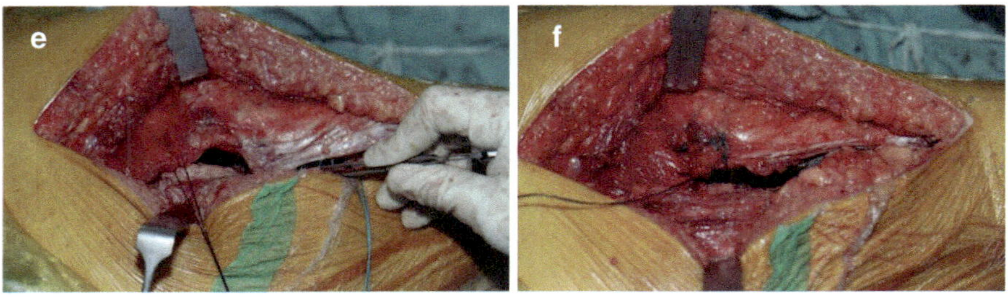

In the final anatomical reconstruction, the vastus lateralis can be attached to the lateral intermuscular septum, and the gluteus maximus is reattached to the prosthesis shaft (Fig. 6e, f).

Suggested Reading

1. Zoccali C, Careri S, Attala D, Florio M, Milano GM, Giordano M. A new proximal femur reconstruction technique after bone tumor resection in a very small patient: an exemplificative case. Children. 2021;8(6):442.
2. Asavamongkolkul A. Implant reconstruction of the proximal femur: modular prosthesis. In: Orthopaedic surgical oncology for bone tumors. Springer Nature Switzerland AG; 2022. p. 143–53.
3. Jamshidi K, Mirkazemi M, Gharedaghi M, et al. Bipolar hemiarthroplasty versus total hip arthroplasty in allograft-prosthesis composite reconstruction of the proximal femur following primary bone tumour resection. Bone Joint J. 2020;102-B(4):524–9.
4. Masterson EL, Ferracini R, Griffin AM, Wunder JS, Bell RS. Capsular replacement with synthetic mesh: effectiveness in preventing postoperative dislocation after wide resection of proximal femoral tumors and prosthetic reconstruction. J Arthroplast. 1998;13(8):860–6.
5. Farid Y, Lin PP, Lewis VO, Yasko AW. Endoprosthetic and allograft-prosthetic composite reconstruction of the proximal femur for bone neoplasms. Clin Orthop Relat Res. 2006;442:223–9.
6. Babis GC, Sakellariou VI, Franklin H. Sim allograft prosthesis composite replacement for bone tumors of the Proxi-Mal femur. In: Master techniques in orthopaedic surgery orthopaedic oncology and complex reconstruction. Lippincott Williams & Wilkins, A Wolters Kluwer; 2011. p. 137–49.
7. Chandrasekar CR, Grimer RJ, Carter SR, Tillman RM, Abudu A, Buckley L. Modular endoprosthetic replacement for tumours of the proximal femur. J Bone Joint Surg Br. 2009;91(1):108–12.
8. Peter FM. Choong megaprosthesis after tumor resection. In: Master techniques in orthopaedic surgery orthopaedic oncology and complex reconstruction. Lippincott Williams & Wilkins, A Wolters Kluwer; 2011. p. 125–37.
9. Donati D, Giacomini S, Gozzi E, Mercuri M. Proximal femur reconstruction by an allograft prosthesis composite. Clin Orthop Relat Res. 2002;394:192–200.
10. Bickels J, Meller I, Henshaw RM, Malawer MM. Reconstruction of hip stability after proximal and total femur resections. Clin Orthop Relat Res. 2000;375:218–30.
11. Calabró T, Van Rooyen R, Piraino I, et al. Reconstruction of the proximal femur with a modular resection prosthesis. Eur J Orthop Surg Traumatol. 2016;26:415–21.
12. Ropars M, Lambotte J-C, Maximen J, Crenn V, Tronchot A, Huten D. Techniques and outcomes of hip abductor reconstruction following tumor resection in adults. Orthop Traumatol Surg Res. 2021;107:1.

Extra-Articular Proximal Femur Resection

Wan Faisham Nu'man Bin Wan Ismail

Introduction

Proximal femur sarcoma with hip joint involvement secondary to direct infiltration or a pathological neck fracture is best managed through extra-articular resection to achieve a negative margin. The hip joint is removed in continuity with the periacetabular structures. 'Type II Pelvic resection' can lead to a complex reconstruction to achieve a stable and functional hip. Furthermore, poor soft tissue attachment to the proximal femur prosthesis and muscle tension to provide a stable hip remains a major challenge to achieve a good functional hip.

Surgical Anatomy

The hip joint capsule is strong and dense and is attached above the acetabular margin 5–6 mm beyond its labrum, in front of the outer labral aspect, and near the acetabular notch, to the transverse acetabular ligament and adjacent rim of the obturator foramen.

The anterior side of the pelvis has nine inner hip muscles: the iliacus, psoas major, psoas minor, obturator externus, obturator internus, superior and inferior gemelli, piriformis, and quadratus femoris muscles.

Rectus femoris attached at the superior acetabulum need to be released for type II pelvic resection.

W. F. N. B. W. Ismail (✉)
Prince Court Medical Center, Kuala Lumpur, Malaysia

Orthopaedic Oncology Reconstructive Unit, Universiti Sains Malaysia, Kubang Kerian, Kelantan, Malaysia

A. Puri, W. F. N. B. W. Ismail (eds.), *Atlas of Orthopedic Oncology Volume 2*,
https://doi.org/10.1007/978-981-95-8962-3_2

Assessment

Extra-articular resection proximal femur with type II periacetabular resection is done in the following cases:

- Direct infiltration of the proximal femur sarcoma to the hip joint and capsule
- Sarcoma with a pathological neck fracture where the fracture hematoma has contaminated the joint
- Prophylaxis stabilization of the neck of the femur in a sarcoma

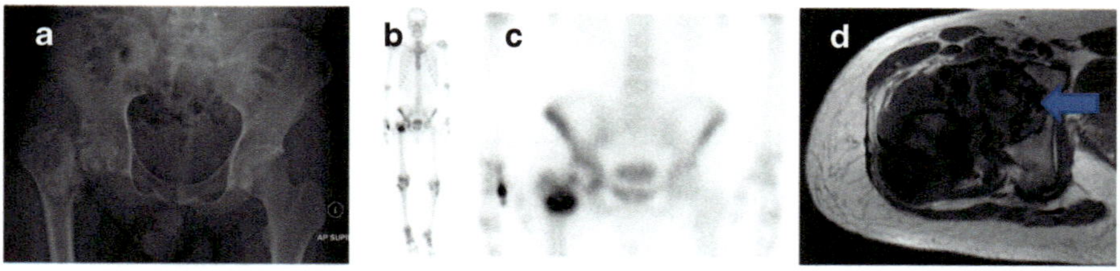

A case of osteosarcoma with a pathological fracture neck of the femur with local contamination to the hip joint. Bone scan revealed that the disease was localized to the proximal femur (Fig. 1a–d).

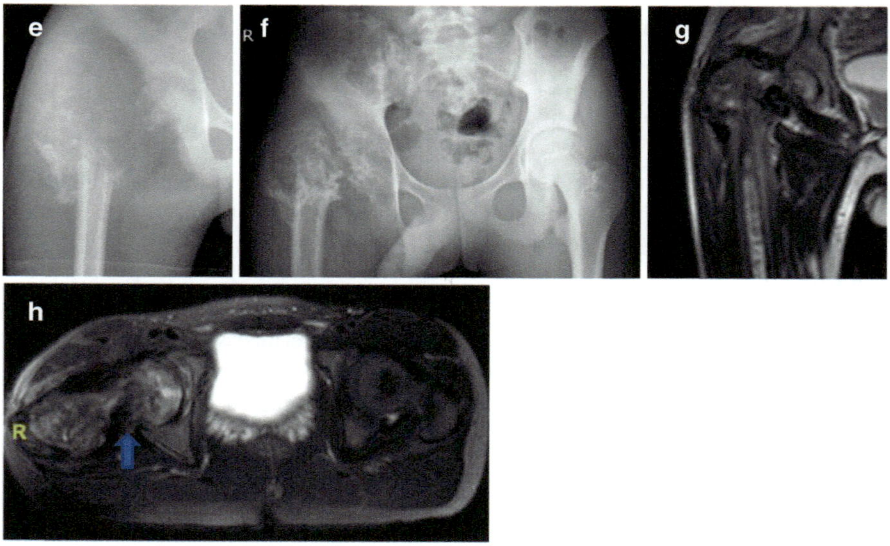

Osteolytic lesion of proximal femur with destruction of the femoral neck and head, which responded well to chemotherapy. The entire hip joint was infiltrated by the sarcoma (Fig. 1e–h).

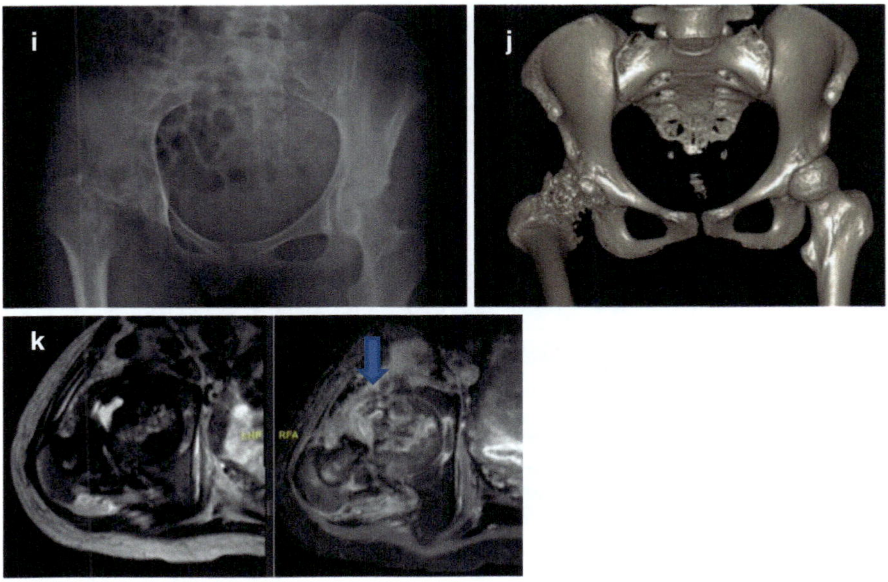

Aggressive osteosarcoma of the proximal femur with early infiltration to the neck and capsule with direct invasion to the acetabulum (Fig. 1i–k).

- Local contamination to the hip joint

Surgical Steps

- Combination of the ilioinguinal and Smith Peterson approaches for mobilization of the anterior femoral neurovascular structures (Fig. 2i, j).
- Distally, the femoral neurovascular structures are mobilized with extensor muscle of the thigh after achieving a good margin at the proximal femur.
- The external iliac vessels together with the iliopsoas tendon are mobilized from the superior pubic rami for medial osteotomy.
- A large posterior myocutaneous flap was developed using the glutei for exploration of the sciatic nerve to the greater sciatic foreman for supra acetabular osteotomy.
- Distally, the pelvic osteotomy is made at the superior part of the ischium after all the short rotators and quadratus femoris muscle are mobilized. Hamstring origins are maintained in the remnant ischium.
- The proximal femur osteotomy is done first, followed by pelvic osteotomy to minimize bleeding and for easy manipulation. The entire hip joint with the intact capsule is removed together with type II pelvic acetabular.

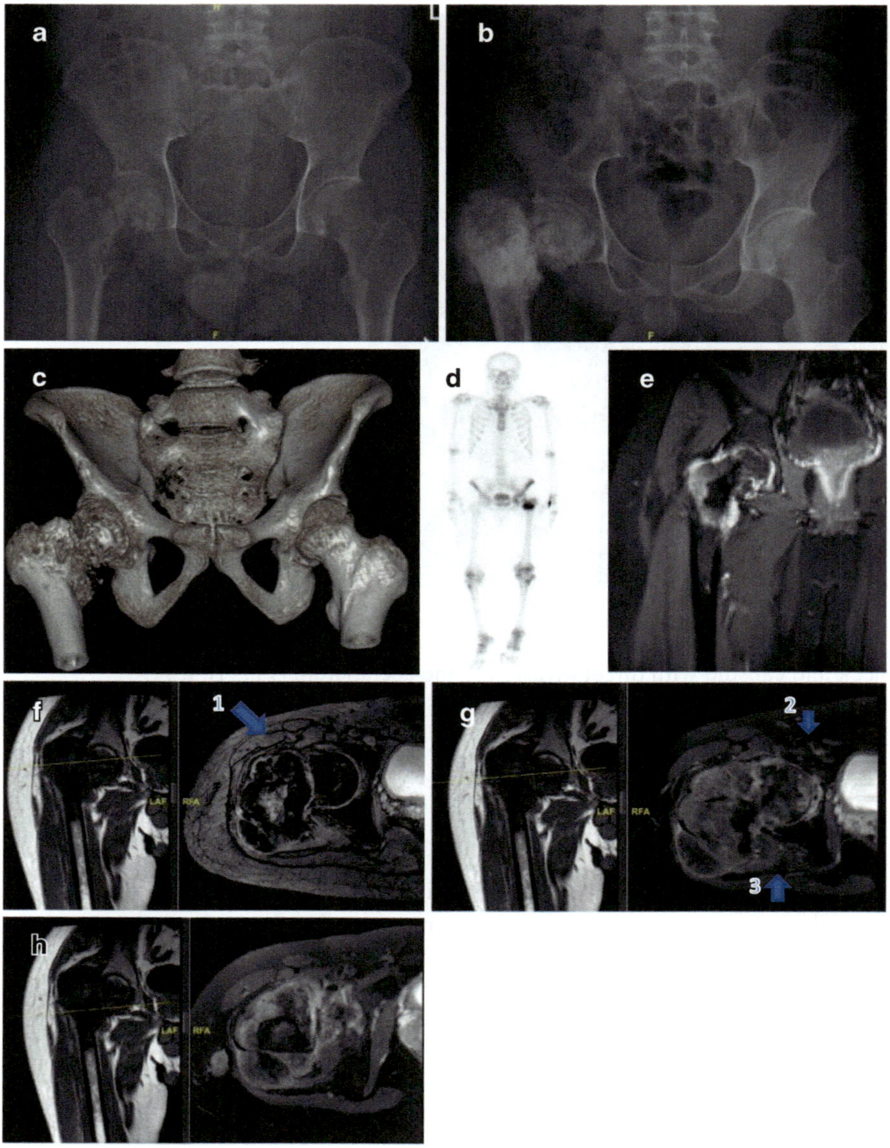

Osteosarcoma with a trans-cervical neck of femur fracture that partially responded to chemotherapy. The hip joint was grossly contaminated, and resection with entire hip joint extra-articular was achieved by a combination of proximal femur and type II pelvic resection (Fig. 2a–h).

1. Sartorius, rectus femoris gluteus medius
2. Femoral vessels
3. Sciatic nerve

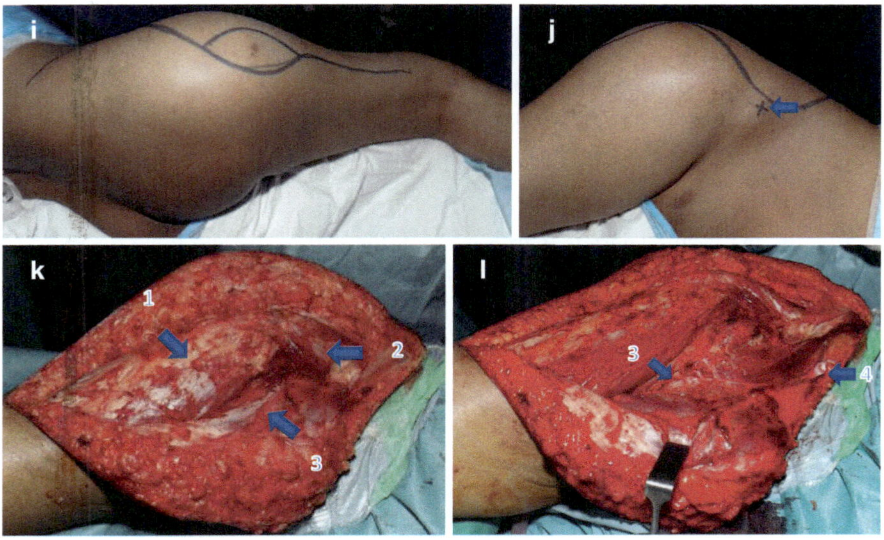

Exploration of the femoral artery and nerve branch to rectus and part of the vastus lateralis. The superior pubic rami are identified by laterally mobilizing the iliopsoas muscle. The iliopsoas tendon is transacted at the level of the acetabulum for a distal oncological margin (Fig. 2k–n).

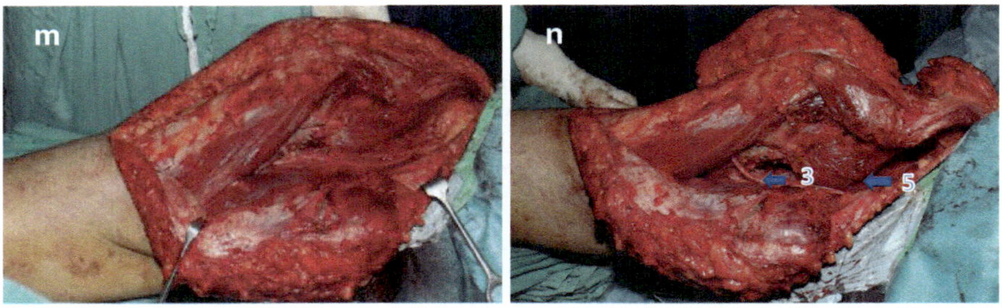

Posterior approach by reflection of the entire gluteus maximus and exploration of the sciatic nerve. Part of the gluteus maximus attached to the proximal femur is removed as part of the oncological margin. Mobilization of the sciatic nerve to the greater sciatic notch. The posterior attachment of adductor brevis and magnus is detached from the proximal femur by internal rotation of the thigh (Fig. 2o, p).

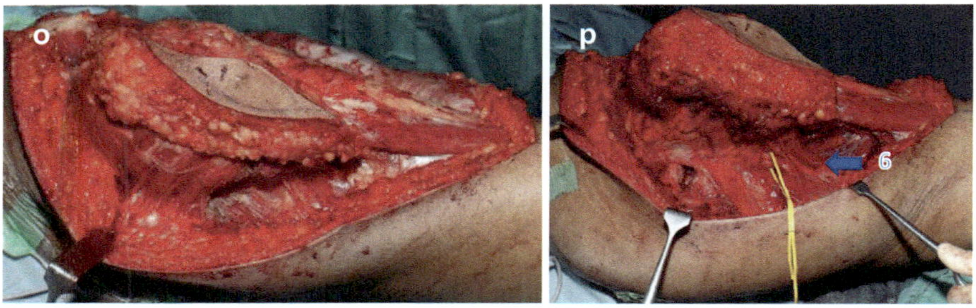

1. Vastus lateralis
2. Gluteus medius
3. Femoral nerve and vessels mobilize medially
4. Inguinal ligament detached from ASIS
5. Iliopsoas muscle and tendon
6. Sciatic nerve

Finally, the vastus lateralis is transected at the soft tissue and bone oncological margin. The osteotomy is marked, guided by an X-ray or image intensifier. Mobilization of the pelvic and proximal femur is done by transecting the sacrotuberus and sacrospinous ligaments (Fig. 2q–t).

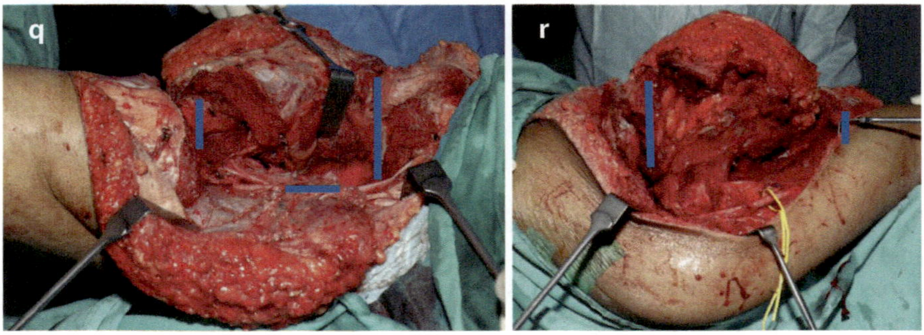

Osteotomy supraacetabular, symphysis pubis and upper femur

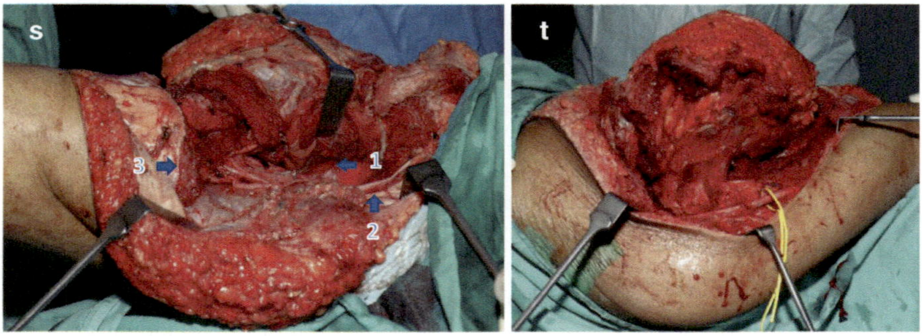

1. Bladder
2. Femoral nerve and vessels
3. Quadriceps margin resection with intact femoral motor nerve

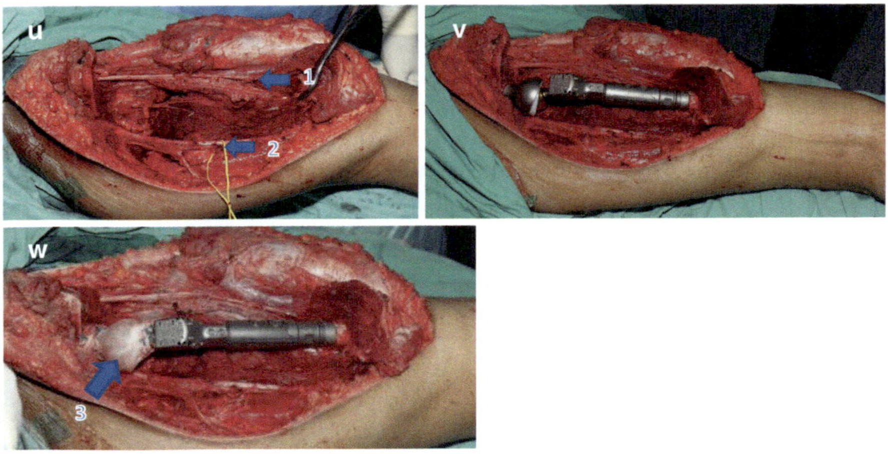

Final resection and reconstruction with an 'ice cream cone acetabulum cup' transfixed to the remnant of the ilium and proximal femur replacement. The hip joint is stabilized with purse-string sutures using a fixation tube (Fig. 2u–w).

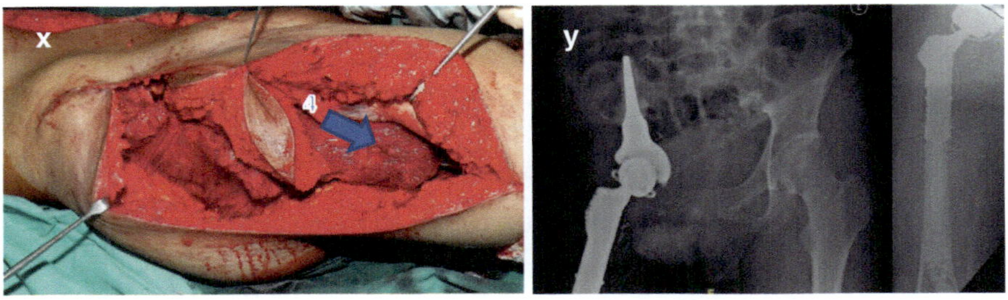

The vertical rectus abdominis muscle flap is used to reconstruct the lateral defect. The gluteus muscle and anterior compartment of the thigh are attached to the prosthesis and flap for anatomical reconstruction. The stability of the hip joint is dependent on the abductor muscle attachment to the proximal femur. In cases of massive soft tissue resection, a constrained acetabulum linear is an option to minimize risk of early dislocation (Fig. 2x, y).

1. Femoral vessels and nerve—continuity to supply quadriceps muscle
2. Sciatic nerve
3. Purse string Trevira tube for hip stability
4. Vertical rectus abdominis rotational flap

Proximal Femur Osteosarcoma with Neck Fracture—Recycle Pelvic with Cryotherapy

In this proximal femur sarcoma, the hip joint is contaminated by a fracture or direct extension to the capsule and surrounding structures. The acetabulum and pelvic bone are rarely involved with the tumour extension (Fig. 3a–d). Sterilizing the contaminated hip joint using extracorporeal radiation or liquid nitrogen and reimplanting the recycle bone is an option.

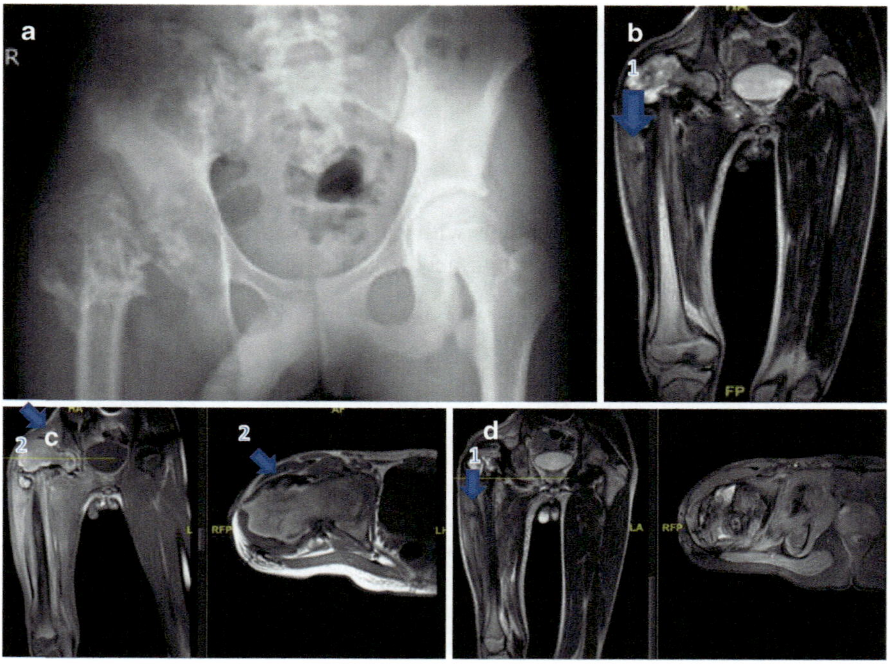

1. Extensive involvement of proximal quadriceps muscle
2. Gluteus medius

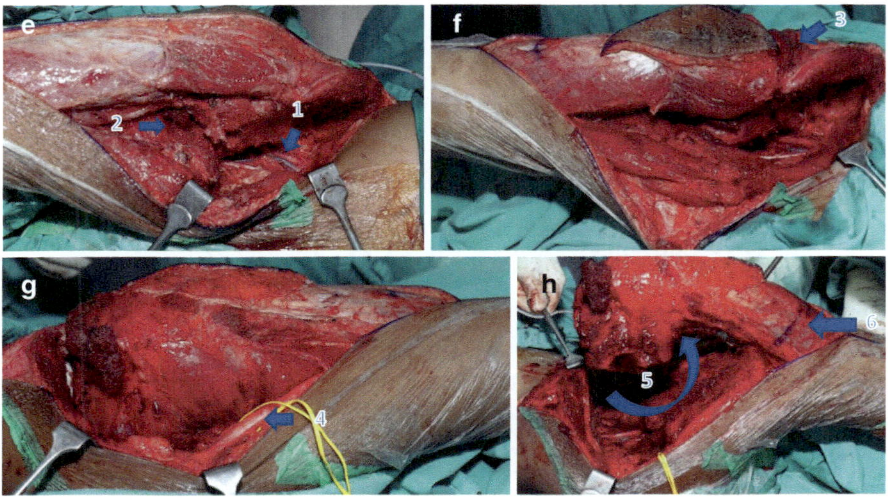

Mobilization of the proximal femur and supracetabular bone for type II resection. Osteotomy done at the supracetabular level, superior pubic rami and superior part of the ischium. The proximal parts of the vastus lateralis and intermedius were included in the surgical margin for oncological clearance (Fig. 3e–h).

1. Femoral nerve and external iliac vessels
2. Adductor longus muscle
3. Gluteus medius resection
4. Sciatic nerve
5. Mobilization of entire peri acetabulum with proximal femur
6. Distal quadriceps muscle margin and femoral osteotomy

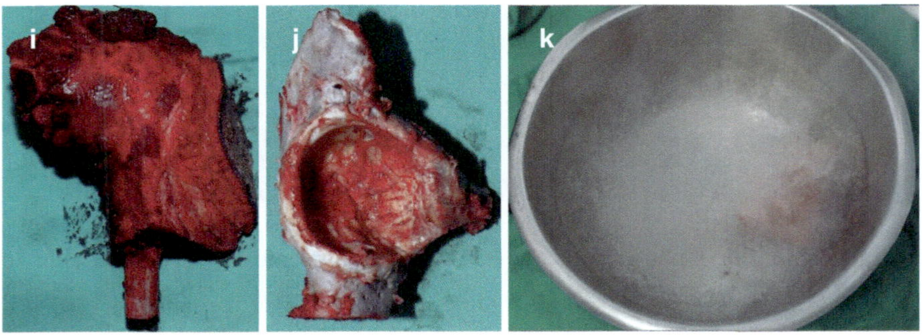

The acetabular bone was cleared of soft tissue attachment and prepared for cryotherapy using liquid nitrogen. Multiple drilling over the bone prevented fracture during the process. The bone is immersed in liquid nitrogen for 20 min (−196°C) and then thawed at room temperature for 15 min and dipped in normal saline for 15 min prior to reimplantation (Fig. 3i–k).

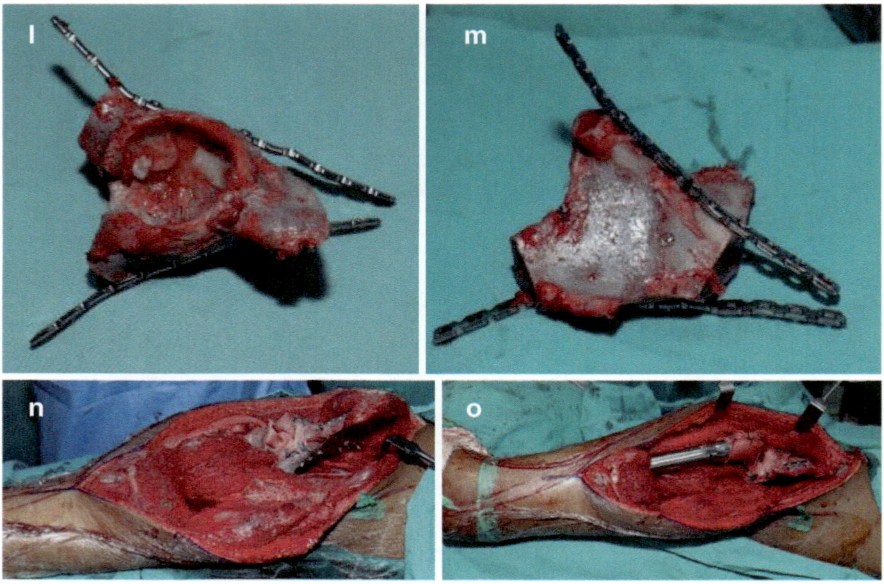

- Pre bending plate for anterior and posterior column stabilization

Process of fixation and stabilization of the recycled bone and stabilization using plate and screw. The proximal femur bone defect was reconstructed with proximal femur endoprosthesis. Hip stability was maintained by purse-string sutures around a trevira tube (Fig. 3l–p). The lateral soft tissue defect was reconstructed with a vascularized latissimus dorsi flap (Fig. 3q–s).

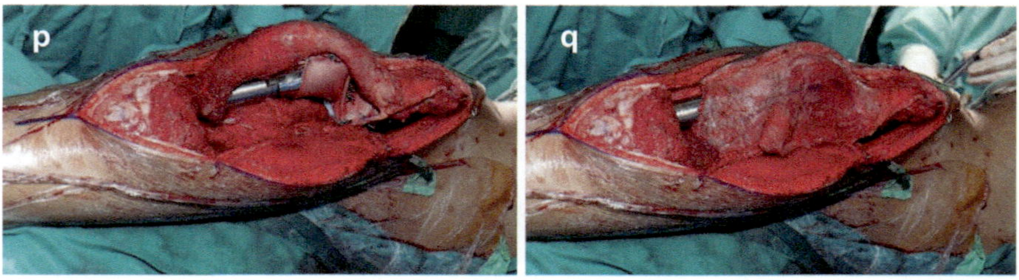

- Latissimus dorsi flap—thoracodorsal vessels anastomosed to end to side to external iliac vessels

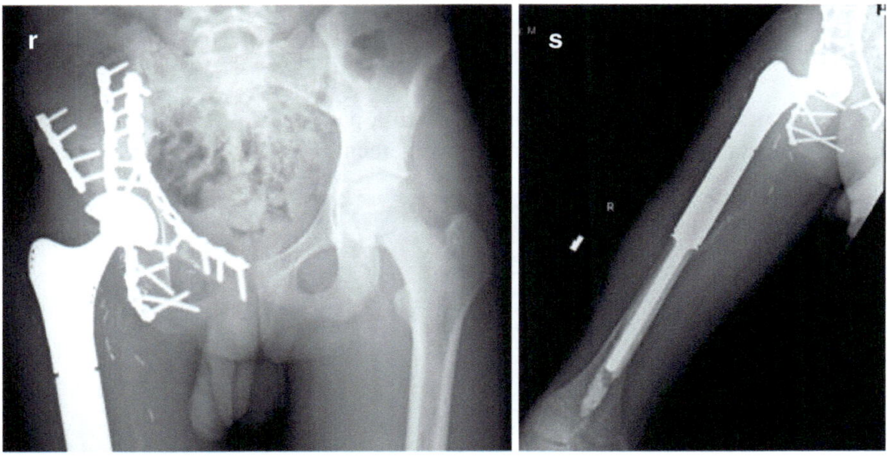

Functional outcome 3 months after surgery, ambulating without support with weakness abductor hip and trendelenburg gait (Fig. 3t–v)

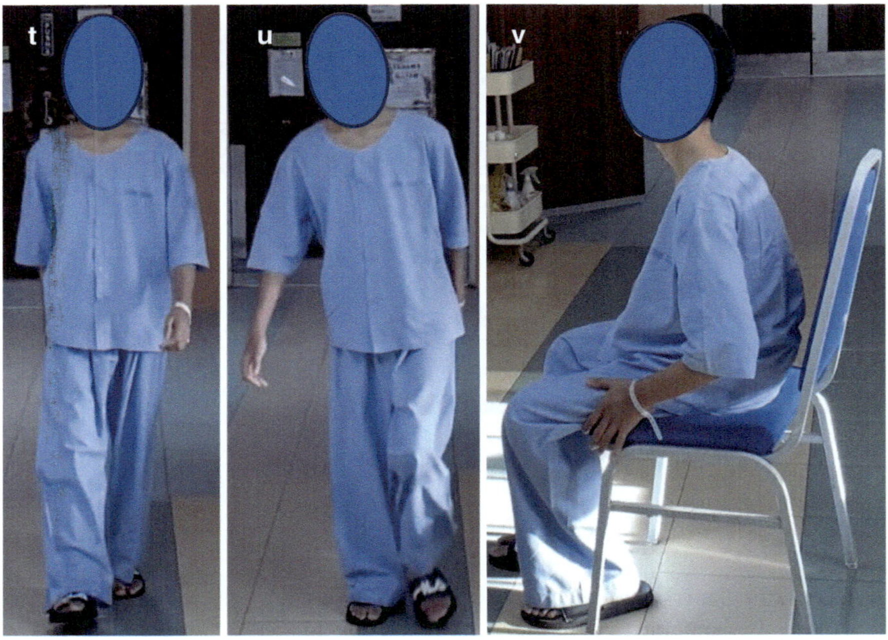

Extra-Articular Resection with Extensive Adductor Involvement

A case of proximal femur osteosarcoma with a pathological fracture of neck and massive medial adductor compartment involvement (Fig. 4a–e).

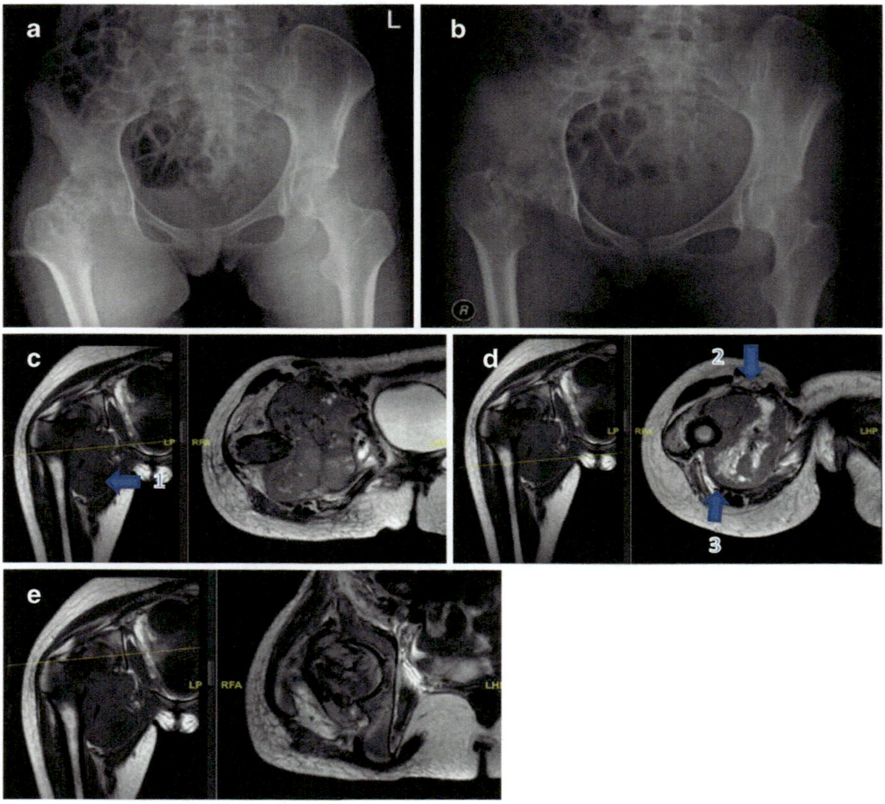

1. Adductor muscle involvement
2. Femoral artery and nerve
3. Sciatic nerve

Extra-articular resection of the proximal femur with the entire adductor resection together with the pubic rami to the symphysis pubis to achieve a wide margin. The vastus lateralis and gluteal region were not involved and maintained and provided good muscle flap to cover the prosthesis and minimize risk of wound break down (Fig. 4f–l)

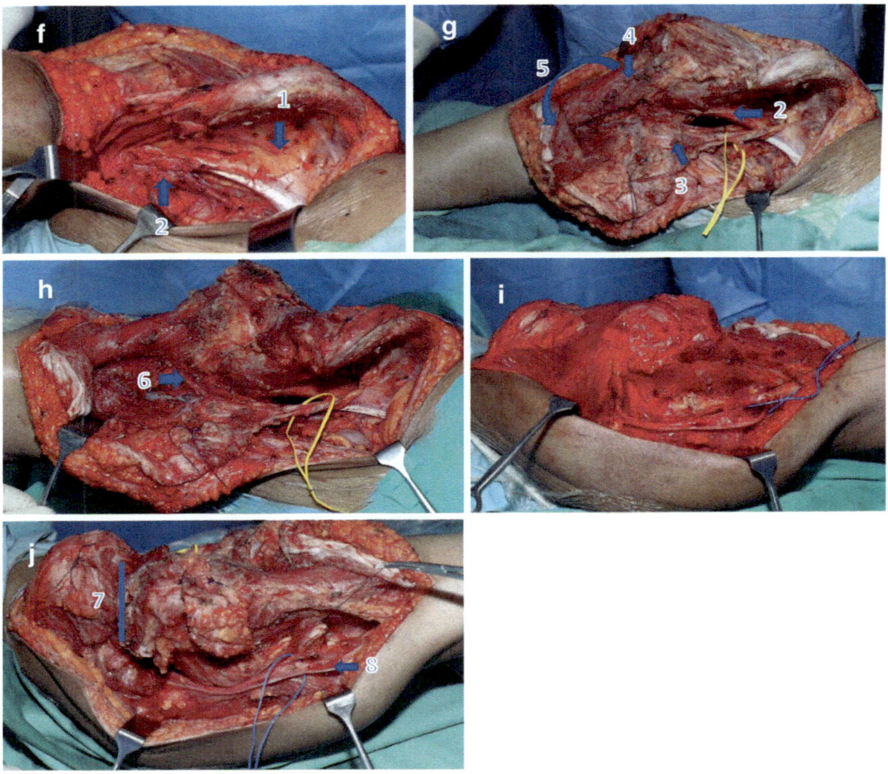

1. Retroperitoneal space
2. Psoas muscle and tendon
3. External iliac vessels and femoral nerve
4. Vastus intermedius
5. Vastus lateralis and rectus mobilize medially together with intact femoral nerve and vessels
6. Profunda femoral artery within adductor tumour extension—ligated
7. Supra acetabulum osteotomy
8. Sciatic nerve

The entire adductor muscle was removed together with the superior and inferior pubic rami at the level of the symphysis pubis. The entire osseous defect was reconstructed with a LUMiC cup and proximal femur replacement. The constrained cup was used as minimal soft tissue was left was for hip stability (Fig. 4m–o)

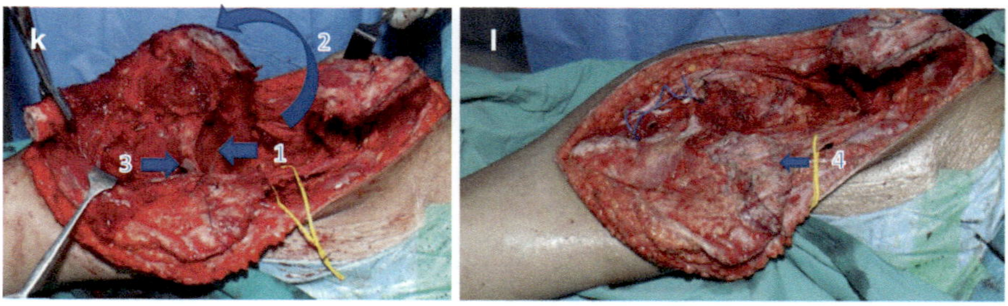

1. Obturator fossae
2. Proximal adductor muscle covering tumour mobilize after symphysis pubis osteotomy
3. Symphysis pubis
4. Femoral nerve with intact motor branch to vastus lateralis and rectus femoris

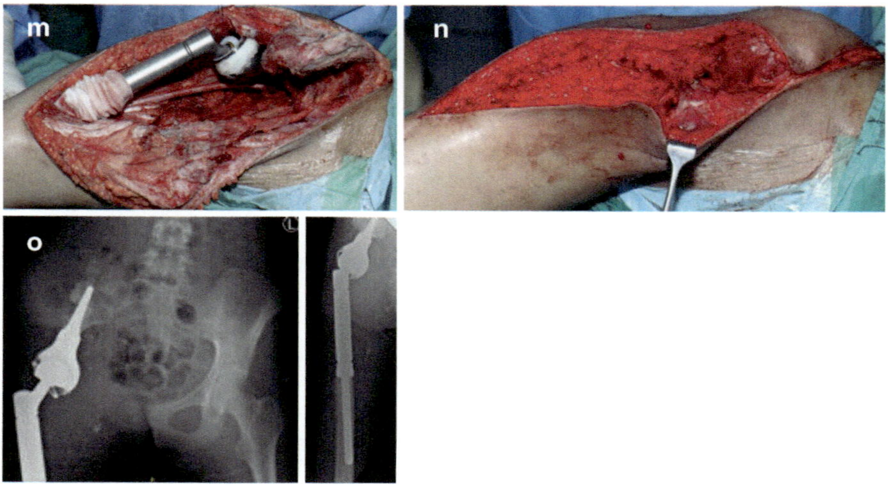

Suggested Reading

1. Li D, Lu X, Guo W, Tang X, Ji T, Yang R. Extra-articular resection is a limb-salvage option for sarcoma involving the hip joint. Int Orthop. 2018;42(3):695–703.
2. Oragui E, Nannaparaju M, Sri-Ram K, Khan W, Hashemi Nejad A, Skinner J. A new technique of endoprosthetic replacement for osteosarcoma of proximal femur with intra-articular extension. Int J Surg Case Rep. 2013;4:10.
3. Manrique J, Schiffman CJ, Chan AD, Olsen D, Thompson MJ. Extra-articular hip resection and reconstruction with custom acetabular resection guide and implants in a case of high-grade spindle cell sarcoma of the proximal femur. JBJS Case Connect. 2020;10:e19.00529.

4. Van Leeuwen RJH, Beck M, Fuchs B. Internal hemipelvectomy through a periacetabular osteotomy combined with an extraarticular (proximal) femur resection using a single posterolateral approach; the surgical technique. J Surg Res. 2022;5(2):305–21.
5. Nakamura S, Kusuzaki K, Murata H, Takeshita H, Hirata M, Hashiguchi S, Hirasawa Y. Extra-articular wide tumor resection and limb reconstruction in malignant bone tumors at the proximal femur. Orthopedics. 2001;24(5):445–7.
6. Fujiwara T, Tsuda Y, Stevenson J, Parry M, Jeys L. Extra-articular resection of the hip joint for pelvic sarcomas: are there any oncological and functional risks compared with intra-articular resection? J Bone Oncol. 2021;31:100401.
7. Fujiwara T, Tsuda Y, Evans S, Stevenson J, Parry M, Jeys L, Abudu A. Extra-articular resection for bone sarcomas involving the hip joint. J Surg Oncol. 2020;121:258–66.
8. Housset V, Anract P, Babinet A, et al. Proximal femur versus acetabular extra-articular resection of the hip joint for primary malignant bone tumors: a retrospective comparative review of 33 cases. World J Surg Oncol. 2022;20:168.
9. Barro V, Velez R, Pacha D, Giralt J, Roca I, Aguirre M. Bernese periacetabular osteotomy in a hip extra-articular resection followed by reconstruction using an extracorporeal irradiated acetabulum autograft with megaprosthesis for proximal femur osteosarcoma in a Pediatric patient. Case Rep Med. 2015;2015:813683.

Total Femur Resection and Replacement

Wan Faisham Nu'man Bin Wan Ismail

Introduction

Total femur replacement is an option for bone tumours of either the proximal or distal femur with extensive intramedullary involvement. Stable reconstruction after resection is challenging owing to the limited length of the remaining bone to anchor a prosthesis after achieving a safe oncologic margin or due to extensive bone loss after revision surgery. Despite major resection and double joint reconstruction, the functional outcome of the limbs remains good. The newer generation of endoprostheses, with modularity, are able to maintain limb length and joint position for optimal muscle balance, patellar tracking, and adductor function for optimum limb functional outcome.

W. F. N. B. W. Ismail (✉)
Prince Court Medical Center, Kuala Lumpur, Malaysia

Orthopaedic Oncology Reconstructive Unit, Universiti Sains Malaysia, Kubang Kerian, Kelantan, Malaysia

A. Puri, W. F. N. B. W. Ismail (eds.), *Atlas of Orthopedic Oncology Volume 2*,
https://doi.org/10.1007/978-981-95-8962-3_3

Surgical Anatomy

Surgical and oncological margins anatomical highlights are described in proximal and distal femur resection. However, understanding muscle coverage attachment for the entire femur is important for resection planning and possibility of tumour extension.

- The vastus intermedius is an important muscle that covers the entire anterior femur from the articularis genu suprapatellar region. This muscle can be removed completely with the femur, especially for distal femur sarcoma.
- Medially, it is attached to the pectineus, adductor brevis, adductor longus and magnus.
- Posteriorly, the entire femur is covered by loose areolar tissue, and the short head of the biceps is attached to the lateral border of the femur.
- The medial and lateral gastrocnemius head are strongly attached to the posterior condyle and have to be released together with the knee ligament for dislocation of the knee joint.
- Proximally, the gluteus maximus, medius and minimus insertion and all the short rotator tendon and iliopsoas are attached.

Assessments

Careful preoperative evaluation for the intramedullary extension and skip lesion is important for the final decision of resecting the entire femur. The indications mainly include:

- Skip lesion intramedullary either too distal or proximal for safe oncological resection (Fig. 1a–g)
- Remnant of the bone for intramedullary stem is too short for stable reconstruction
- Revision for prior endoprosthesis of femur with significantly poor bone stock for reconstruction (Fig. 1h, i)

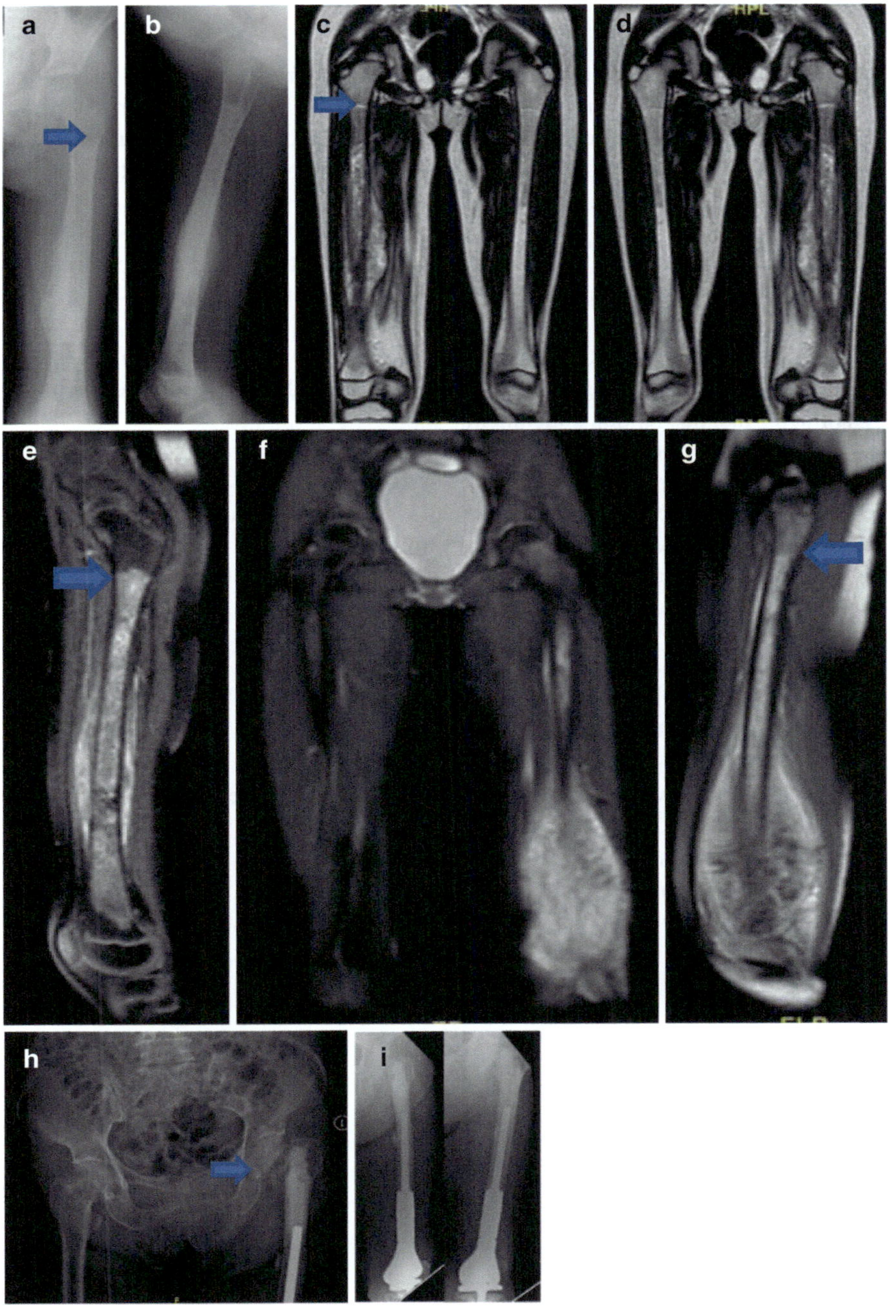
a
b
c
d
e
f
g
h
i

Surgical Steps

Resection of the entire femur depends on initial tumour presentation: either proximal or distal femur. The surgical margin is based on primary tumour extension. Proximal or distal intramedullary extension is resected with periosteum and soft tissue margin. Remnant of soft tissue is important for soft tissue reconstruction and stability and function of the hip and knee.

- A direct extensile lateral approach from the hip joint to the lateral epicondyle and curve to the patella tuberosity is important for tibial tray preparation of prosthesis fitting.
- Mobilisation of the femoral popliteal neurovascular structures through a lateral approach and progressing medially to the subsartorial opening after releasing the adductor magnus tendon attachment.
- The vastus intermedius is included in the margin for most cases and above it for mobilising the entire quadriceps.
- The short head biceps is released from the lateral side to mobilise the entire hamstring and separate the sciatic nerve from the femur.
- Proximal and distal release of the muscle and tendon attachment as described in the initial topic based on primary sites of sarcoma.

Osteosarcoma Distal Femur with Extensive Intramedullary Involvement

A 15-year-old boy with distal femur osteosarcoma and extensive proximal intramedullary extension. Post-neoadjuvant chemotherapy showed calcification of the intramedullary extension to the proximal femur, and total femur resection was decided. The superior part of the vastus intermedius showed tumour extension and had to be resected completely in total with the femur (Fig. 2a–g).

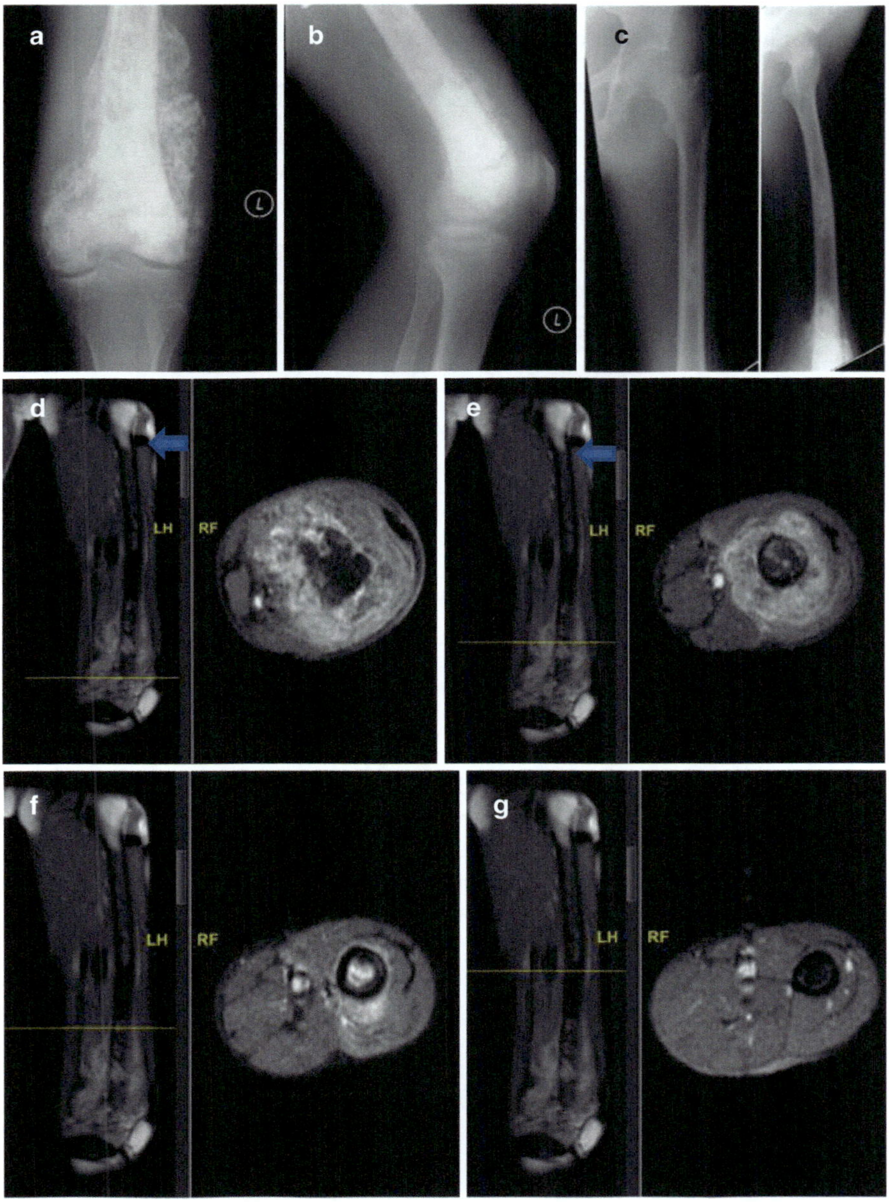

Total femur resection is approached through a direct lateral incision from the knee to the hip joint. The popliteal neurovascular structures are approached by detaching the lateral gastrocnemius and short head of the biceps. The subsartorial opening of the adductor magnus can be released once the knee joint is dislocated and the entire soft tissue is detached from the distal femur. The vastus intermedius is removed in total for clear oncological margin (Fig. 2h–k).

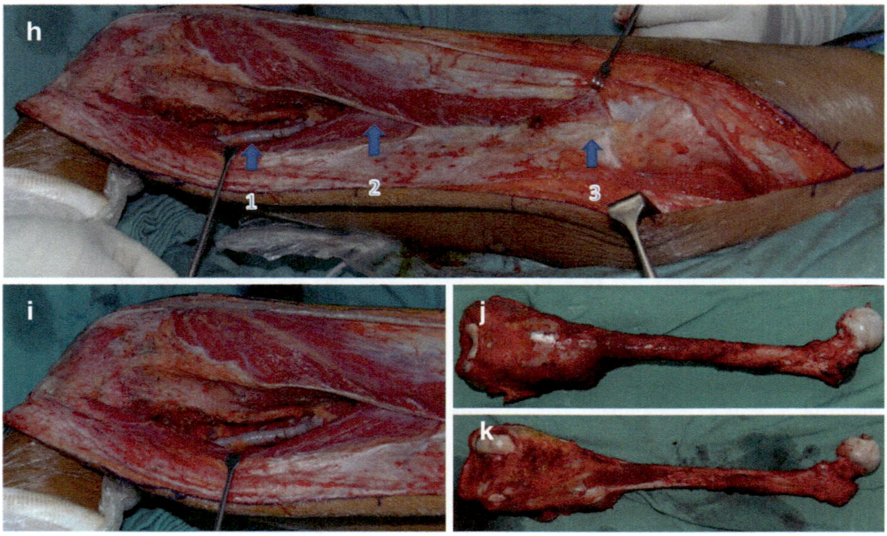

1. Femoral artery
2. Short head biceps femoris
3. Gluteus maximus tendon insertion

The vastus lateralis is reflected medially with the rectus and vastus medialis. However, the intermedius muscle was retained as the cuff of the oncological margin. The proximal hip muscle was detached as close to the bone as possible while dislocating the hip for subsequent reconstruction. The hip capsule was maintained for reconstruction and stability of the femoral head endoprosthesis.

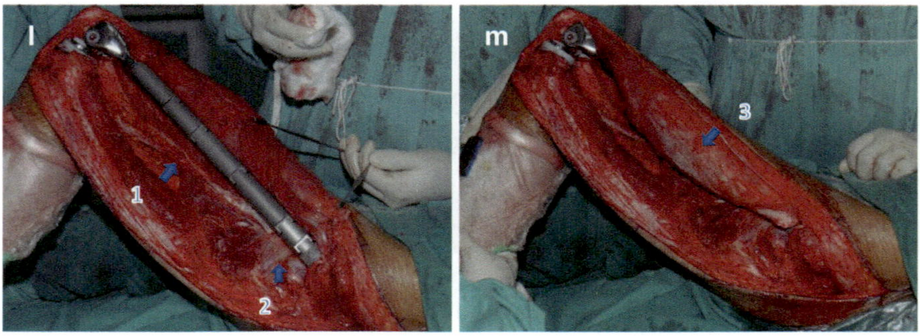

1. Adductor magnus canal opening
2. First perforator below the gluteus maximus insertion
3. Vastus lateralis

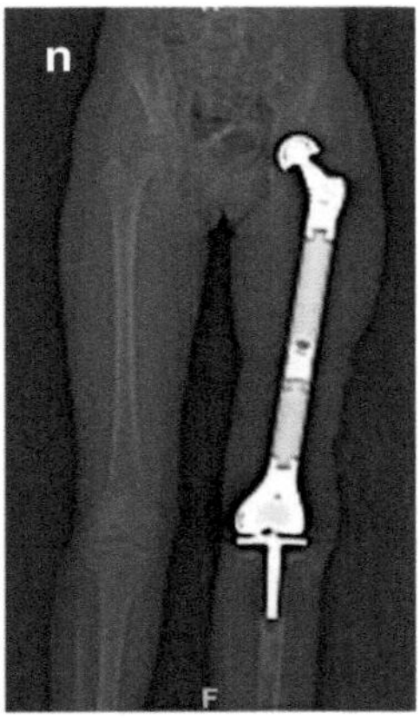

Stability of both the hip and knee joint is important for immediate and long-term function of the limb. The proximal femur and hip joint were reconstructed with bipolar hip replacement with purse-string sutures around the capsule and gluteus medius reattachment to the endoprosthesis trochanter. Knee stability is provided by rotating the hinge endoprosthesis. Limb length was carefully adjusted by the modular prosthesis body, and the muscle must be closed anatomically to achieve good tension for better function (Fig. 2l–n).

Osteosarcoma Distal Femur with Extensive Soft Tissue and Intramedullary Involvement

In cases where massive soft tissue resection is required to achieve a good surgical margin, a free latissimus dorsi flap is an option to minimise wound dehiscence, contracture and knee stiffness. The latissimus dorsi allows flexible closure, good padding around the knee and patella alignment and stability.

MRI image of distal femur osteosarcoma with extensive soft tissue involvement (Fig. 3a–e)

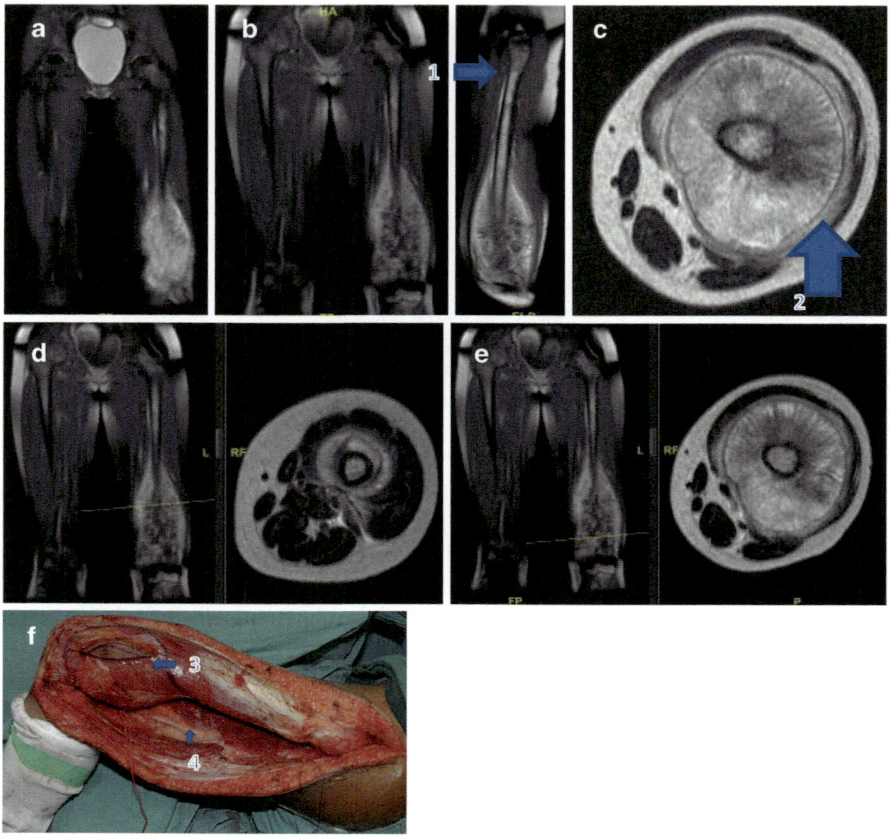

1. Intramedullary extension to proximal femur
2. Vastus lateralis with no clear border with tumour
3. Plan resection vastus lateralis
4. Sciatic nerve

The vastus lateralis and intermedius was include as distal femur surgical margin. The intermuscular plane and spaces between vastus intermedius and rectus and vastus medialis are a good anatomical boundary against tumour extension (Fig. 3f–i). Remnant of the rectus femoris is not adequate for prosthesis covers. However, it is good as anti-gravity function for ambulation (Fig. 3j–m).

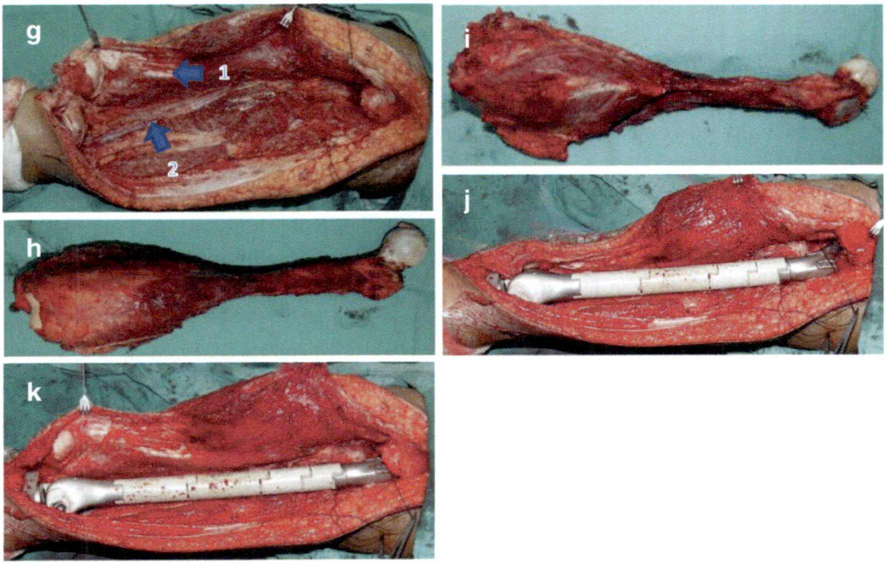

Patency of the vessels is accessed prior to reconstructive procedures. Trial prosthesis with correct limb length, femoral head size and muscle tension prior to definitive endoprosthesis implantation (Fig. 3g–k).

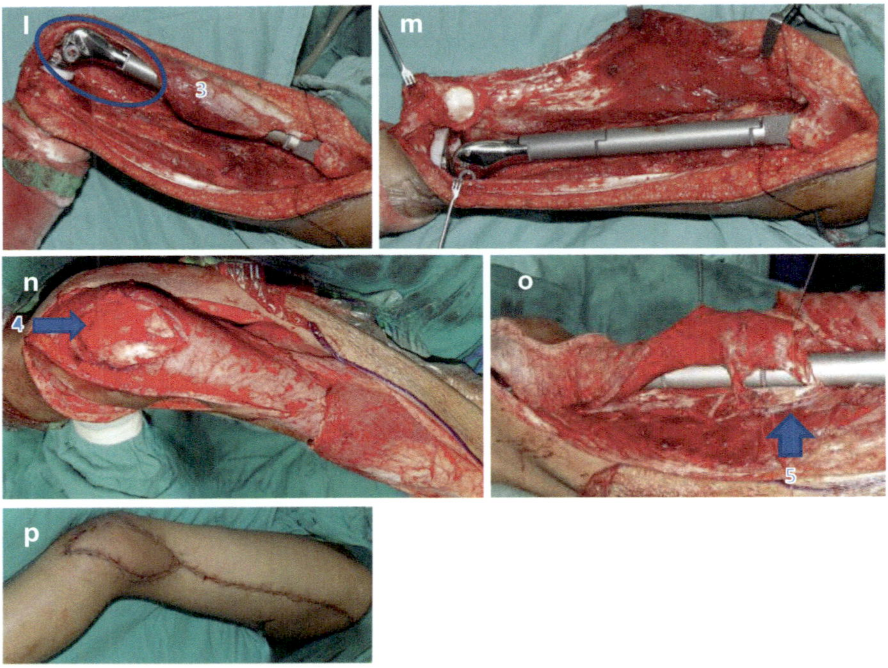

1. Rectus femoris tendon
2. Femoral vessels
3. Exposed prosthesis—vastus lateralis resection
4. Split distal latissimus dorsi
5. Thoraco dorsal vessels anastomosed end to side with superficial femoral vessels

The latissimus dorsi muscle provides lateral soft tissue covers of the prosthesis, and additional reconstruction was done by motorising the thoracodorsal nerve to the motor branch of the vastus medialis, which can provide augmentation of the weak quadriceps. Attaching the latissimus dorsi to the remaining quadratus femoris and the proximal tibia with good tension is important for augmentation of quadriceps strength. It also provides soft tissue reconstruction for the medial lateral stability of patella. Splitting latissimus dorsi flap at the distal mid fibre and position the patella at the centre, while the remnant of latissimus dorsi was suture to provide tension and stability. Stabilisation the patella provides better tracking and stability (Fig. 3n–p).

Pathological Fracture with Intramedullary Contamination with Nailing Procedures

A 17-year-old with a history of mid shaft femur fracture developed osteosarcoma distal femur 3 years later. In view of the intramedullary implant and extensive involvement distal femur, resection of the total femur with soft tissue resection of the entire medial and lateral distal femur over screw tip area was planned (Fig. 4a–h).

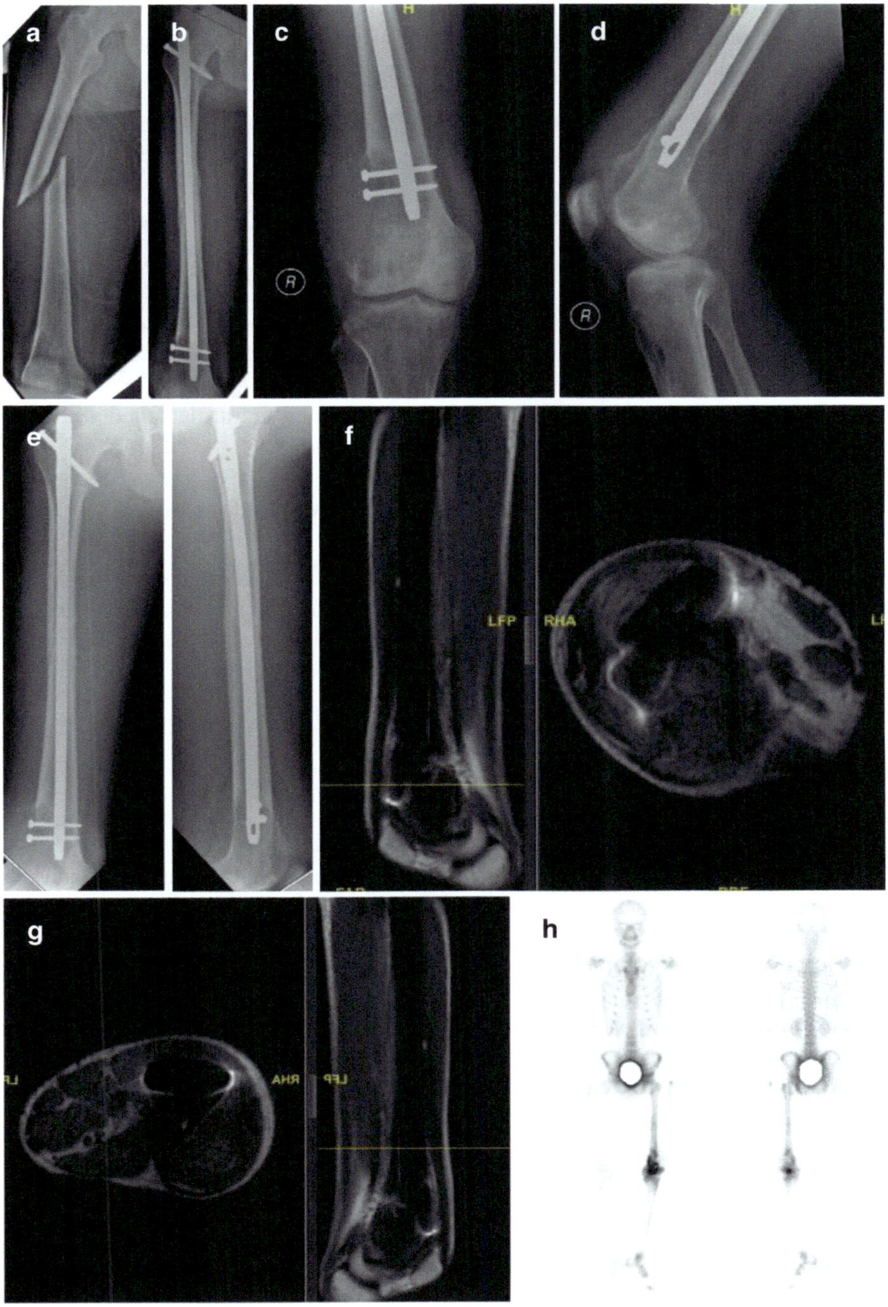
a
b
c
d
e
f
g
h

MRI evaluation was complicated with significance metal interference and not suitable for surgical planning. He responded well to chemotherapy, and the bone scan showed that the disease was localised (Fig. 4f, g).

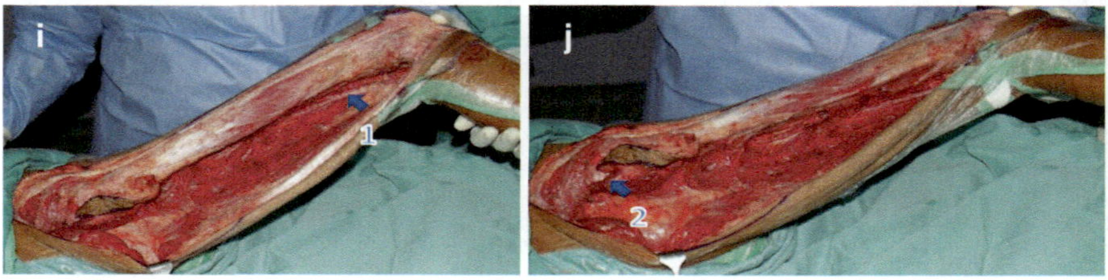

1. Superficial femoral vessels
2. Soft tissue attachment to the trochanter and proximal femur detached with cuff of tissue as contamination during nail insertion
3. Adductor magnus and sub sartorial opening
4. Patella with rectus femoris—other quadriceps were include as margin

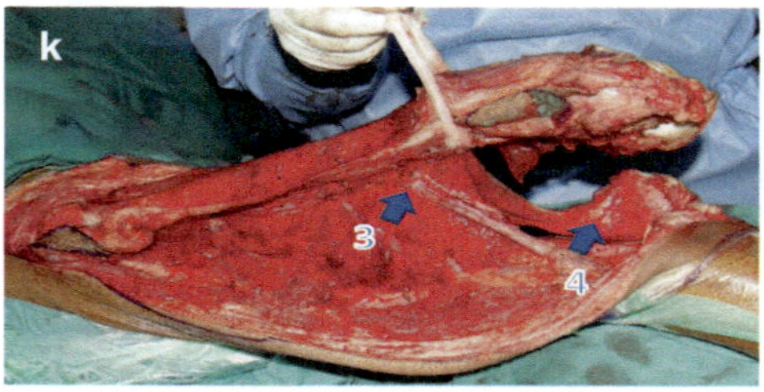

The femoral vessels passed from medial compartment to posterior at the subsartorial hiatus of the adductor magnus tendon. Exploration from the distal lateral side distally usually cannot reach the medial courses of this vessels. Within the subsartorial canal, detachment of the knee ligament and dislocation help explore the vessels and ensure the tumour margin. A direct lateral approach also provides better access for proximal resection (Fig. 4i–k).

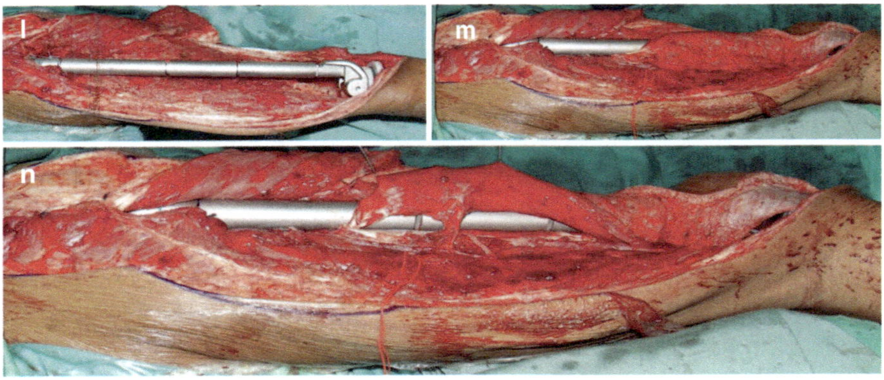

The latissimus dorsi muscle flap provides soft tissue reconstruction for the medial and lateral coverage of prosthesis and stability of patella (Fig. 4l–n).

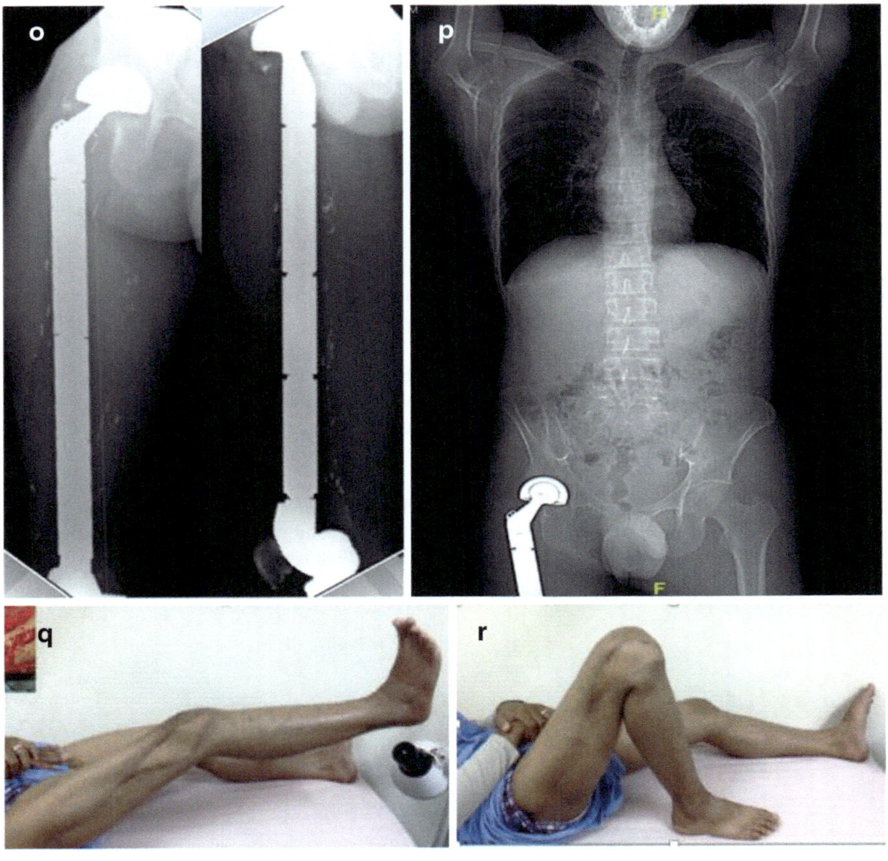

He has been disease free for 8 years. The range of knee motion is acceptable with good function; however, the extensor weakness remained with extensor lag (Fig. 4o–r)

Acknowledgement The author thanks Professor Zulmi Wan, Dr. Nor Azman Mat Zin, Dr. Syurahbil Abdul Halim, for their contributions and team member for managing the patients in this chapter.

The author also thanks Professor Wan Azman Wan Sulaiman, Professor Arman Zaharil Mat Saad and Professor Ahmad Sukari Halim from the plastic reconstructive unit at Universiti Sains Malaysia and MSU Medical Centre, Management and Science University for their contributions and team member for managing the patients. All plastic reconstructive and microsurgery surgical procedures were performed by the team members.

Suggested Reading

1. Adzhar AL, Faisham WI, Zulmi W, Azman WS, Sahran Y, Syurahbil AH, Nor-Azman MZ. Long-term outcome of total femur replacement. Malays Orthop J. 2023;17(2):21–7.
2. Faisham WI, Zulmi W, Halim AS. Modular endoprosthetic replacement after total femur resection for malignant bone tumor. Med J Malaysia. 2005;60(Suppl C):45–8.
3. Gonzalez MR, Inchaustegui ML, Layme J, Ruiz-Arellanos K, Larios F, Pretell-Mazzini J. Postoperative outcomes of total femur replacement in oncologic and non-oncologic patients: a systematic review of the literature. J Arthroplast. 2023;39:1624–1631.e2.
4. Innocenti M, Abed YY, Beltrami G, Delcroix L, Balatri A, Capanna R. Quadriceps muscle reconstruction with free functioning latissimus dorsi muscle flap after oncological resection. Microsurgery. 2009;29(30):189–98.
5. Kakimoto T, Matsumine A, Asanuma K, Matsubara T, Nakamura T, Sudo A. The clinical outcomes of total femur prosthesis in patients with musculoskeletal tumors. SICOT-J. 2019;5:23.
6. Kalra S, Abudu A, Murata H, Grimer RJ, Tillman RM, Carter SR. Total femur replacement: primary procedure for the treatment of malignant tumours of the femur. Eur J Surg Oncol. 2010;36(4):378–83.
7. Muratori F, Mondanelli N, Prifti X, Scoccianti G, Roselli G, Frenos F, et al. Total femur prosthesis in oncological and not oncological series. Survival and failures. J Orthop. 2019;17:215–20.
8. Puri A, Gulia A, Chan WH. Functional and oncologic outcomes after excision of the total femur in primary bone tumors: results with a low cost total femur prosthesis. Indian J Orthop. 2012;46:470–4.
9. Sevelda F, Schuh R, Hofstaetter JG, Schinhan M, Windhager R, Funovics PT. Total femur replacement after tumor resection: limb salvage usually achieved but complications and failures are common. Clin Orthop Relat Res. 2015;473:2079–87.

Distal Femur Resection and Reconstruction

Wan Faisham Nu'man Bin Wan Ismail

Introduction

The knee is the most frequent site of primary bone tumours. A majority of the tumours arising in the knee can be treated with limb sparing surgery. Resection of a malignant distal femur tumour is reliable, safe and reconstruction with an endoprosthesis which enables immediate weight bearing, maintenance of joint mobility and early return to activities. Functional outcomes are generally good to excellent with good range of knee motion enabling activities of daily living.

Amputation should be reserved for tumours with multi-compartment soft tissue involvement and/or major neurovascular involvement with a high risk of local recurrence.

Surgical Anatomy

Anatomical structures overlying the distal femur sarcoma limit tumour progression and are important for planning good quality margins:

- Distal femur joint cartilage protects against direct infiltration of the knee joint.
- Vastus intermedius muscle covers the suprapatellar anterior distal femur and its broad tendon protects rectus femoris, part of vastus medialis and lateralis muscle.
- Loose areolar tissue posteriorly protects the popliteal vessels, tibial and peroneal nerve, and long hamstring tendon against direct infiltration.

W. F. N. B. W. Ismail (✉)
Prince Court Medical Center, Kuala Lumpur, Malaysia

Orthopaedic Oncology Reconstructive Unit, Universiti Sains Malaysia, Kubang Kerian, Kelantan, Malaysia

A. Puri, W. F. N. B. W. Ismail (eds.), *Atlas of Orthopedic Oncology Volume 2*, https://doi.org/10.1007/978-981-95-8962-3_4

Possible direct infiltration from distal femur sarcoma can occur through

- Ligaments of the knee—ACL, PCL LCL and MCL
- Short head of biceps over the distal femur
- Both heads of gastrocnemius

Femoral vessels pass through the saphenous opening of 'adductor magnus' and enter the popliteal space joining the tibial nerve and subsequently run above the soleus to the deep compartment of the leg. These structures together with the major nerve must be mobilised free for limb salvage surgery.

Assessment

Surgical planning is based on tumour extension, neuro-vascular anatomy and soft tissue extension particularly the relation with respect to anatomical barriers. Assessment of tumour extension in a distal femur malignant bone tumour is extremely important to achieve adequate oncological clearance and maintaining enough muscle for good functional outcome. Assessment with an MRI of the relevant anatomical structures mentioned earlier is the key to plan resection achieving wide resection margins around the distal femur.

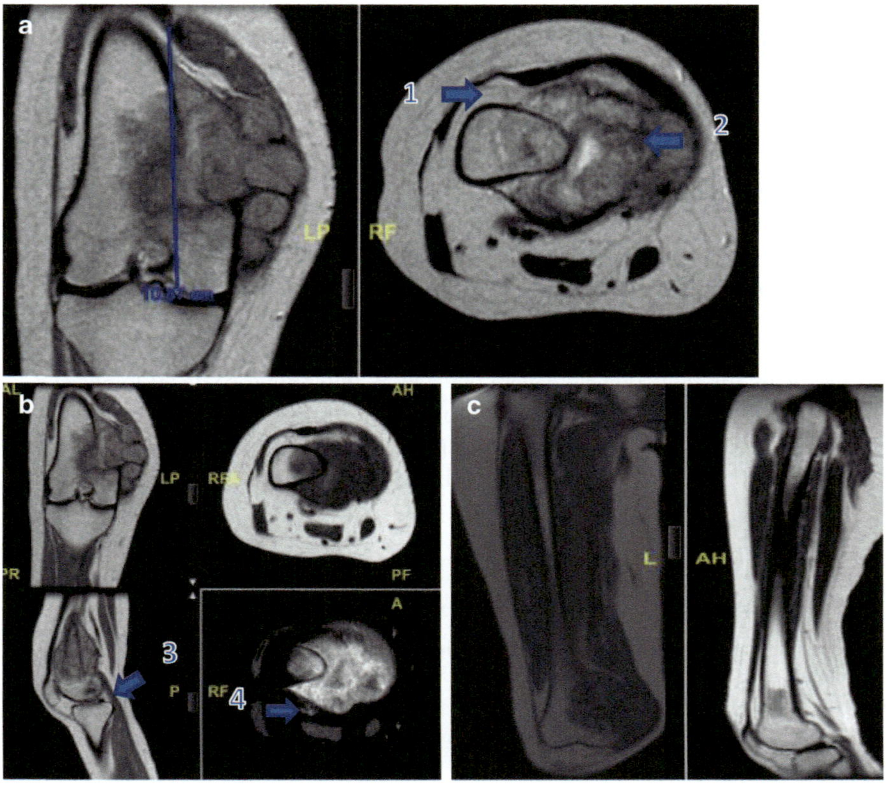

1. Vastus medialis
2. Supra patella fat covering distal femur and intermedius muscle
3. Medial gastrocnemius attachment
4. Popliteal vessels

Distal femur osteosarcoma with extension to the vastus medialis muscle, demonstrating a good response to chemotherapy. The vastus lateralis and posterior popliteal structures were free of tumour. Wide margins were achieved by removing a cuff of vastus medialis together with vastus intermedius and popliteal fat tissues. Menisci and all the ligaments were resected at the tibia attachment for better intra-articular oncological clearance. It is important to evaluate the entire femur on T1 weighted image for intramedullary skip lesions (Fig. 1a–c).

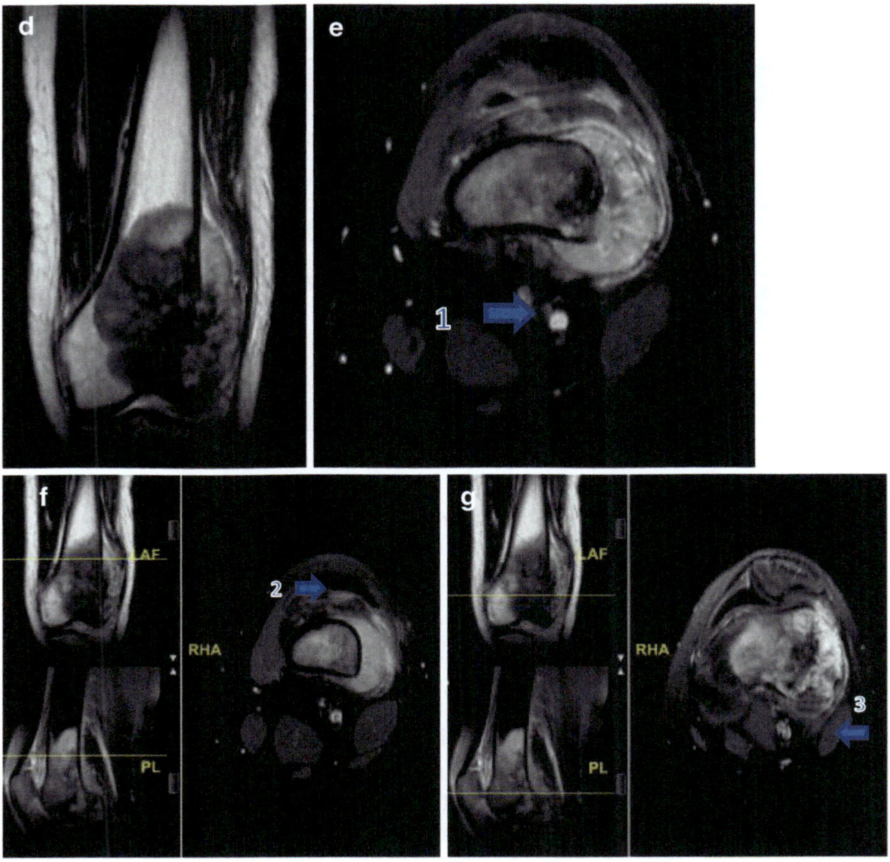

1. Popliteal vessels
2. Rectus femoris tendon
3. Biceps femoris long head

Distal femur malignant tumour with lateral extension to the vastus lateralis necessitating careful MRI evaluation for tumour extension of lateral gastrocnemius tendon, origin of short head biceps femoris and peroneal nerve to achieve oncological clearance (Fig. 1d–g).

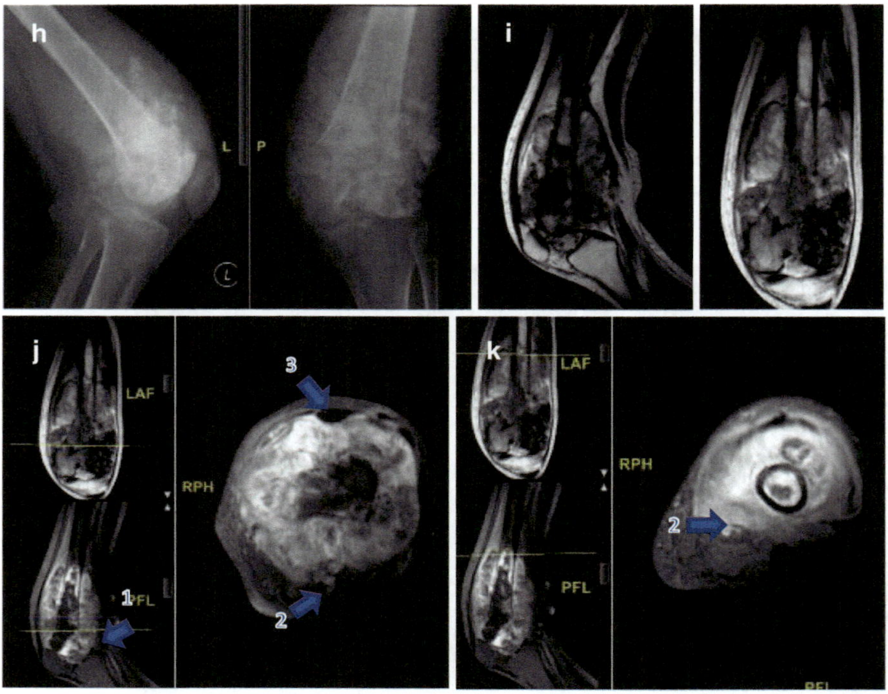

1. Medial gastrocnemius muscle insertion
2. Popliteal and femoral vessels
3. Rectus femoris tendon

Osteosarcoma distal femur with involvement of surrounding tissue and posterior compartment. MRI demonstrated that the knee joint was involved, and entire quadriceps compartment was involved directly by invasion of sarcoma. The short head of biceps origin was also involved. The tendon of rectus femoris can be preserved to serve as the main extensor, and the neurovascular structures can be separated (Fig. 1h–k). Though amputation is an option, limb salvage surgery can be considered with careful dissection of major vessels and nerves, extra-articular resection and free tissue transfer to augment quadriceps function.

Principles of Reconstruction in Distal Femur Sarcoma

The main aim of reconstruction is to achieve a stable, painless, mobile knee for early weight bearing and ambulation. These can be achieved by:

1. Stable osseous reconstruction
   - A modular replacement system is an option for stable knee function and its modularity offers accommodating for different lengths of resection
   - Allograft prosthesis (semi constrained knee) for early knee function; however, delayed full weight bearing ambulation is advised until junctional union occurs
   - Osteoarticular allograft with medial lateral and posterior ligament reinforcement—this type of reconstruction needs protection until ligament healing and junctional allograft union—in our opinion, this is only suitable for paediatric reconstructions
2. Restoration of quadriceps continuity and function as an antigravity muscle for walking
   - Vastus intermedius muscle is frequently excised for oncological boundaries, and the remaining vastus medialis, lateralis and rectus femoris are strong extensors for knee extension function
   - In large tumours if a major part of quadriceps must be removed due to tumour infiltration, the options available are:
     - Mobilisation of sartorius muscle/gracilis/medial gastrocnemius muscle on the medial side
     - Mobilisation of biceps femoris on the lateral side
     - Free tissue transfer using latissimus dorsi muscle with motorised thoracodorsal nerve to the remnant branch to vastus medialis
3. Flexibility of soft tissue cover for good knee function
   - Soft tissue cover over prosthesis and flexible reconstruction is the most important aspect to prevent wound breakdown and permit early mobile knee function. This can be achieved with principles similar for the extensor mechanism

Surgical Steps

Medial Approach

Exploration of popliteal vessels via a medial approach is the standard procedure. The medial approach utilising a longitudinal incision curved distally to the patella tubercle enables exploration of femoral and popliteal vessels and knee resection. Biopsy scar is included in the excision as part of the surgical margin. The adductor magnus opening is freed for mobilisation of femoral vessels and proximal exploration. Medial gastrocnemius tendon is detached to mobilise the vessels distally for safer resection (Fig. 2a, b).

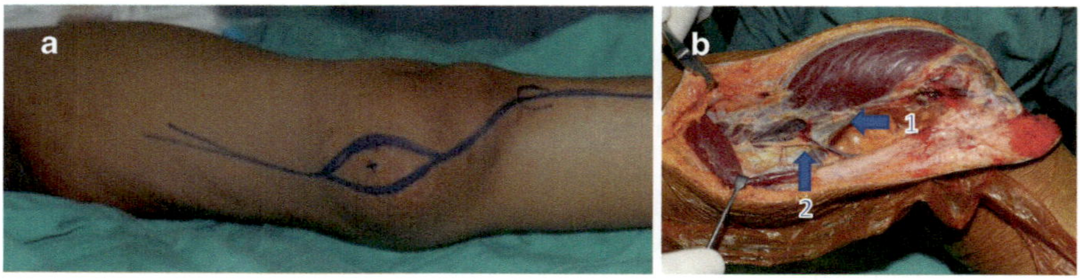

Saphenous nerve exits from the subsartorial canal above the adductor opening and subsequently joins the saphenous vein. It should be identified and protected to prevent injury and numbness over the medial leg (Fig. 2b).

1. Adductor magnus tendon insertion (adductor hiatus)
2. Saphenous nerve

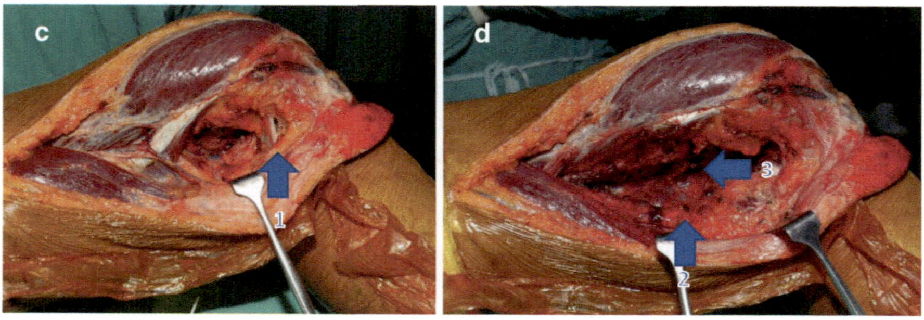

1. Medial gastrocnemius tendon
2. Popliteal vessels
3. Short head of biceps muscle attached to the lateral femoral condyle

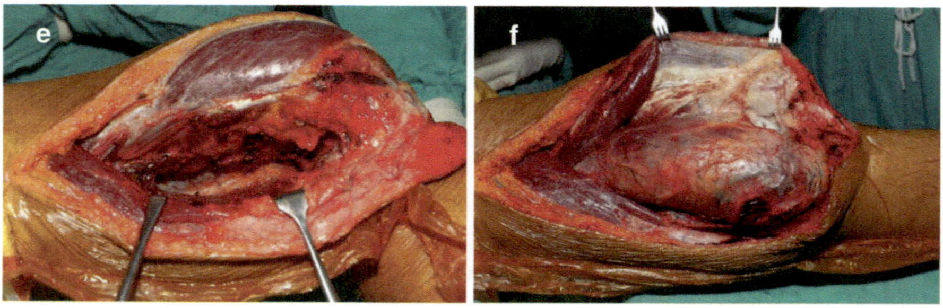

Medial gastrocnemius head and adductor magnus is detached from distal femur for complete exploration of the entire popliteal artery. The short head of biceps origin is identified for determination of postero-lateral surgical margin (Fig. 2d, e).

Plane is created between vastus medialis and intermedius for surgical margin. Patella and patella tendon is mobilised laterally to visualise the anterior margin (Fig. 2f, g).

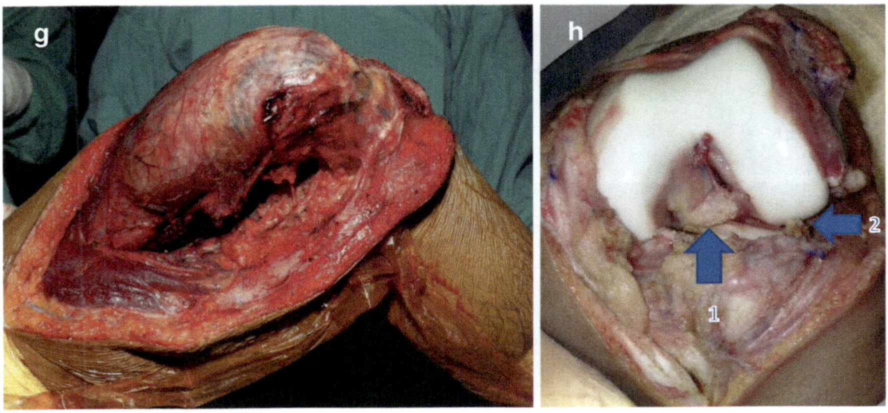

Resection completed by transection of intra-articular ligament ACL, PCL and collateral ligament from the tibia with meniscus as intra-articular margin (Fig. 2h). Bony osteotomy was performed at the level 3–5 cm from marrow involvement

1. Anterior cruciate ligament transacted
2. Medial subluxation after cutting the medial collateral and ACL

The prepatellar fat pad was mobilised for visualisation of the joint structures. The medial collateral ligament was transacted to open the medial joint line, the anterior cruciate ligament was detached to the tibial insertion, and it will destabilise the knee for external rotation and detached remaining capsule, posterior cruciate ligament and lateral collateral ligament.

Lateral Approach

For a sarcoma involving the lateral compartment or involving a long segment of resection, it is preferable to approach it via a lateral longitudinal incision. The plane is in between biceps femoris and vastus lateralis (Fig. 3a, b). Peroneal nerve and subsequently popliteal vessels exploration and mobilisation distally below joint line is achieved for safe posterior capsule transection after anterior intra-articular resection (Fig. 3c).

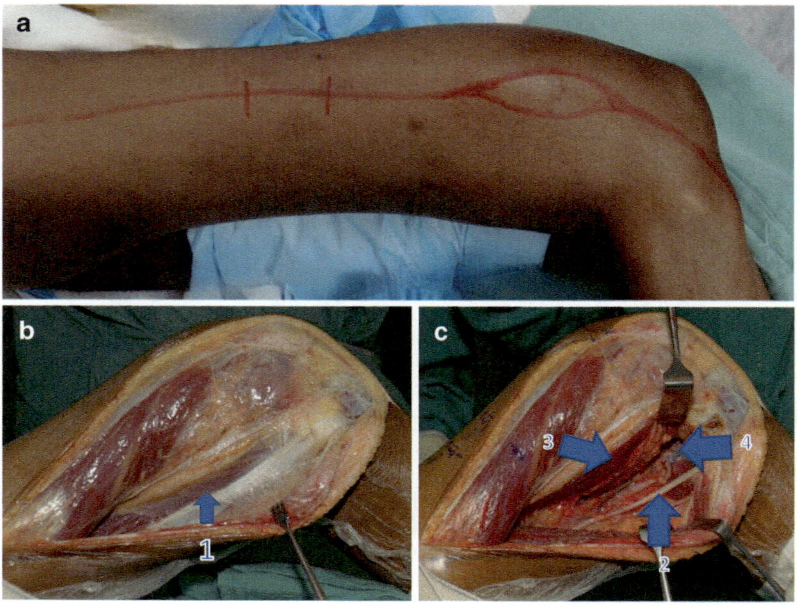

1. Biceps femoris muscle and tendon
2. Peroneal nerve
3. Remnant of short head of biceps as a margin
4. Popliteal vessels

Short head of biceps and lateral gastrocnemius tendon are detached for exploration of popliteal vessels and nerve (Fig. 3c, d).

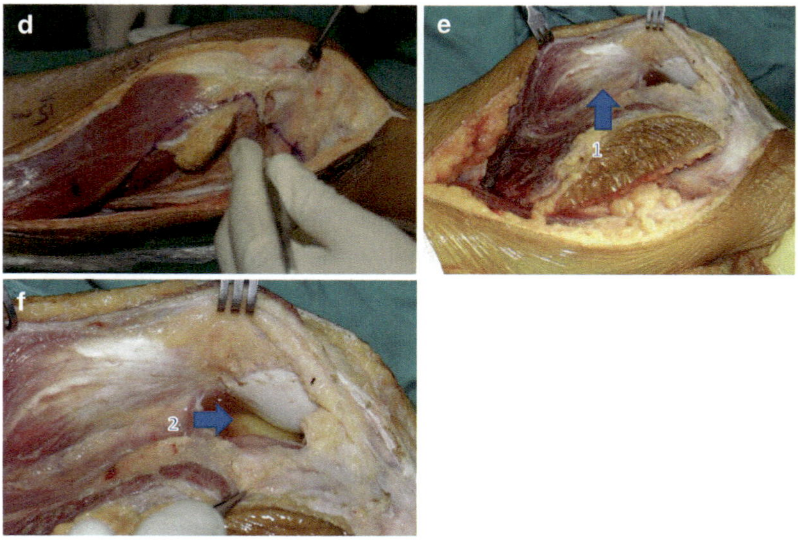

1. Elevation vastus lateralis and rectus femoris from vastus intermedius
2. Clear synovial fluid after lateral arthrotomy

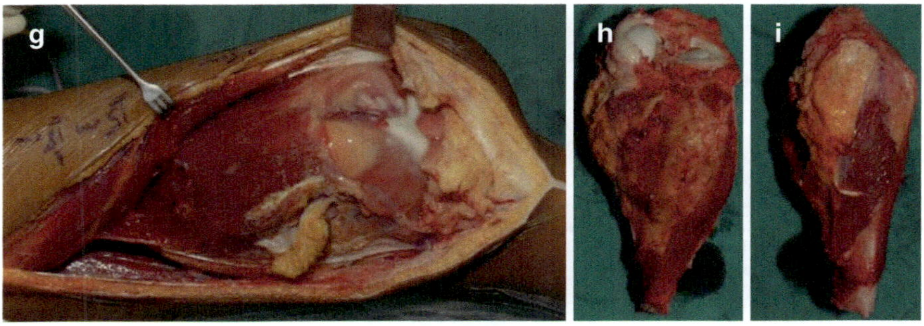

Vastus lateralis and biopsy scar with margin are included in resection plane created above the vastus intermedius for wide surgical margins. The plane continues medially between vastus intermedius and rectus femoris after lateral capsulotomy. Assessment of synovial fluid for hemarthrosis and joint involvement helps minimise the incidence of tumour contamination (Fig. 3e–i).

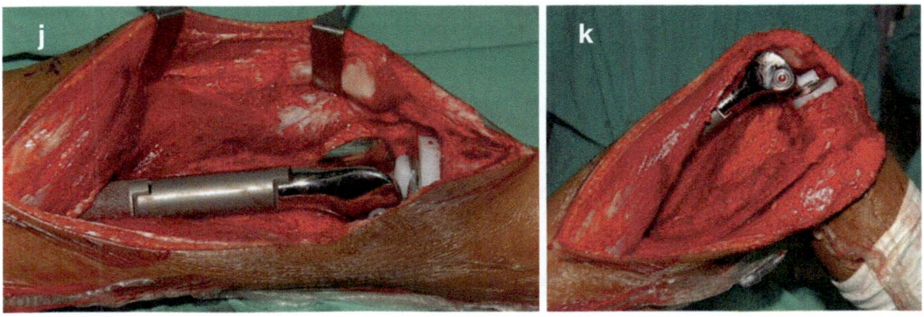

Final bone reconstruction with endoprosthesis replacement (Fig. 3j, k).

In cases where the femoral and popliteal neurovascular bundles are in close proximity to the resection margin particularly around the adductor magnus opening, medial mobilisation of the femoral vessels is only possible after intra-articular resection and dislocation of the knee. The adductor magnus tendon attachment must be transacted and the popliteal neurovascular bundle traced superiorly (Fig. 3l–s).

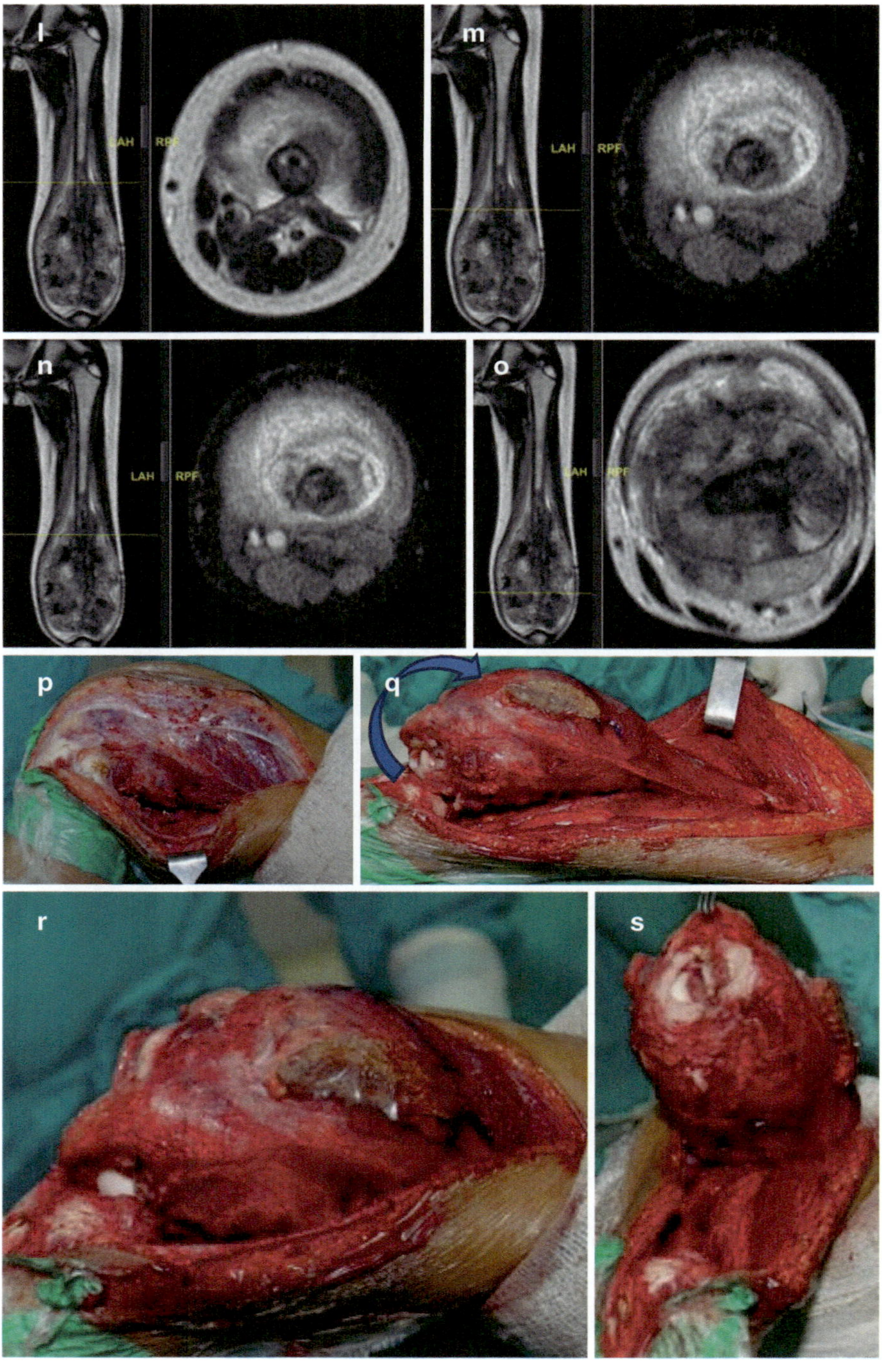
l
LAH
RPF
m
LAH
RPF
n
LAH
RPF
o
LAH
RPF
p
q
r
s

Distal Femur Osteosarcoma with Vastus Medialis Involvement

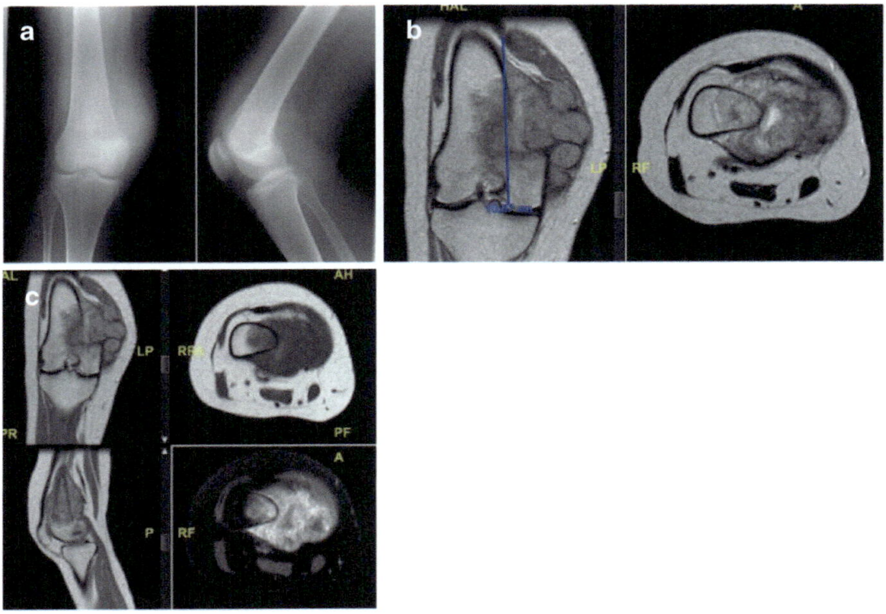

Distal femur osteosarcoma with extension to the vastus medialis muscle, good response to chemotherapy. The vastus lateralis and posterior popliteal structure was free of tumour (Fig. 4a–c). Wide margin achieved by excising cuff of vastus medialis together with vastus intermedius and popliteal fat tissues. Meniscus and all the ligaments were resected at the tibia attachment for better intra-articular oncological clearance (Fig. 4d, e).

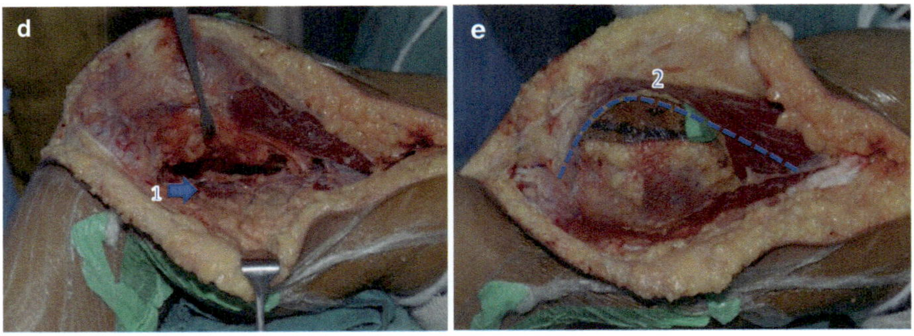

1. Popliteal vessels
2. Vastus medialis resection margin
3. Vastus intermedius
4. Lateral intermuscular septum

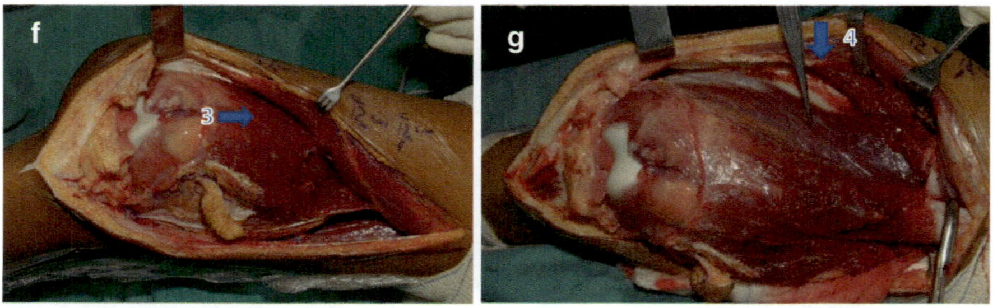

The entire extensor muscles are released from tumour with attached intermedius group. Periosteum is stripped circumferentially before osteotomy (Fig. 4f, g).

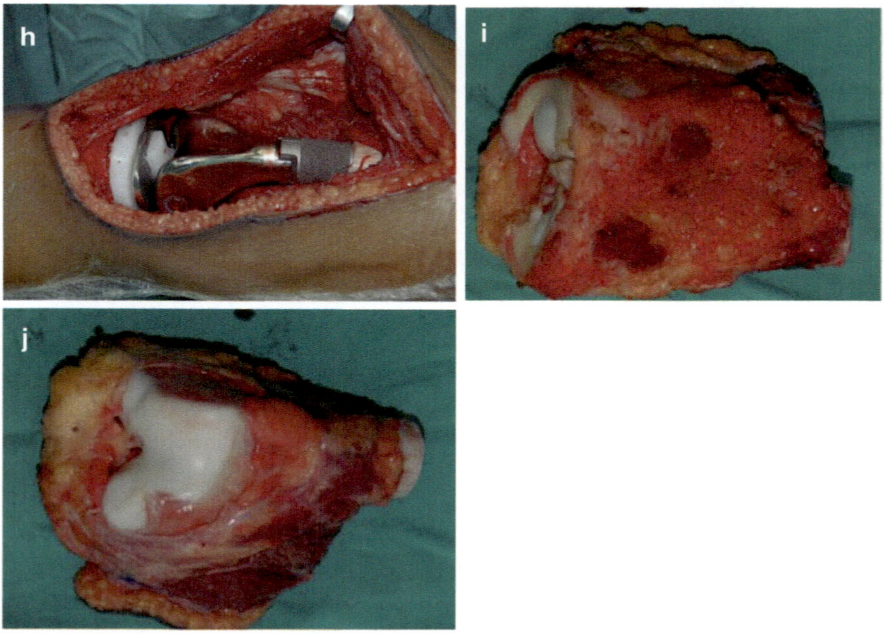

Endoprosthesis design with small condyle and less prominence allows tissue closure without tension in majority of cases despite removal of medial tissue (Fig. 4h–j).

Osteosarcoma with Postero-Medial Extra-Osseous Extension

Massive tumour infiltration of the vastus medialis and intermedius compartment needs extensive resection for oncological clearance. A free flap, particularly a latissimus dorsi flap, is indicated for flexible closure to minimise wound break down and better knee motion.

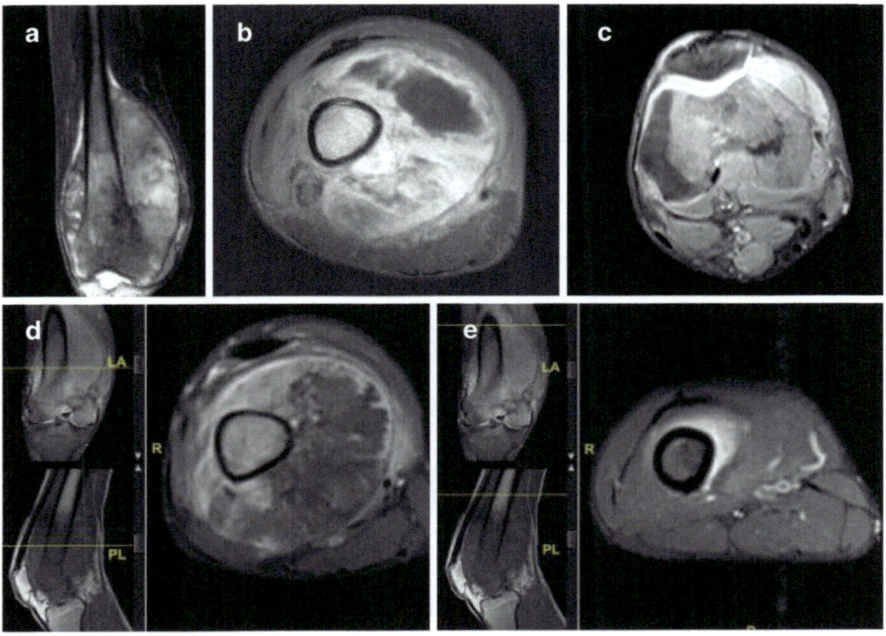

Proximal boundary of soft tissue and marrow extension must be confirmed by careful evaluation of coronal, sagittal and axial slices (Fig. 5a–e).

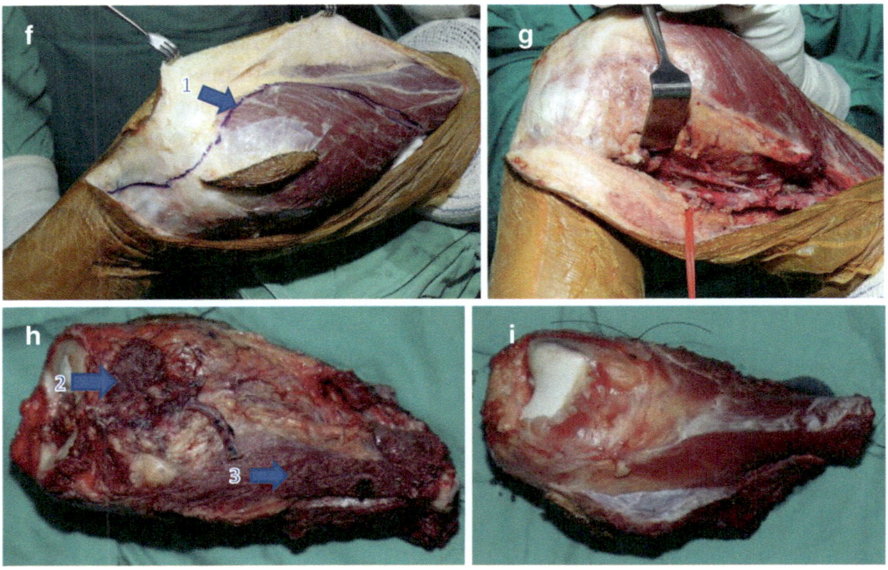

1. Resection margin of vastus medialis
2. Medial gastrocnemius origin
3. Short head biceps femoris origin at distal femur

Major part of vastus medialis, intermedius and medial parapatellar tissue were resected up to the rectus femoris compartment. The medial gastrocnemius tendon and muscle attachment, short head of biceps femoris origin and part of the vein were include in the tumour margin (Fig. 5f–i). The medial tissue defect is reconstructed with a free latissimus dorsi flap (Fig. 5j, k).

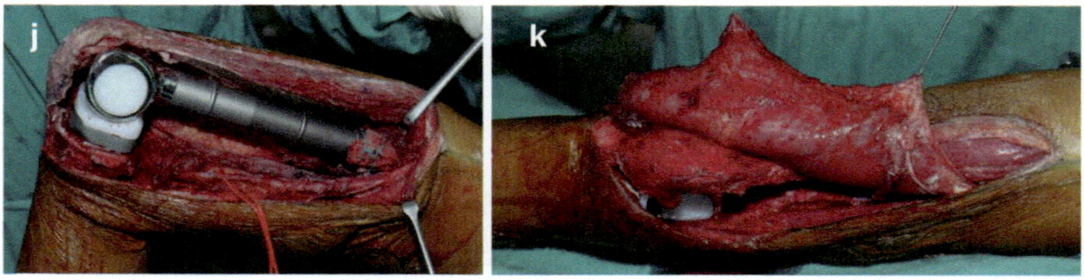

Osteosarcoma with Postero-Lateral Extra-Osseous Extension

Tumour with posterior popliteal extension will push the neurovascular bundle superficially and rarely infiltrate and affect the peroneal nerve. The MRI evaluation of vessels is important for limb salvage surgery; however, evaluation of peroneal nerve can be occasionally difficult. Exploration of distal peroneal nerve through its anatomical courses will minimise iatrogenic injuries. Tumour that infiltrates to the vastus lateralis and posterolateral area is best approached through lateral approach by exploring the common peroneal nerve first. The femoral and popliteal artery with tibial nerve are easily accessed after proximal femoral osteotomy and knee disarticulation by flipping the entire tumour medially.

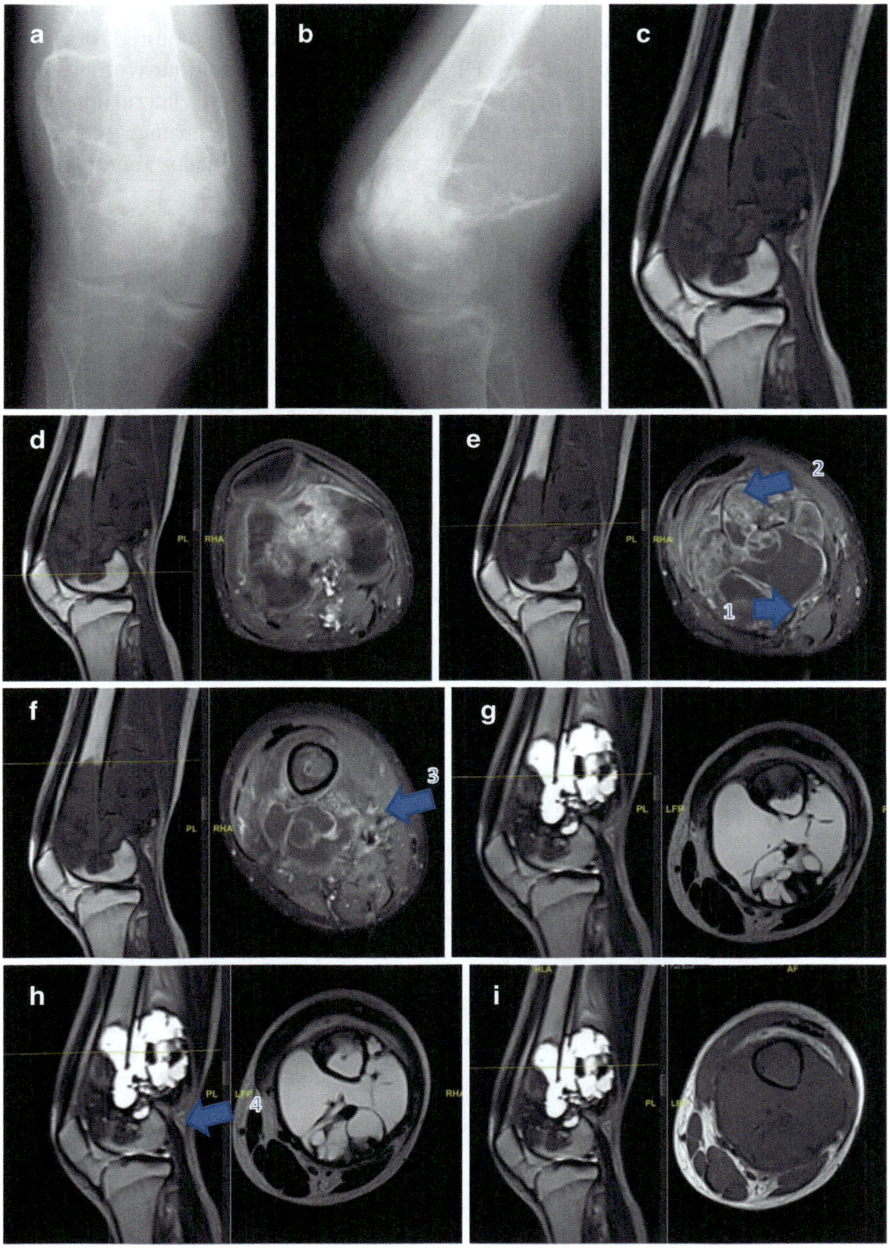

1. Popliteal vessels and tibial nerve
2. Vastus intermedius tumour extension
3. Femoral vessels
4. Medial gastrocnemius tendon

Careful MRI evaluation to preclude tumour extension to lateral gastrocnemius tendon, origin of short head biceps femoris and peroneal nerve is required for ensuring oncological clearance (Fig. 6a–i). Distal femur malignant tumour with posterolateral extension to the vastus lateralis is best approached through a lateral approach. The tumour extension can be well controlled to prevent local recurrence with a cuff of muscle margin especially vastus lateralis and short head of biceps (Fig. 6j–m).

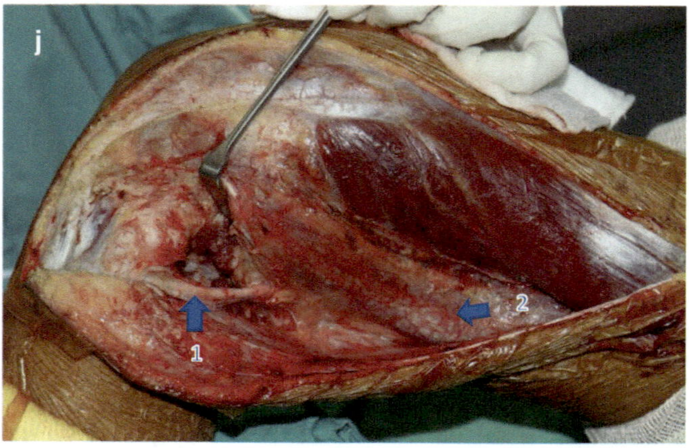

1. peroneal nerve exploration
2. Biceps femoris

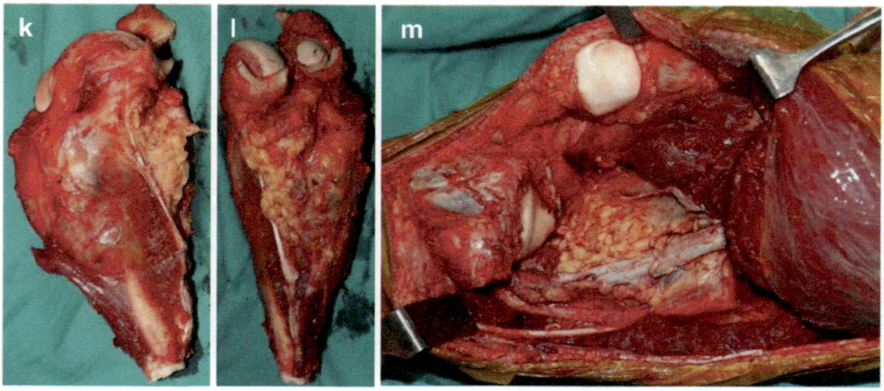

Extra-Articular Resections

When there is an extension or infiltration into the knee joint, the risk of contamination and recurrence is high in case an intra-articular resection is attempted. An extra-articular resection describes a resection of a distal femur sarcoma with surrounding involved tissue without opening the knee joint. To maintain the extensor mechanism of the knee with an extra-articular resection, surgical technique requires a patella osteotomy above the synovial line combined with a proximal tibia resection below the capsular attachment.

Distal femur osteosarcoma with knee joint involvement requires extra articular resection for adequate oncological margins (Fig. 7a–f).

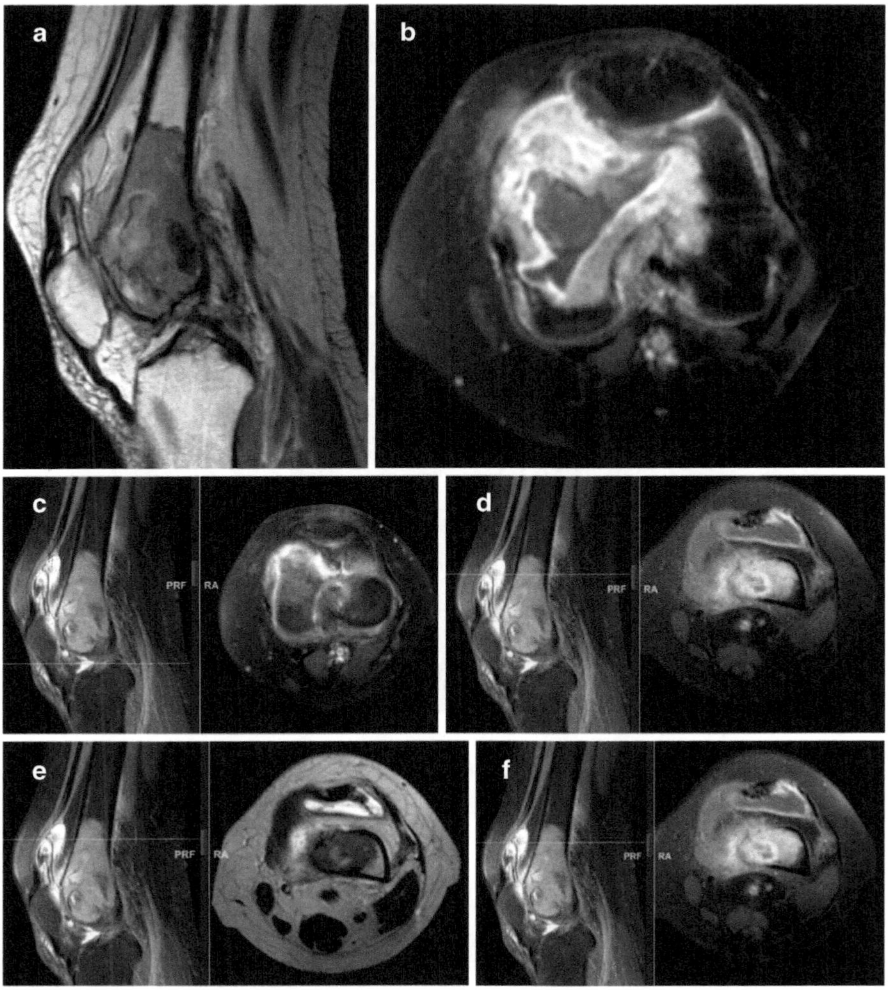

Distal femur osteosarcoma with intra-articular extension, the synovial fluid and tissue contaminated from hematoma and direct infiltration of patella surface from lateral condyle of femur. The vastus medialis and lateralis were free from tumour extension. Extra-articular resection of distal femur with entire knee joint is the only option to minimised contamination and achieve oncological clearance.

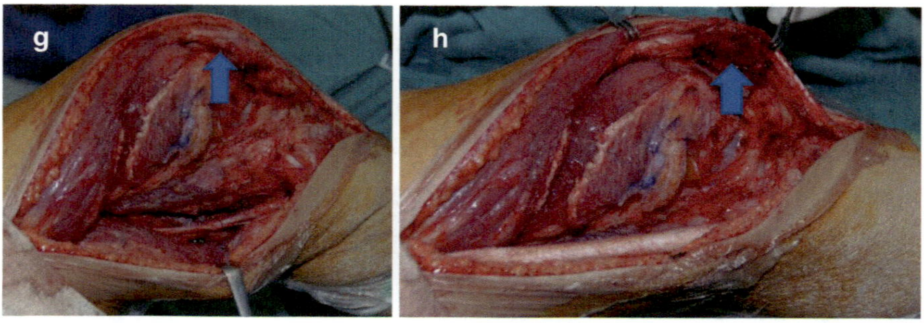

Mobilising the patella tendon distally and quadriceps tendon superiorly for a uniform cut of patella. Image-intensifier guidance can help to prevent an excessive cut (Fig. 7g–i).

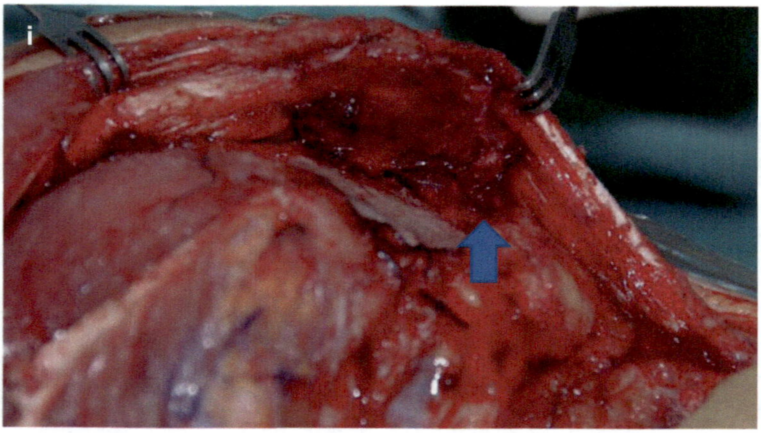

- Identification of medial patella surface by clearing the parapatellar tissue; partial patella osteotomy leaves the patellar articular surface along with the distal femur enabling oncological clearance (Fig. 7l).

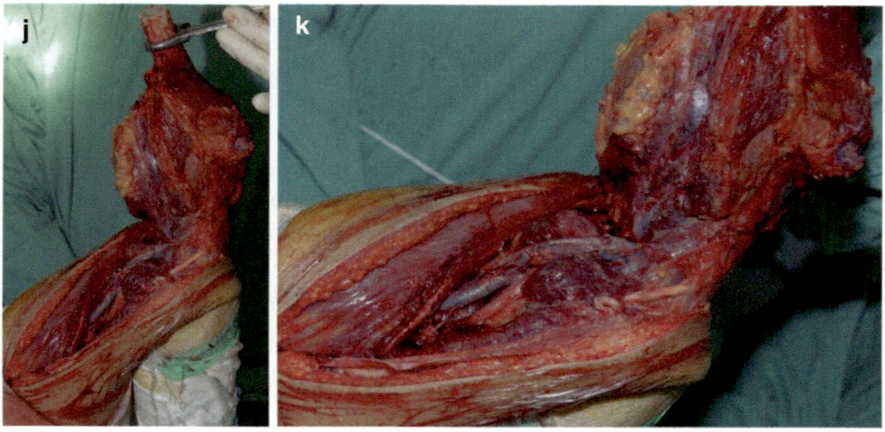

Posterior neuro-vascular is dissected and protected for proximal tibial osteotomy below the capsular attachment. The entire distal femur tumour is removed together with the intra-articular part of patella and proximal tibial to prevent a tumour breach at the knee joint (Fig. 7j–n).

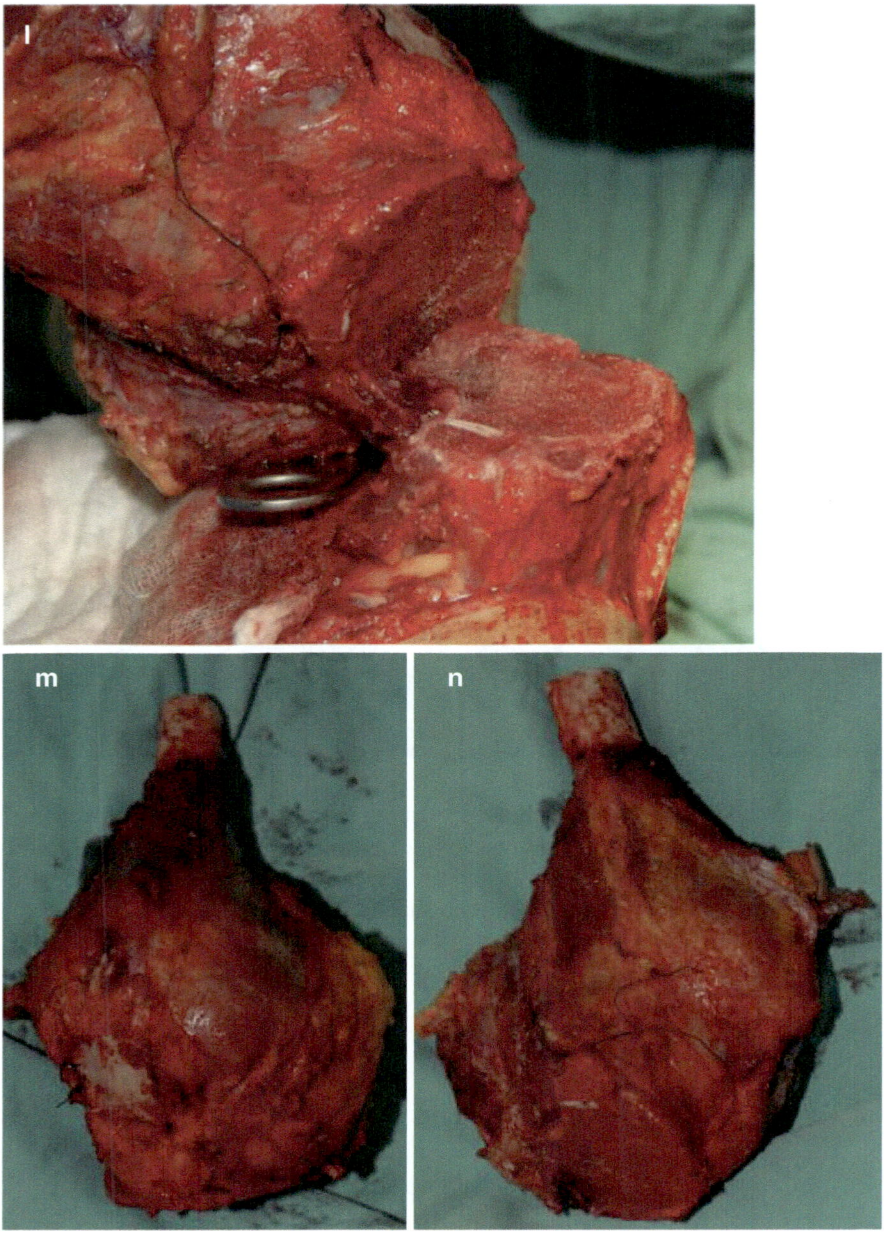

Extra-Articular Resection with Latissimus Dorsi Flap Reconstruction

Intra-articular extension of a tumour requires a conventional extra-articular resection with en bloc removal of the knee including extensor apparatus. Usually it occurs in extensive tumours with direct intra-articular extension, poor responders to chemotherapy, intra-articular fracture into the joint or previous intra-articular 'whoops' contamination surgery.

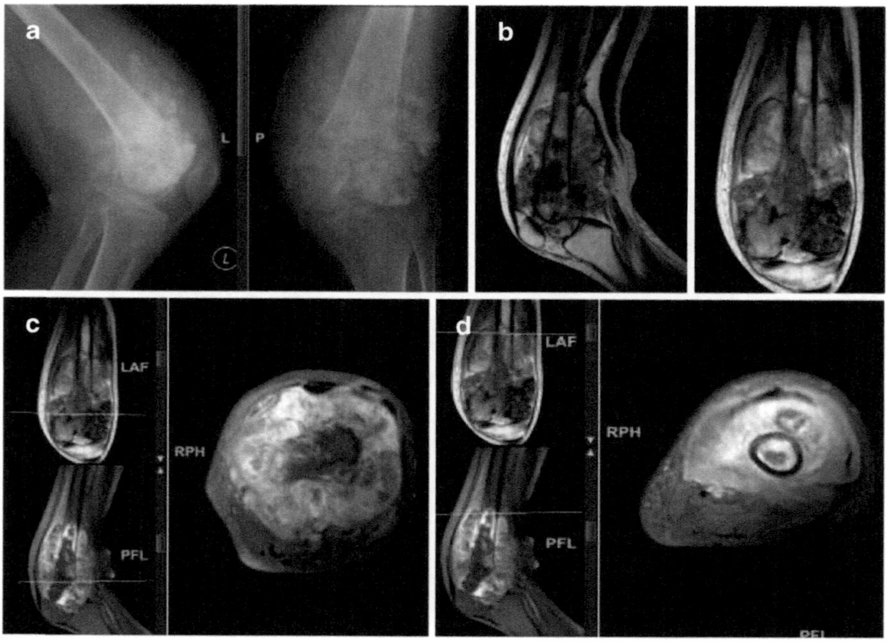

MRI revealed knee joint was breached and the vastus lateralis, intermedius and medialis were involved. The short head of biceps origin in the distal femur was also involved; however, the vessels were intact. The main extensor that could be preserved was the tendon of rectus femoris, superficial surface of patella and patella tendon (Fig. 8a–d).

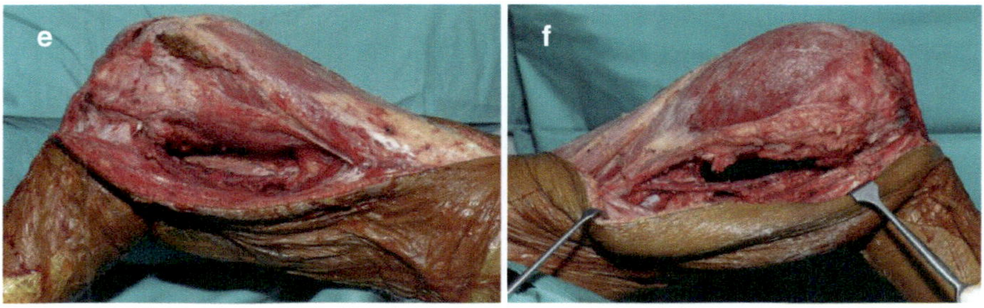

Exploration of peroneal nerve from lateral side and the entire subcutaneous flap was mobilised medially for entire quadriceps exposure (Fig. 8e, f).

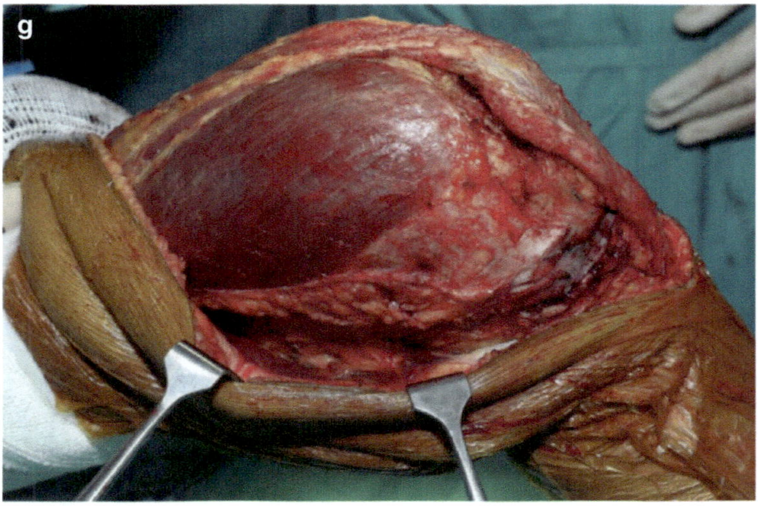

Medial and lateral subcutaneous flap for visualisation of anterior surface of patella. The quadricep tendon, mainly rectus, was elevated superiorly and the patella tendon inferiorly for visualisation of entire anterior surface of patella. The patella surface and retinacular were left intact to be excised en bloc with the tumour (Fig. 8g) The entire quadriceps was detached from the tumour, and proximal femur osteotomy helped to control the tibia osteotomy margin. Image guidance can be used for tibial resection (Fig. 8h–k).

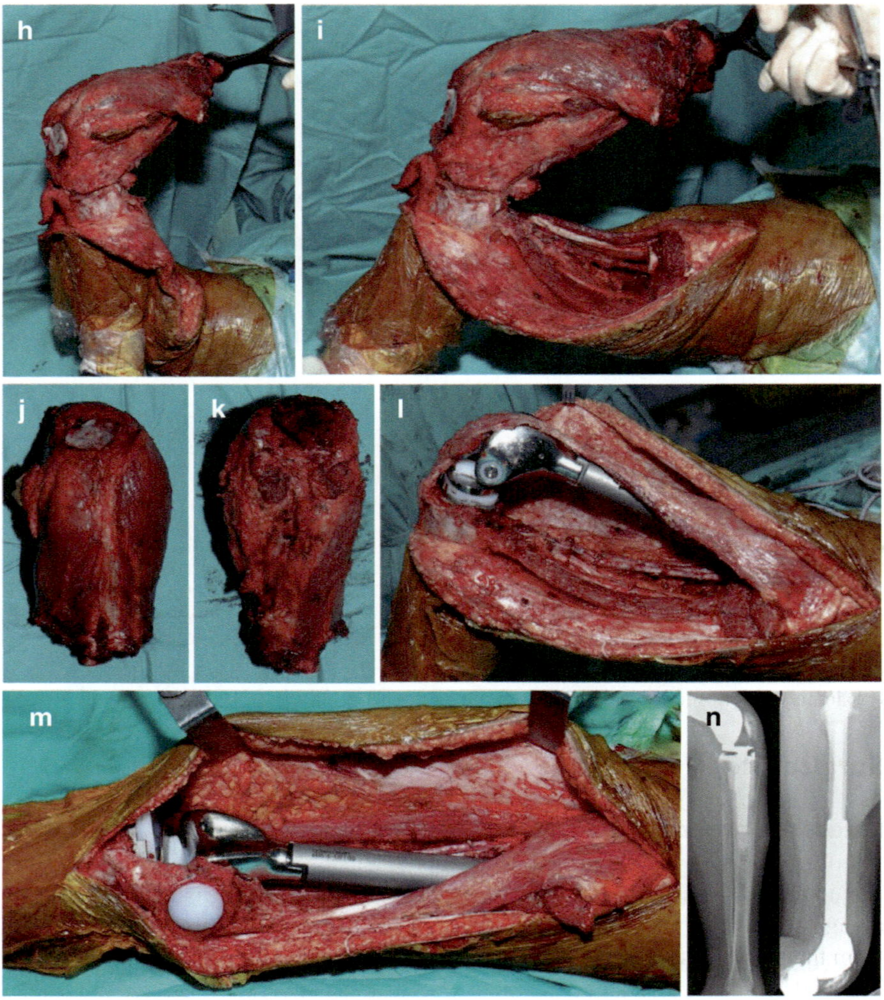

Reconstruction with cemented endoprosthesis. Patella button was inserted over the exposed patella surface after patellar osteotomy during extra-articular resection. Extensive tissue loss was managed with free latissimus dorsi flap motorised by the remnant nerve to the vastus medialis enabling better extensor function (Fig. 8l–p).

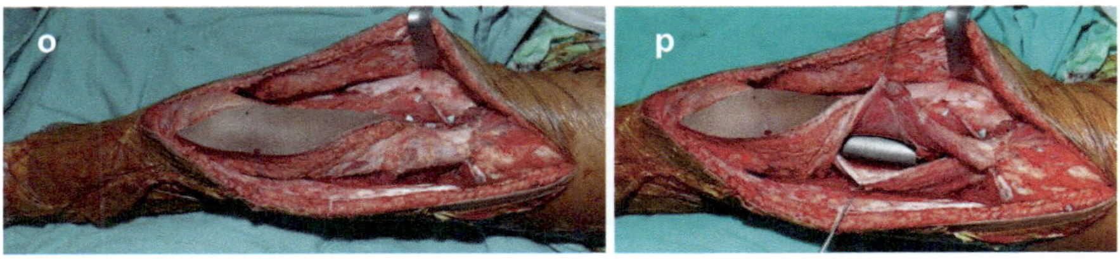

Pathological Fractures and Limb Salvage in Osteosarcoma

Recent literature demonstrates that pathological fracture has no influence on overall survival, and limb salvage surgery is considered a safe option with no significant increase in risk of local recurrence. Response to adjuvant chemotherapy, healing of fracture and calcification/ossification of entire fracture hematoma are few indicators for attempting limb salvage following a pathological fracture.

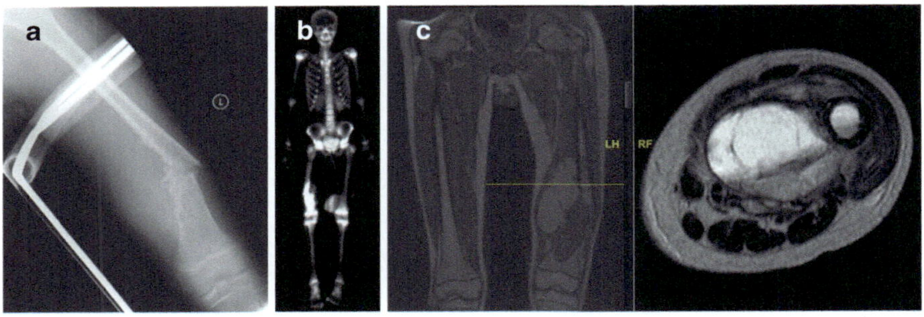

Fracture united following four cycles of neo-adjuvant chemotherapy, but the soft tissue around hematoma was still cystic covered by vastus intermedius and medialis. Dynamic MRI showed necrosis following chemotherapy (Fig. 9a–g).

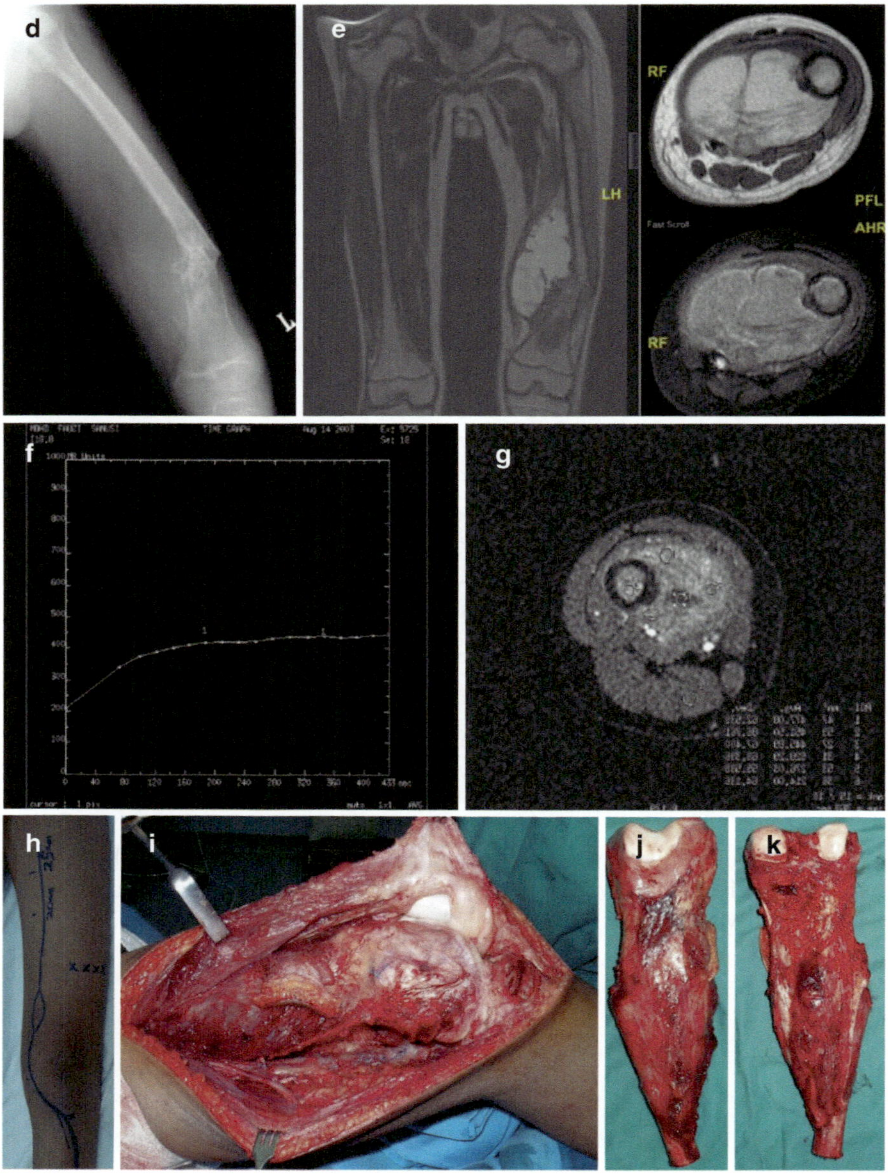

Resection with good margin without hematoma contamination is possible when there is good chemotherapy response (Fig. 9h–k).

Important Tips in Distal Femur Reconstruction When Reconstructing with a Megaprosthesis

Preservation of patella height to prevent repetitive irritation of the patella is important; else it will lead to weakness of quadriceps function, chronic effusion and pain. The inferior border of patella must be clear from the polyethylene bushing and other component (Fig. 10a–c).

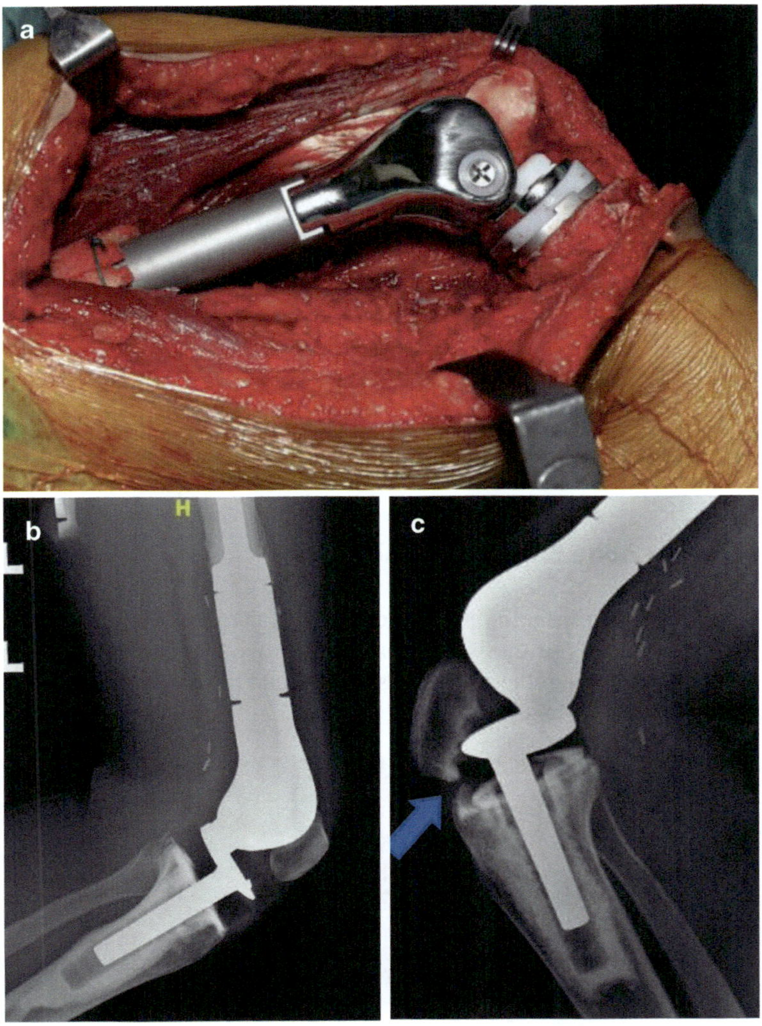

Reconstruction with distal femur endoprosthesis, inferior border of patella has to be above the prosthesis bushing to prevent chronic irritation. Joint line elevation caused chronic irritation to the patella and subsequent bony erosion. Patella height has to be evaluated during trial with knee flexion of 100° (Fig. 10d–f).

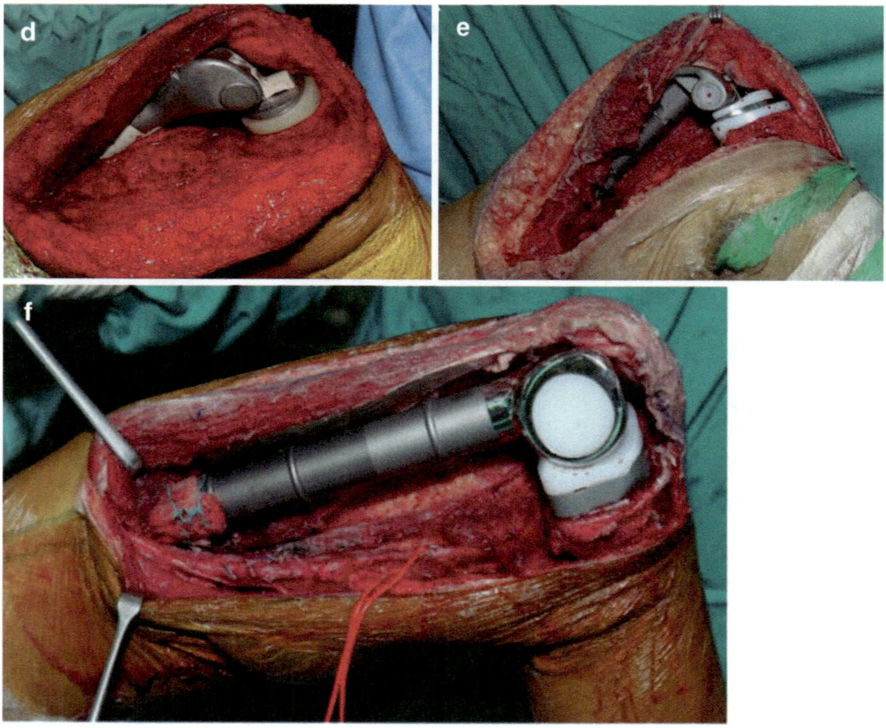

Extra Cortical Bone Bridge Interface (EBBI)

A bone graft at the prosthesis bone junction for a cemented implant will induce bone integration at the prosthesis junction and improve long term survival and prevent early stem loosening. Pieces of excised proximal tibial condyle can be used as a source of graft (Fig. 11a–d).

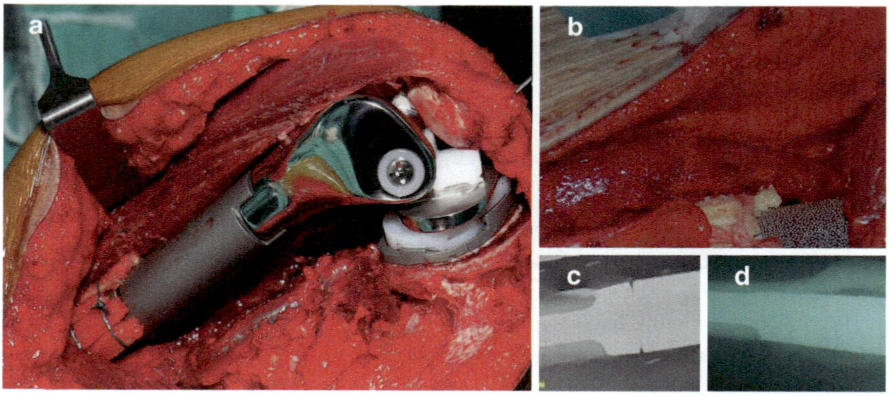

All polyethylene or metal back for tibia? Both have equal long-term survival provided that all polyethylene must be cemented to the entire stem (Fig. 12a–d).

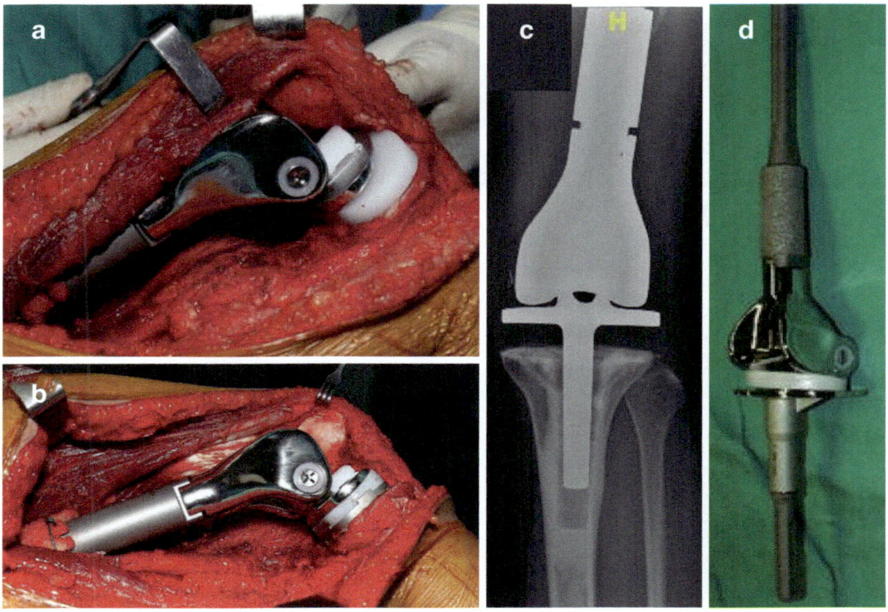

Options for Osseous Reconstructions Other than Megaprosthesis

Reconstruction with Allograft Prosthesis Composite

Allograft prosthesis composites (APC) constitutes a revision type prosthesis inserted inside the skeletal allograft mainly cemented and connected to remaining bone with osteosynthesis. For immediate stability, fixed and rotating hinge knee endoprosthesis is used (Fig. 13a–c).

APC is an option for reconstruction:

- Remaining proximal femur is not adequate for stem fixation after resection.
- Young patient where further revision surgeries may be required.

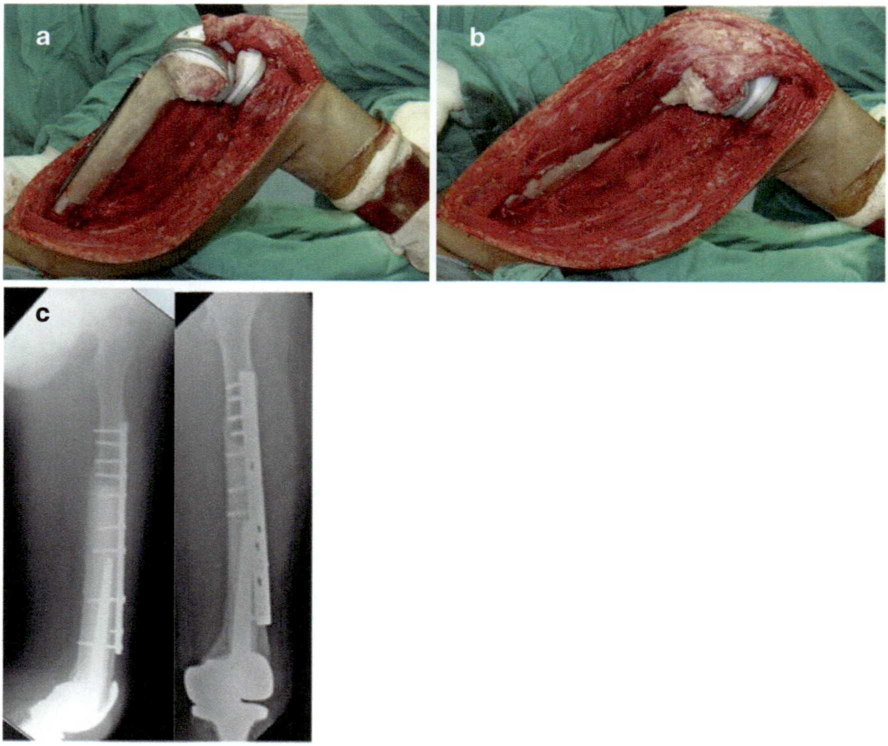

Osteosarcoma with extensive intramedullary and soft tissue extension, and final resection was at subtrochanteric region which was not adequate for stem fixation. Long segment allograft with hinge prosthesis and connected to remaining proximal femur with plate and screw. Plate has to interface the stem over metaphyseal to prevent fracture (Fig. 13d–i).

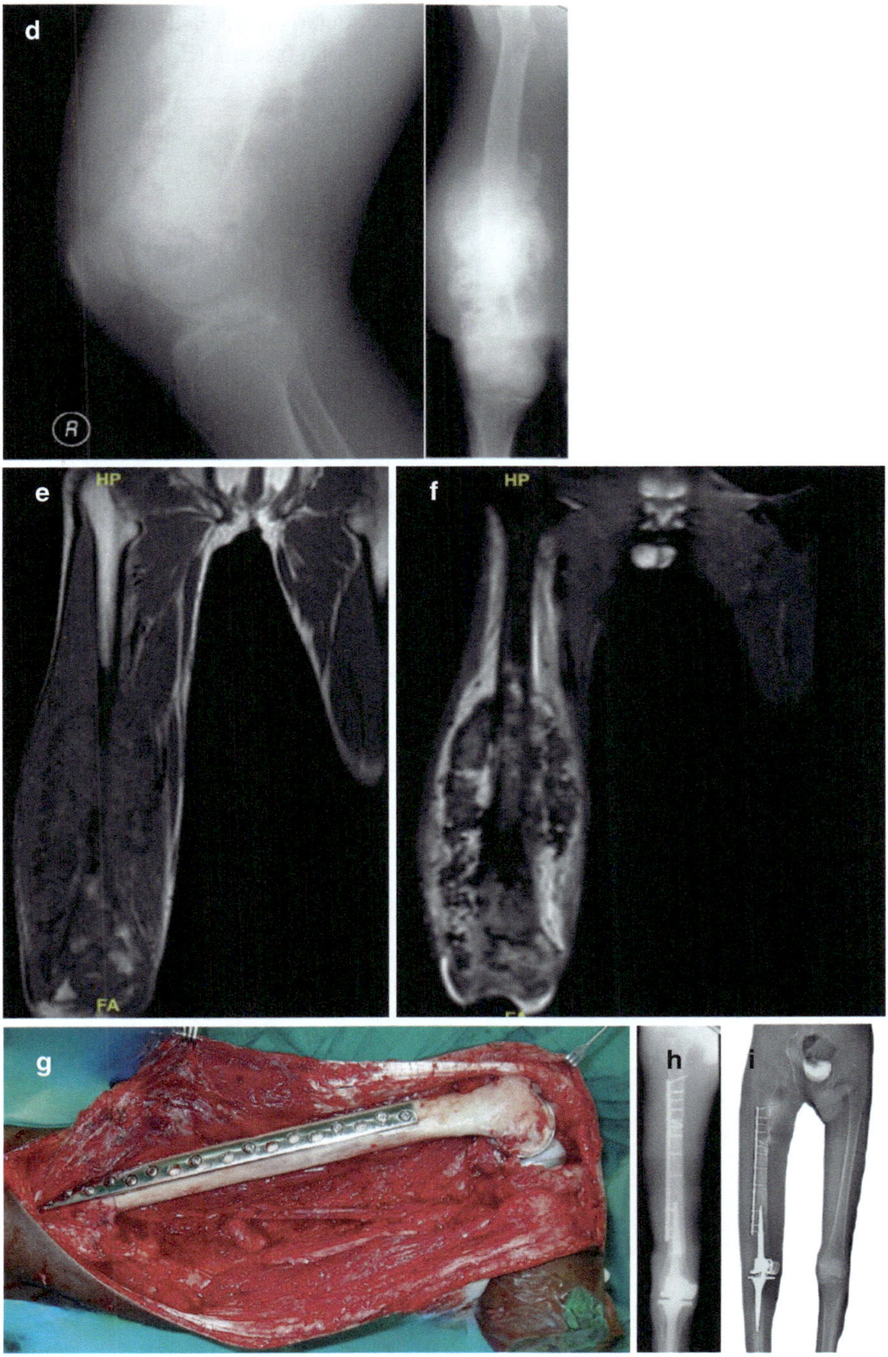
d
R
e
HP
FA
f
HP
g
h
i

Combination of an allograft prosthesis with vascularised fibula to enhance better incorporation and prevent long-term disintegration and fracture (Fig. 13j–m).

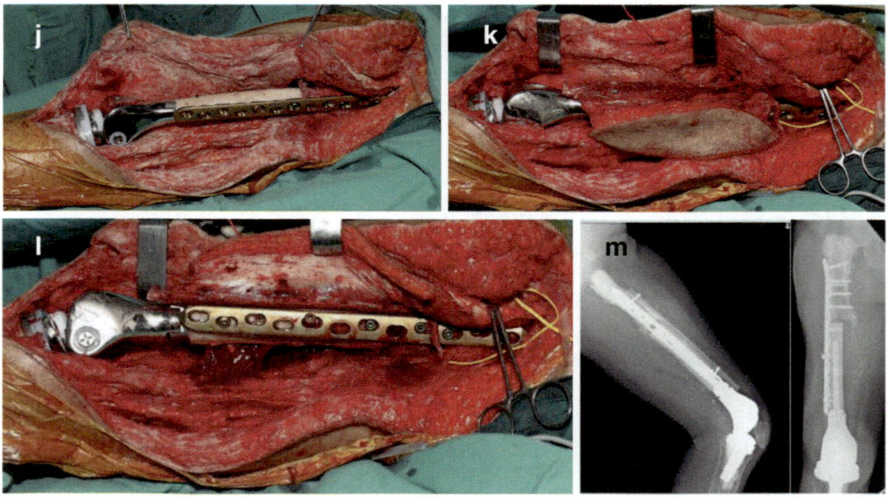

Paediatric Distal Femur Reconstruction

Allograft reconstruction of distal femur tumour by reconstruction of medial and lateral collateral ligaments and posterior capsule to remaining capsule of allograft. Suitable for paediatric age reconstructions as preserves the physeal plate of tibia (Fig. 14a–d).

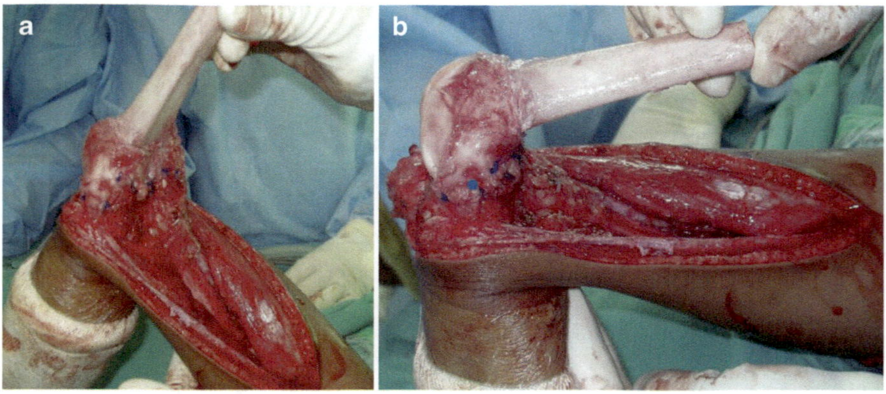

The stability and mobility of the knee joint are evaluated before osseous stabilisation.

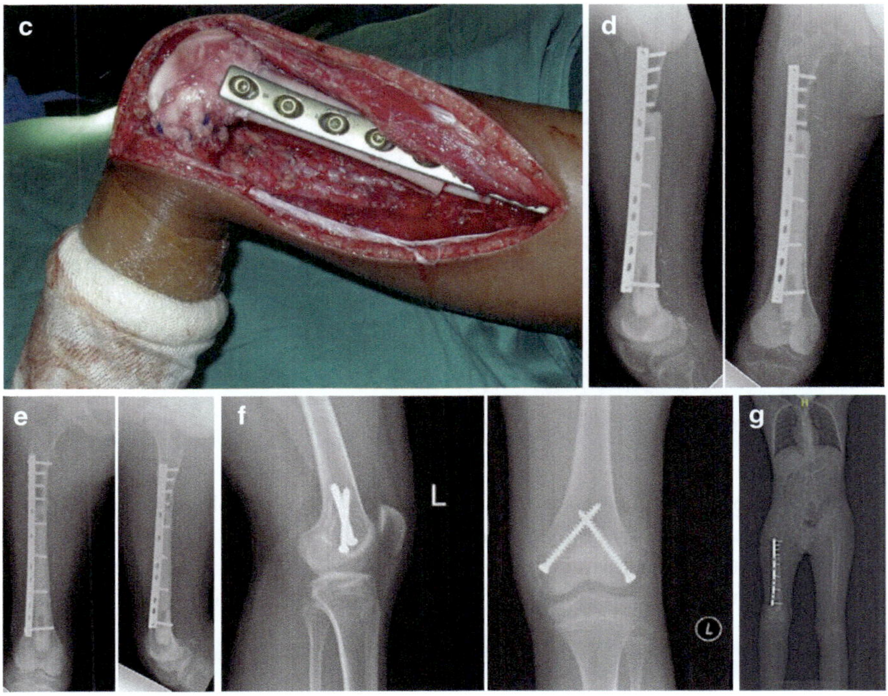

The allograft was bigger and mismatched with tibia for knee joint articulation; the longitudinal growth of the recipient bone equalised the medial lateral joint size. The limb length discrepancy growth was managed with contralateral distal femur epiphysiodesis (Fig. 14e–g).

Combination Allograft Hemicondylar Prosthesis Replacement

This technique utilised the smallest size of partial knee replacement to accommodate mismatched large osteo-articular allograft reconstruction for young patient. Stability of knee joint provided by multiple anchor suture which was fixed to both epicondylar femur for medial and lateral collateral stability. Posterior capsules were attached by multiple anchor suture to the posterior femoral allograft condyle. The anterior stability provided by quadriceps, patella, patella tendon soft tissue closure.

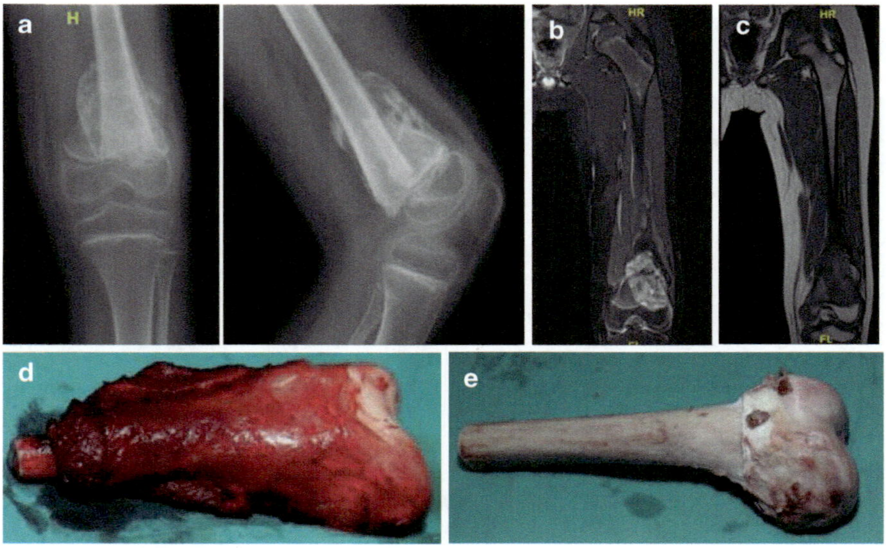

Osteosarcoma distal femur in 9 years old boy with pathological fracture thru physeal plate responded well to chemotherapy (Fig. 15a–c). Osteoarticular allograft not suitable due to size mismatched. The smallest hemicondylar prosthesis used to create better match size to the tibia articular surface (Fig. 15f–i).

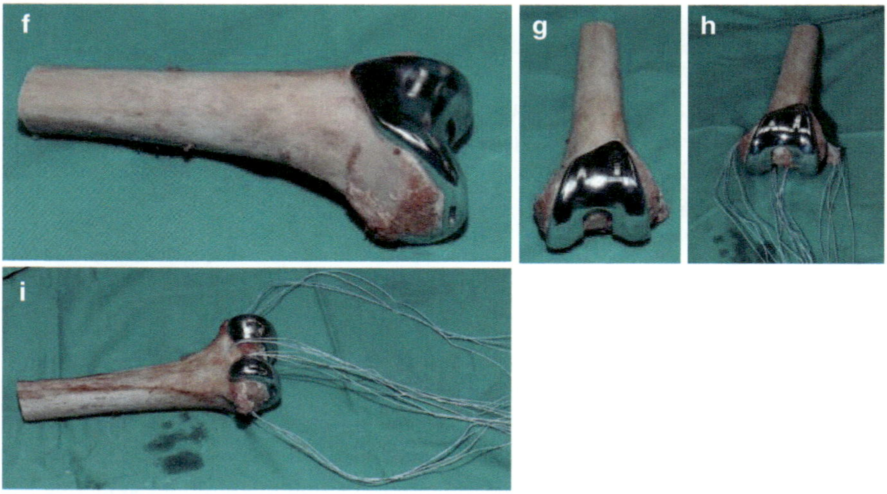

Stability tested through knee range of motion after tightened the anchor suture to the remaining collateral ligament and posterior capsule (Fig. 15j–n).

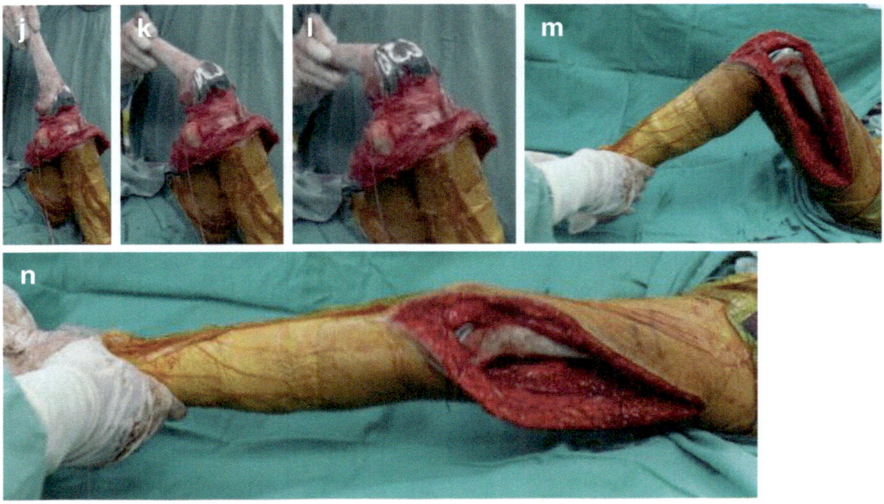

The allograft host junction healing enhanced by intramedullary slot of host bone to allograft 'Kumpta technique' and final anticipated limb length discrepancy managed by contralateral distal femur epiphysiodesis (Fig. 15o–s).

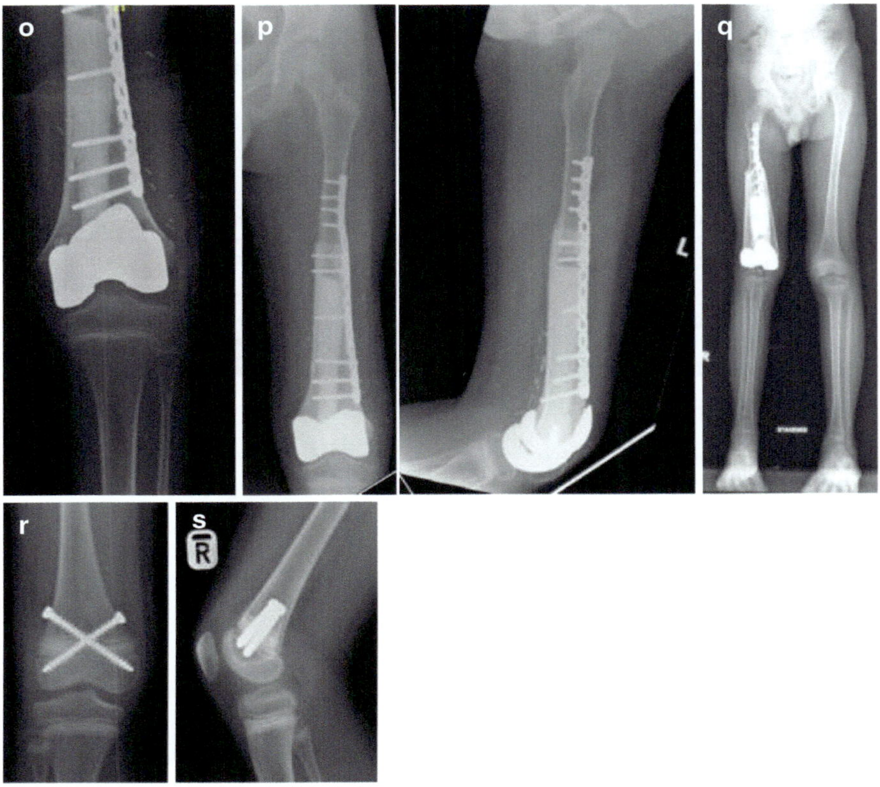

Intercalary Physeal Preservation Distal Femur Reconstruction

Intercalary Allograft Reconstruction

Osteosarcoma mid-shaft femur with spared distal femur growth plate was reconstructed with intercalary allograft. The proximal junction complicated with nonunion and collapse with implant failure. The vascularised fibula graft was used to splint the posterior medial segment to prevent further collapse and induced union, and the allograft was maintained. There is total incorporation of vascularised graft to allograft, and long-term biological incorporation was anticipated.

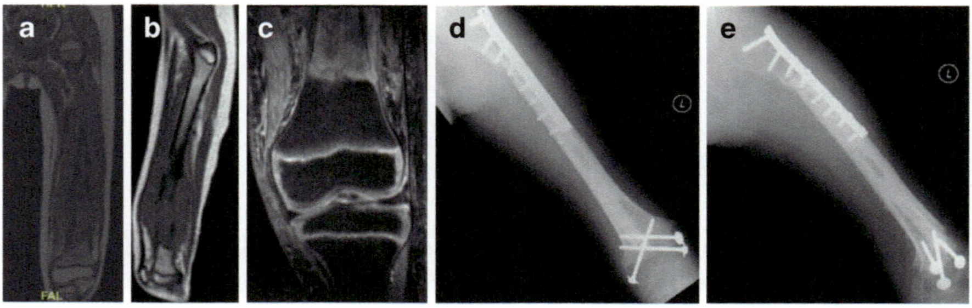

Osteosarcoma in 10-year-old girl was managed by intercalary resection with preservation of epiphyseal part, reconstructed with cemented allograft and fixed with multiple screw distally and DCP plate for proximal stability (Fig. 16a–e).

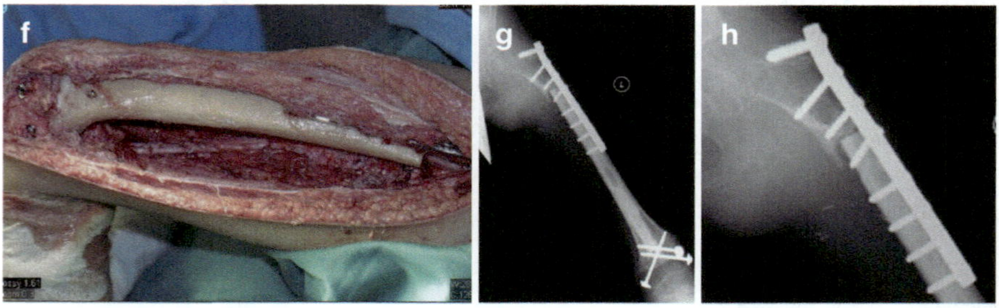

Junctional non-union and late collapse of metaphyseal area of allograft is known complication for failure this method of reconstruction. Salvage procedures with vascularised fibula graft to prevent further collapse and improve union. Long plate for stabilisation protection of entire allograft is also an option to prevent late failure and collapse (Fig. 16f–h).

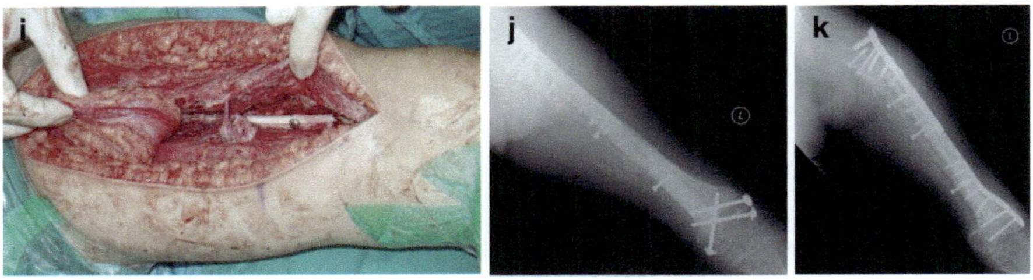

Non-union and collapse of the medial allograft lead to varus deformity of proximal fragment. On lay vascularised fibula graft over the posterior medial femur. Full incorporation and retain of reconstruction 10 years after primary reconstructive surgery (Fig. 16i–k).

Intercalary Allograft Fibula Composite Reconstruction

Intracalary osteosarcoma mid shaft femur in 8-year-old girl responding well to chemotherapy. The resection margin was predetermines by MRI and allograft fibula composite reconstruction was used for long term biological outcome (Fig. 17a–e). Long distal femur locking plate was used, and contralateral distal femur epiphysiodesis was planned.

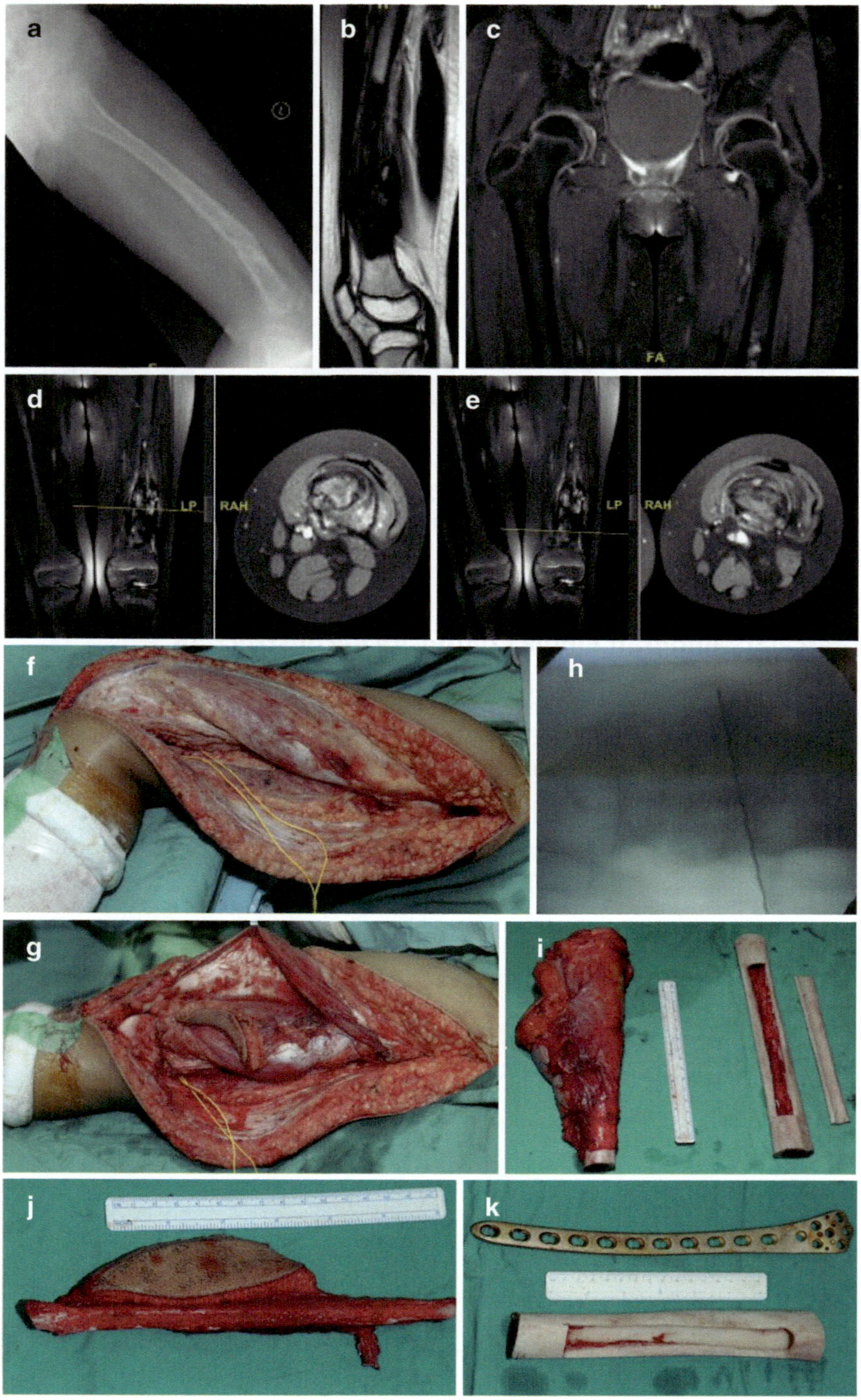
a
b
c
FA
d
LP
RAH
e
LP
RAH
f
h
g
i
j
k

Resection through lateral approach whereby the entire vastus intermedius and partial vastus medialis was include in the margin. Image intra-operative was confirmed prior to bone resection. The intra-operative planning of allograft, vascularised fibula graft, and plate 'Capanna method'. The peroneal vessels was anastomosis to remnant branch to vastus intermedius (Fig. 17f–m).

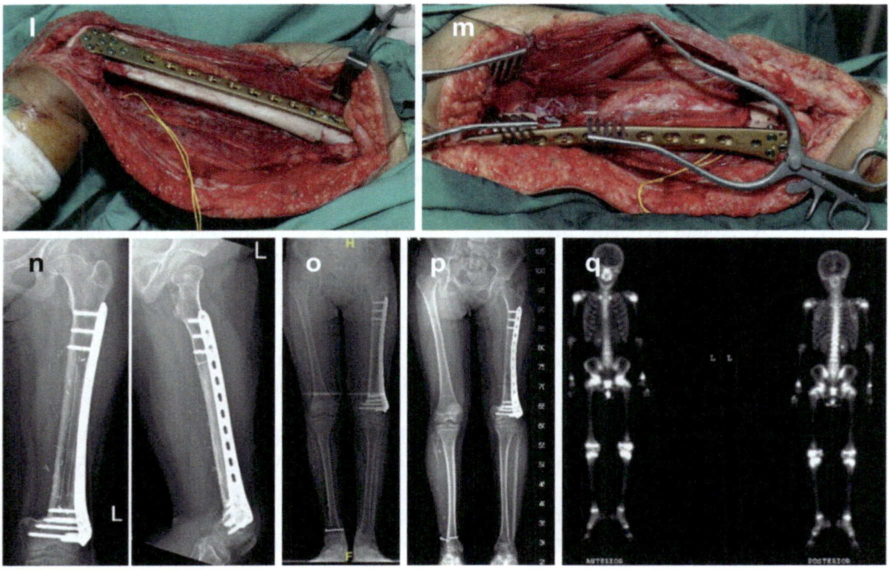

Radiograph showed full incorporation of graft, and scanogram at the age of 10 and 13 revealed 3 cm shortening; however, patient comfortable with shoe raised. Total incorporation and revascularisation of graft was elicited on staging bone scan 3 years later (Fig. 17n–q).

Acknowledgement The author thanks Professor Zulmi Wan, Dr. Nor Azman Mat Zin, Dr. Syurahbil Abdul Halim, for their contributions and team member for managing the patients in this chapter.

The author thanks Professor Wan Azman Wan Sulaiman, Professor Arman Zaharil Mat Saad and Professor Ahmad Sukari Halim from the plastic reconstructive unit at Universiti Sains Malaysia and MSU Medical Centre, Management and Science University for their contributions and team member for managing the patients. All plastic reconstructive and microsurgery surgical procedures were performed by the team members.

The author also thank Professor Ismail Munajat, Dr. Emil Fazliq Mohd and Professor Abdul Razak Sulaiman for managing limb length discrepancy in pediatric sarcoma patient using contralateral epiphysiodesis methods.

Suggested Reading

1. D'Arienzo A, Colangeli S, Andreani L, Mani O, Capanna R. Biological reconstruction of the distal femur – I: massive allograft and inlaid free vascular fibula. In: Orthopaedic surgical oncology for bone tumors. Switzerland: Springer Nature; 2022.
2. Shahril AR, Nawaz AH, Azman MZN, Zulmi W, Faisham WI. Early functional outcome of resection and replacement for primary tumor of the knee. Malaysian Orthop J. 2013;7:30–5.
3. Gautam D, Malhotra R. Megaprosthesis versus allograft prosthesis composite for massive skeletal defects. J Clin Orthop Trauma. 2018;9:63–80.
4. Muscolo DL, Ayerza MA, Aponte-Tinao LA. Distal femur allograft prosthetic composite. In: Master techniques in orthopaedic surgery orthopaedic oncology and complex reconstruction. Lippincott Williams & Wilkins, A Wolters Kluwer; 2011. p. 209–15.
5. Campanacci DA, Scanferla R, Muratori F. Biological reconstruction of the distal femur - resurfacing allograft-prosthesis composite. In: Orthopedic Surgical Oncology For Bone Tumors. Switzerland: Springer Nature; 2022.
6. Myers GJC, Abudu AT, Carter SR, Tillman RM, Grimer RJ. Endoprosthetic replacement of the distal femur for bone tumours long-term results. Bone Joint Surg. 2007;89-B:4.
7. Hardes J, Henrichs MP, Gosheger G, Gebert C, Höll S, Dieckmann R, Hauschild G, Streitbürger A. Endoprosthetic replacement after extra-articular resection of bone and soft-tissue tumours around the knee. Bone Joint J. 2013;95-B:1425–31.
8. Eckardt JJ, Malawer MM, Sickels J, Kiatsevi P. Distal femoral resections with endoprosthesis replacement operative technique in orthopaedic surgical oncology. Lippincott Williams & Wilkins, A Wolters Kluwer; 2012.
9. Weber KL. Megaprosthesis of the Distal Femur. In: Master techniques in orthopaedic surgery orthopaedic oncology and complex reconstruction. Lippincott Williams & Wilkins, A Wolters Kluwer; 2011. p. 183–201.
10. Innocenti M, Abed YY, Beltrami G, Delcroix L, Balatri A, Capanna R. Quadriceps muscle reconstruction with free functioning latissimus. Microsurgery. 2009;9:189–98.
11. Aponte-Tinao LA, Fartalli GL, Ayerza MA, Muscolo DL. Distal femur osteoarticular allograft. In: Master techniques in orthopaedic surgery orthopaedic oncology and complex reconstruction. Lippincott Williams & Wilkins, A Wolters Kluwer; 2011. p. 201–9.
12. Zwolak P, Kühnel SP, Fuchs B. Extraarticular knee resection for sarcomas with preservation of the extensor mechanism: surgical technique and review of cases. Clin Orthop Relat Res. 2011;469(1):51–256.
13. Choong PFM, Pang G. Surgical management of lower limb sarcomas sarcoma a practical guide to multidisciplinary management. Springer Nature Singapore Pte Ltd; 2021.
14. Capanna R, Scoccianti G, Campanacci DA, Beltrami G, De Biase P. Extraarticular knee resection with prosthesis - proximal tibia-extensor apparatus allograft for tumors invading the knee. Clin Orthop Relat Res. 2011;469:2905–14.
15. Nakamura S, Kusuzaki K, Murata H, Takeshita H, Hirata M, Hashiguchi S, Hirasawa Y. Extra-articular wide tumor resection and limb reconstruction in malignant bone tumors invading the knee joint. Oncol Rep. 2001;8:365–8.

Proximal Tibial Resection and Reconstruction

Wan Faisham Nu'man Bin Wan Ismail, Muhamad Naseh Sajadi Budi, Muhammad Phetrus Johan, Istan Irmansyah Irsan, Vivek Ajit Singh, Azura Mansor, and Nor Faissal Yasin

Introduction

Resections and reconstruction of the proximal tibia are challenging as the patella attachment and function of the extensor mechanism need to be maintained. Proximal tibial sarcoma has a unique anatomical relation with major trifurcation of vessels and the posterior tibial nerve, superior tibiofibular joint and common peroneal nerve and needs proper evaluation and surgical steps for limb salvage procedures. Understanding and advancement of biological techniques and the use of composite synthetic material for tendon attachment for patella tendon reattachment and gastrocnemius reinforcement have improved the functional outcome of the extensor mechanism.

W. F. N. B. W. Ismail (✉)
Prince Court Medical Center, Kuala Lumpur, Malaysia

Orthopaedic Oncology Reconstructive Unit, Universiti Sains Malaysia, Kubang Kerian, Kelantan, Malaysia

M. N. S. Budi
Department Orthopaedic and Traumatology, Hasan Sadikin General Hospital, Padjadjaran University, Bandung, Indonesia

M. P. Johan
Department Orthopaedics and Traumatology, Faculty of Medicine, Hasanuddin University, Makassar, Indonesia

I. I. Irsan
Department of Orthopaedic Surgery, Saiful Anwar Hospital, Brawijaya University, Malang, Indonesia

V. A. Singh · A. Mansor · N. F. Yasin
Department of Orthopaedic Surgery, Faculty of Medicine, University Malaya, Kuala Lumpur, Malaysia

A. Puri, W. F. N. B. W. Ismail (eds.), *Atlas of Orthopedic Oncology Volume 2*,
https://doi.org/10.1007/978-981-95-8962-3_5

Surgical Anatomy

Anatomical barriers against tumour extension for proximal tibial malignant tumours are:

- The tumour rarely infiltrates and involves the knee joint. However, direct infiltration to the cruciate ligament and capsule are possible and need careful evaluation.
- The popliteus muscle is a barrier to protect the major popliteal neurovascular structures and its trifurcation.
- The tibialis posterior and flexor digitorum longus muscles originate from the proximal tibia and must be included in the surgical margin. They have segmental supply from posterior tibial nerve, and the function can still be retained even if the proximal portion is resected.
- The tibialis anterior muscle and other leg extensors in the anterior compartment.
- Thick periosteum, especially in children, prevents subcutaneous and skin infiltration.
- The proximal tibia fibula joint and its cartilage does not cover the tibia fibula attachment and direct joint infiltration is possible through the pericapsular tissue.

The entire medial aspect of the tibia is in a subcutaneous location, and the periosteum is the only anatomical barrier. If direct infiltration to the subcutaneous fat occurs, it must be included as a margin. Preservation of the medial septocutaneous blood vessels, mobilization of the gastrocnemius for prosthesis cover, flexible closure and split skin grafting significantly minimize wound dehiscence and chances of secondary infection.

Assessment of the tendon and ligament insertion over the proximal tibial for infiltration of the tumour is important for adequate oncological clearance. Assessment of the patella tendon and level of resection are important aspects to consider achieving oncological clearance as well as reconstruction of the extensor mechanism. The proximal tibia fibula joint is frequently involved in lateral tumour extension, and it is best to resect it in total with the proximal tibia for better oncological margins. Anserina's bursa and its tendon attachment might be contaminated by the medial extension of the tumour. Distal medial tumour extension will medially infiltrate the soleus line and attachment of common flexor origin, particularly the tibialis posterior and flexor digitorum and hallucis. Assessment of tumour extension to the muscle origin and attachment and cuff of the normal tissue must be included to ensure a wide oncological margin.

Assessment

Systemic assessment of the pulmonary CT and bone scan is mandatary for staging prior to surgical intervention.

The important structures to be critically evaluated before resection are:

- Knee joint: cruciate and collateral attachment and joint fluid/haematoma
- Tibia fibula joint
- Posterior: the popliteus muscle, neurovascular structures, origin of the deep posterior muscle and joint capsule
- Anterior: the tibialis anterior, anterior tibial vessels and tibial tubercle for patella attachment
- Medial: subcutaneous tissue and skin infiltration, anserine bursa and tendon attachment and soleus line attachment

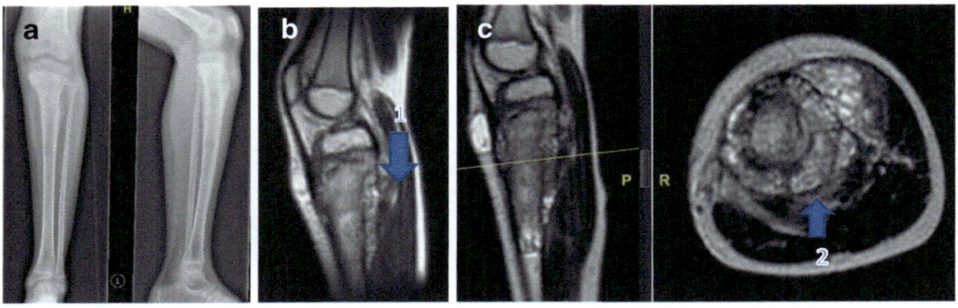

1. Popliteus muscle
2. Deep posterior compartment origin

The popliteus muscle, which acts as a barrier for posterior tumour extension and protects the neurovascular structures, is the first structure to be infiltrated posteriorly. The anterior tibial muscle is also infiltrated by the tumour and had to be completely removed for a surgical margin (Fig. 1a–c).

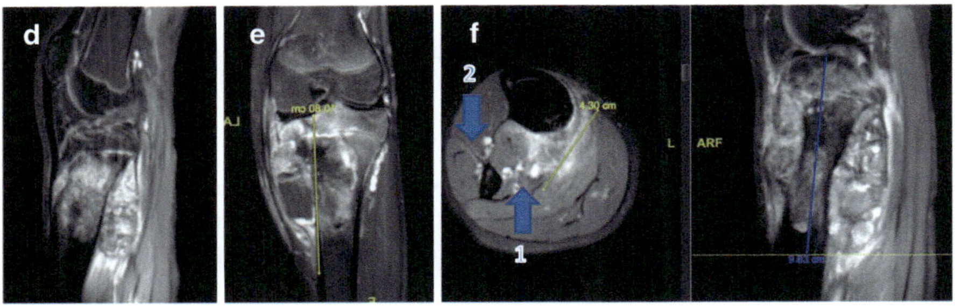

1. Posterior tibial and peroneal vessels
2. Anterior tibial vessels

The anterior soft tissue extension was very minimal, and the patella tendon was spared. The posterior soft tissue involvement was mainly over the medial soleus, popliteus muscle and proximal part of the deep flexors. The medial collateral ligament and soft tissue that covered the medial joint was oedematous and had to be completely removed over the femoral attachment for a better oncological margin. MRI evaluation showed only an 8 cm marrow extension; however, the posterior soft tissue and periosteum involvement were up to 11 cm (Fig. 1d–f).

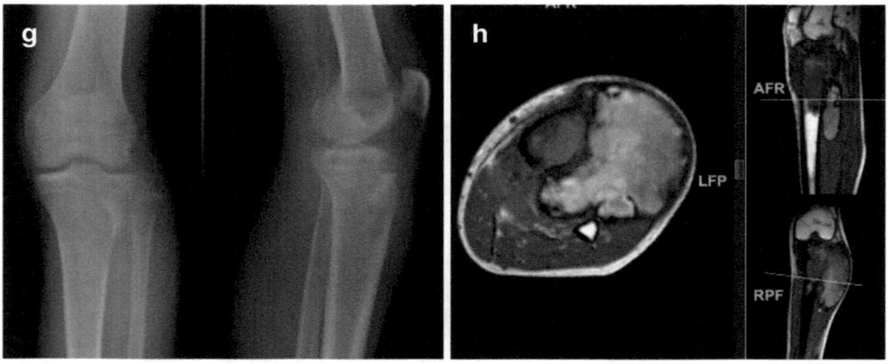

In tumours that involve the anterior muscle compartment, post-operative foot drop and loss of ankle dorsiflexion are to be expected (Fig. 1g, h).

Surgical Steps

Proximal tibial resection surgical steps:

- Medial exploration of the popliteal vessels, trifurcation and mobilization of the posterior tibial artery and tibial peroneal trunk. This includes (Fig. 2a):
  - Medial gastrocnemius mobilization from medial border of tibia
  - Mobilization of the soleus attachment at the soleal line
- Assessment of patella tendon and mobilization from tibial tuberosity with good margin

In cases with superior extension to the popliteal space, medial gastrocnemius mobilization and tendon release from the distal femur are important for better visualization and exploration of neurovascular structures. It is important to maintain the branch of vascular supply to medial gastrocnemius for the rotational flap to cover the prosthesis. In cases with proximal tibiofibular joint extension particularly in lateral proximal tibial sarcomas, the peroneal nerve at the fibula neck must be explored prior to proximal fibula osteotomy as the proximal fibula joint along with the proximal tibia fibula joint is included as surgical margin.

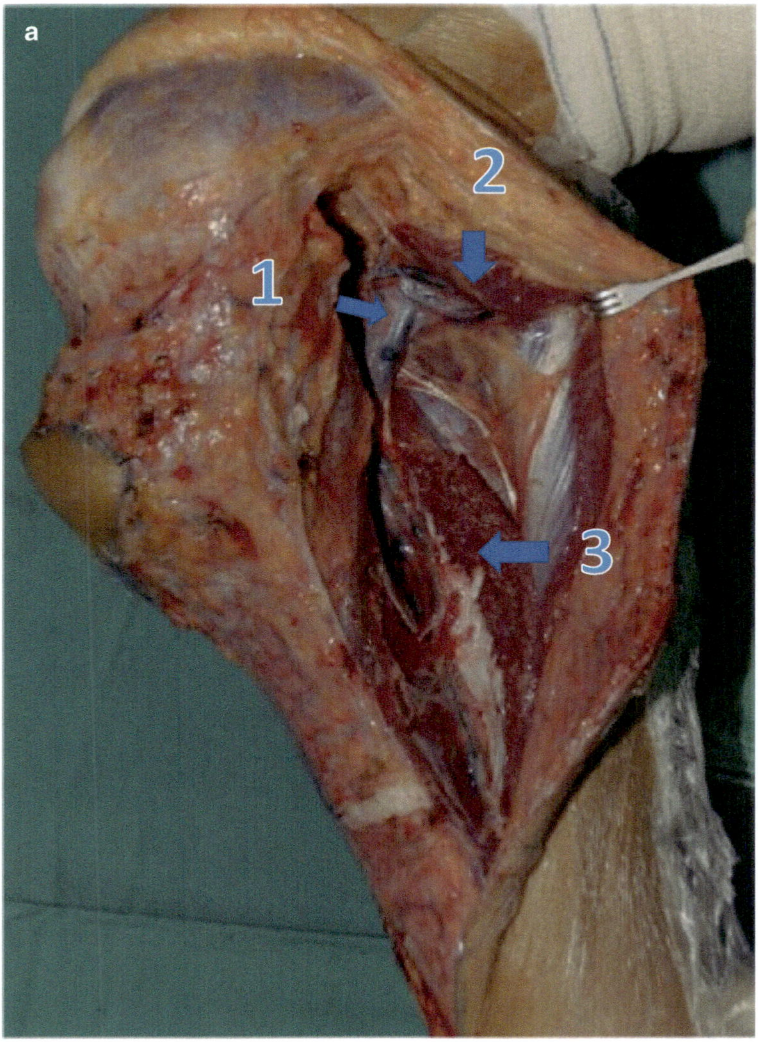

1. Popliteal vessels and its trifurcation
2. Medial sural vessels: branch to medial gastrocnemius
3. Soleal line (soleus insertion at the medial tibial)

Surgical steps of Proximal Tibial Resection

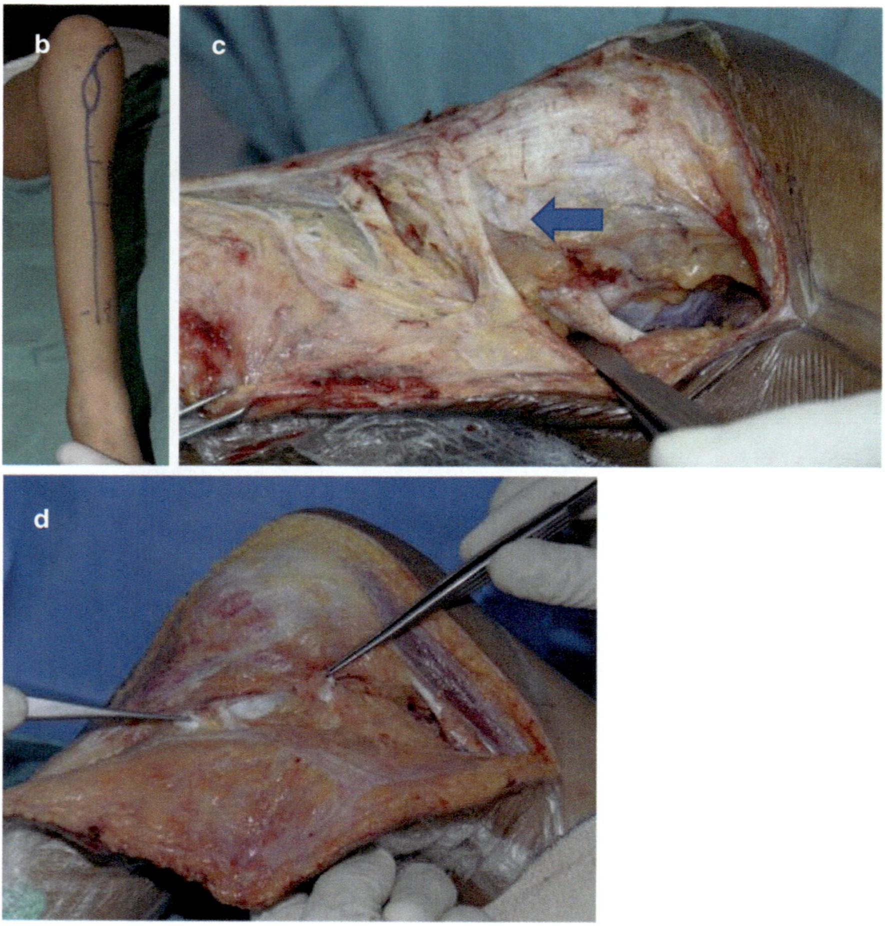

Arrow—anserinus bursae tendon: sartorius, gracilis and semitendinosus

All the tendons attached to the anserinus bursa are detached for medial exposure (Fig. 2b–d).

Exploration of the popliteal vessels to the trifurcation and tibial peroneal trunk. The soleus is detached at the soleal line of the medial tibia according to its oncological margin. The knee is flexed to relax the vessel from the point where the anterior tibial branch will cross anteriorly (Fig. 2e, f).

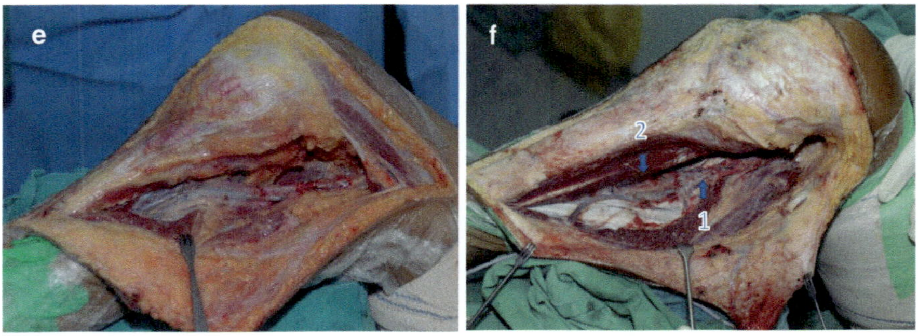

1. Tibial peroneal trunk vessels
2. Deep posterior compartment muscle: tibialis posterior

A lateral flap is created for exploration of the common peroneal nerve below the biceps tendon attachment over the fibula head. The peroneal nerve is elevated with motor unit of the anterior compartment of the leg. The soft tissue oncological margin is guided by the MRI extension of the tumour (Fig. 2g, h)

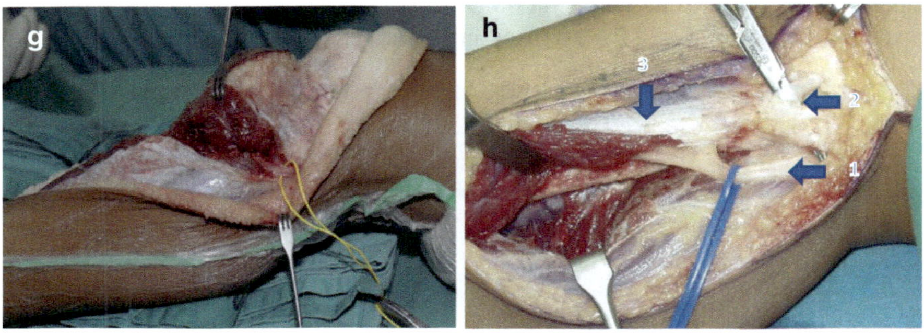

1. Peroneal nerve
2. Lateral collateral ligament and biceps femoris tendon insertion at the fibular head
3. Tibialis anterior muscle

The proximal branch of the peroneal nerve provides proprioception to the joint and supplies the tibialis anterior. The main motor branch will supply the muscles of the anterior and peroneal compartments. The superficial sensory peroneal nerve lies more laterally.

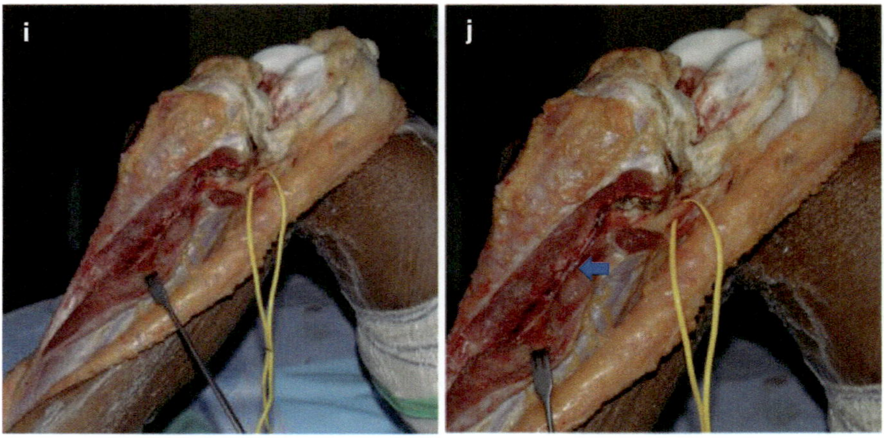

Arrow—superficial 'cutaneous branch' of peroneal nerve

The patella tendon and iliotibial band attachment at Gerdy's tubercle are detached from the tibia. The joint is inspected for hemarthrosis and involvement before intra-articular circumferential resection of the capsule above the meniscus. The tibialis anterior is detached from the lateral tibial border up to the intermuscular septum to maintain the motor unit of the extensor ankle and toe (Fig. 2i, j).

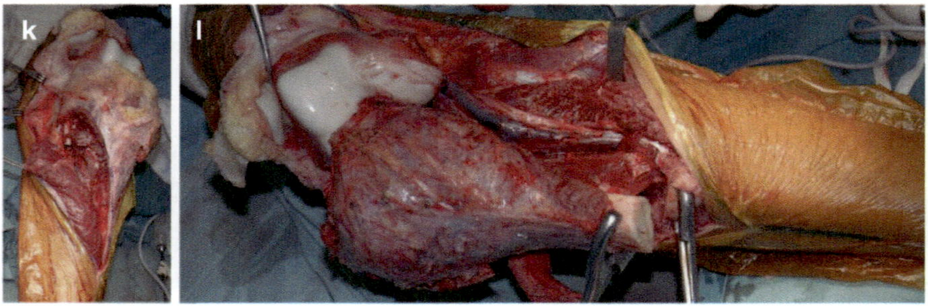

Osteotomy over the fibula neck is performed below the peroneal nerve. Distal osteotomy of the tibia with lateral rotation allows for visualization of the trifurcation to clear the posterior tibial vessels and free the anterior tibial vessels. In cases with massive anterior compartment involvement, the anterior tibial artery must be sacrificed (Fig. 2k, l).

The gastrocnemius flap is important for reconstruction of the extensor mechanism and soft tissue cover over the anteromedial subcutaneous area to minimize skin dehiscence and infection. Blood supply to the medial gastrocnemius, which is from a branch of the popliteal artery above the trifurcation, must be maintained and kinks should be prevented during the entire procedure (Fig. 2m–o).

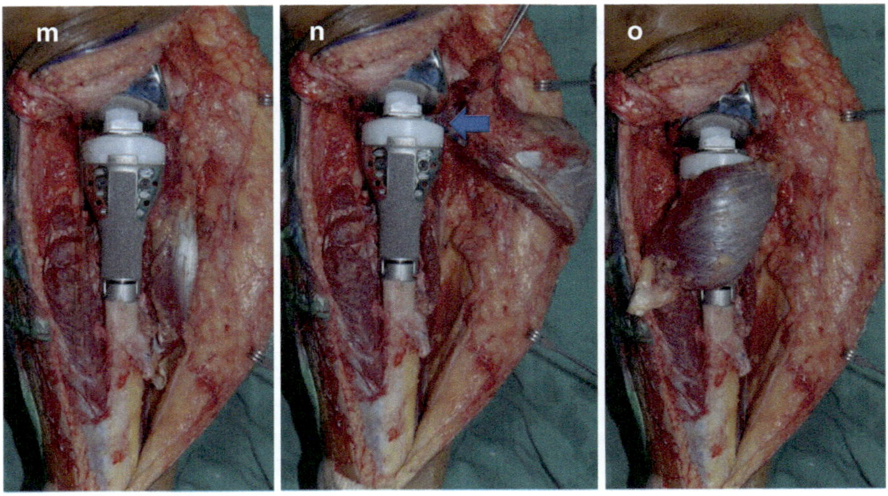

Arrow—medial sural artery (branch to gastrocnemius muscle) must be preserved and protected

The medial gastrocnemius is mobilized to reattach the extensor mechanism and cover the entire prosthesis. The soleus muscle is sutured to the medial border of the gastrocnemius and the extensor compartment muscle to the lateral border of the gastrocnemius (Fig. 2p, q).

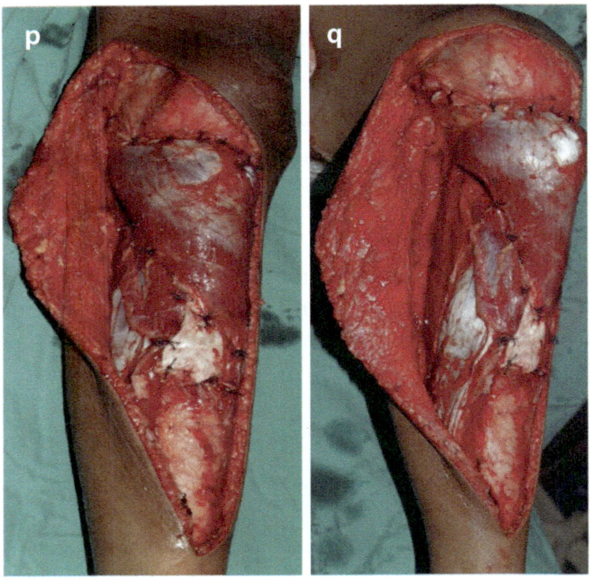

Proximal Tibia Osteosarcoma with Involvement of the Proximal Tibia Fibular Joint

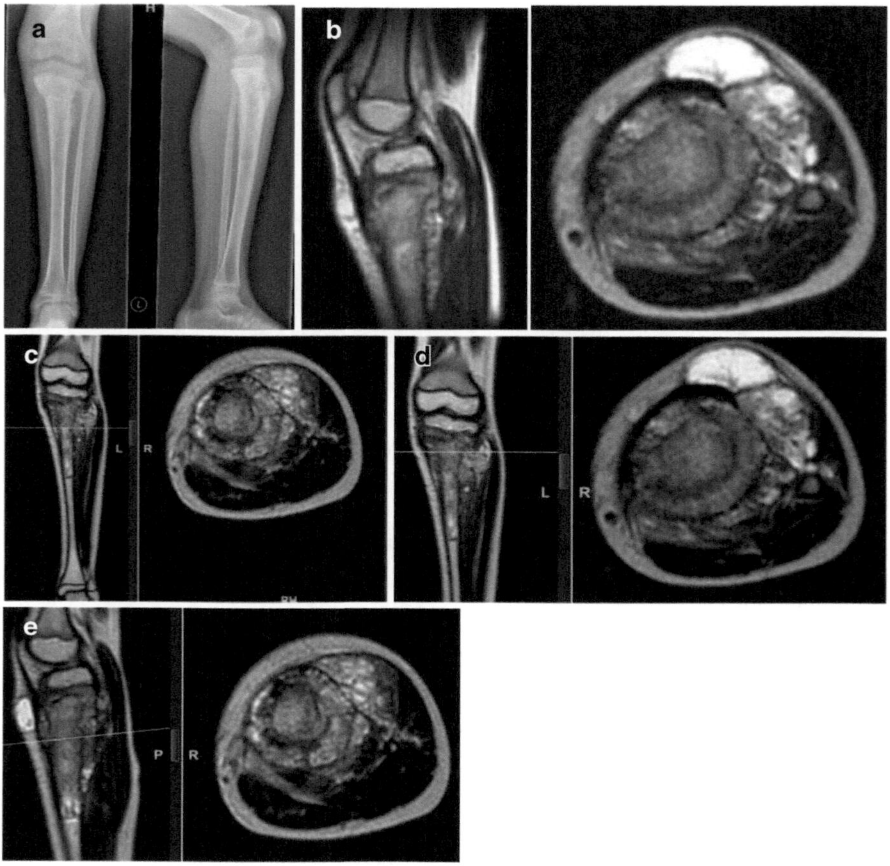

Although MRI showed direct infiltration to the popliteus muscle, the posterior neurovascular structures remained free. The tibialis anterior and part of the anterior compartment muscle were involved and pushed by the anterior tumour extension (Fig. 3a–e).

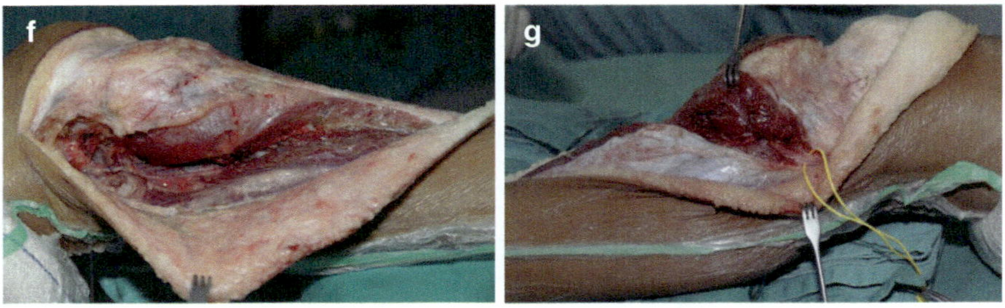

The popliteus muscle acts as a barrier for posterior tumour extension and protects the neurovascular structures. The entire extensor compartment was mobilised from the tibia with the intact motor unit of the peroneal nerve while the tibialis anterior extensor muscle was removed as part of the surgical margin due to infiltration (Fig. 3f–i).

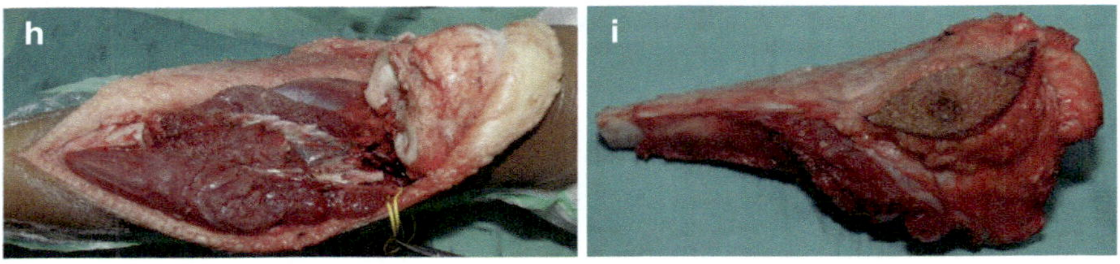

Proximal Tibia Osteosarcoma with Postero-medial Extension

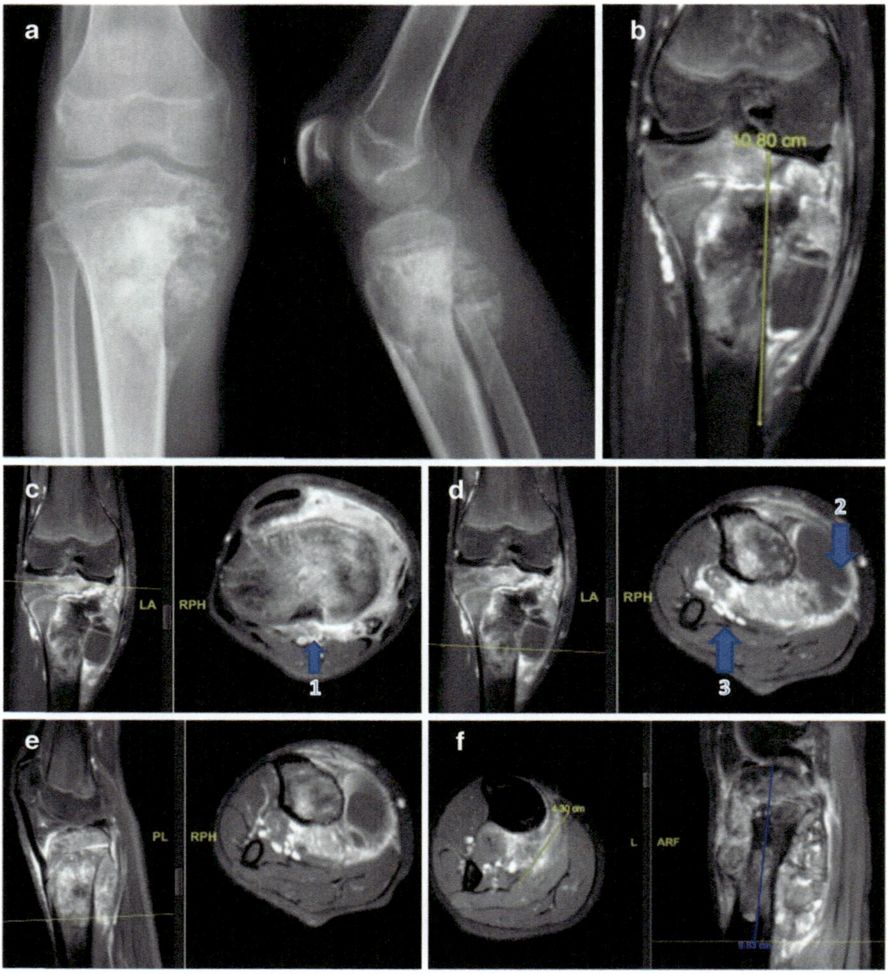

1. Popliteal vessels protected by involved popliteus
2. Postero medial extension of the sarcoma
3. Tibialis posterior and peroneal vessels pushed laterally and not involved

The MRI evaluation showed an 8 cm marrow extension; however, the posterior soft tissue and periosteum involvement was up to 11 cm. The anterior soft tissue extension was very minimal, and the patella tendon attachment was spared. The posterior soft tissue involvement was mainly over the medial soleus, popliteus muscle and proximal part of the deep flexors (Fig. 4a–f). The medial collateral and soft tissue that covered the medial joint was oedematous and had to be completely removed over the femoral attachment for a better oncological margin.

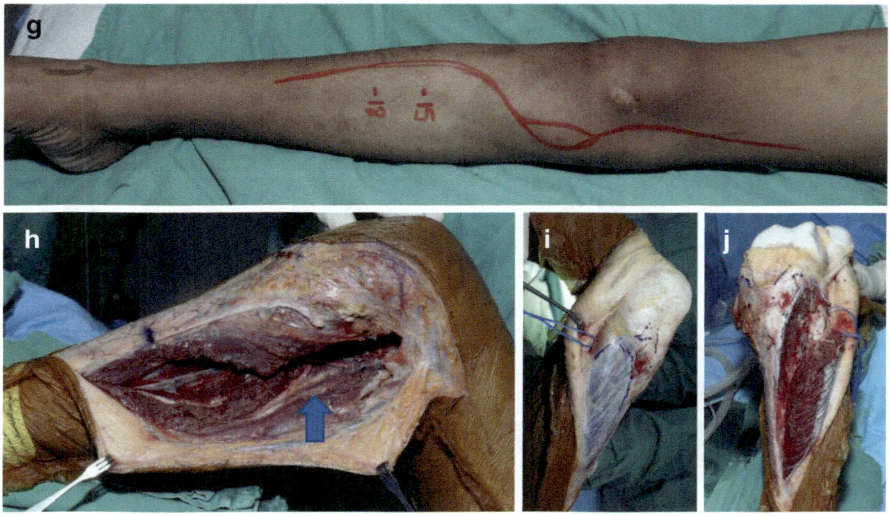

Arrow—Posterior medial extension of the tumour covered by soleus attachment, popliteus and deep posterior muscle

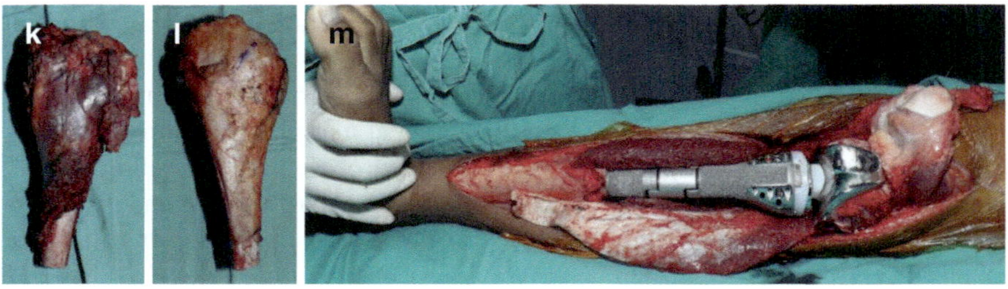

The tissue over the posterior-medial extension, which had tumour involvement, and the deep posterior compartment and superior part of the soleus were completely removed. There was no anterior muscle involvement; however, the proximal tibia-fibula joint was involved and had to be resected (Fig. 4g–m).

Sarcoma with Extensive Circumferential Involvement

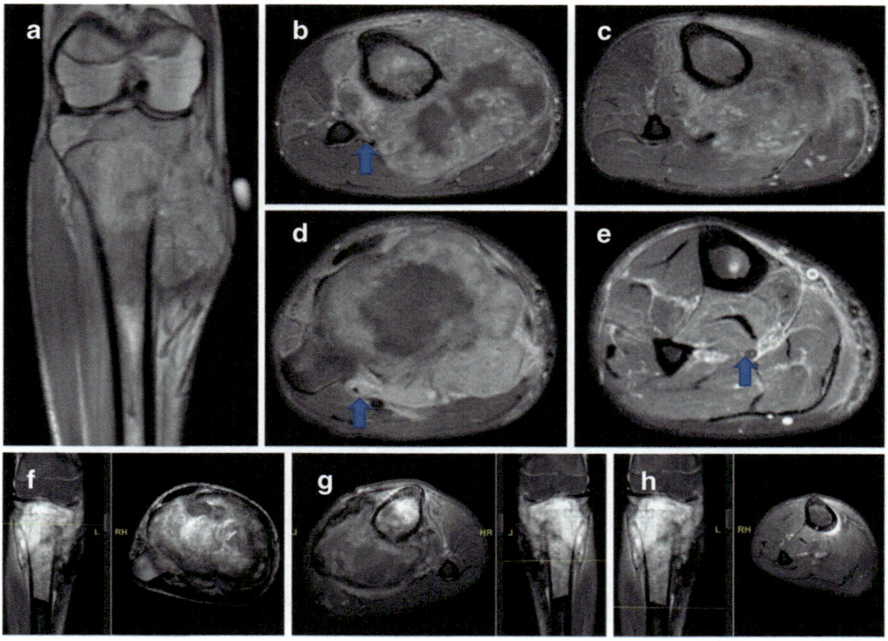

Arrows—The tibialis posterior vessels were pushed laterally and remained patent throughout their course

More extensive involvement over the proximal posterior medial area needs a proper MRI evaluation of the soleus for oncological margins. The popliteal artery and its trifurcation will be pushed laterally, and neurovascular exploration is challenging. The MRI also demonstrated the popliteal vessels trifurcation and main posterior tibial and anterior tibial vessels and evaluation of the posterior soft tissue extension (Fig. 5a–h).

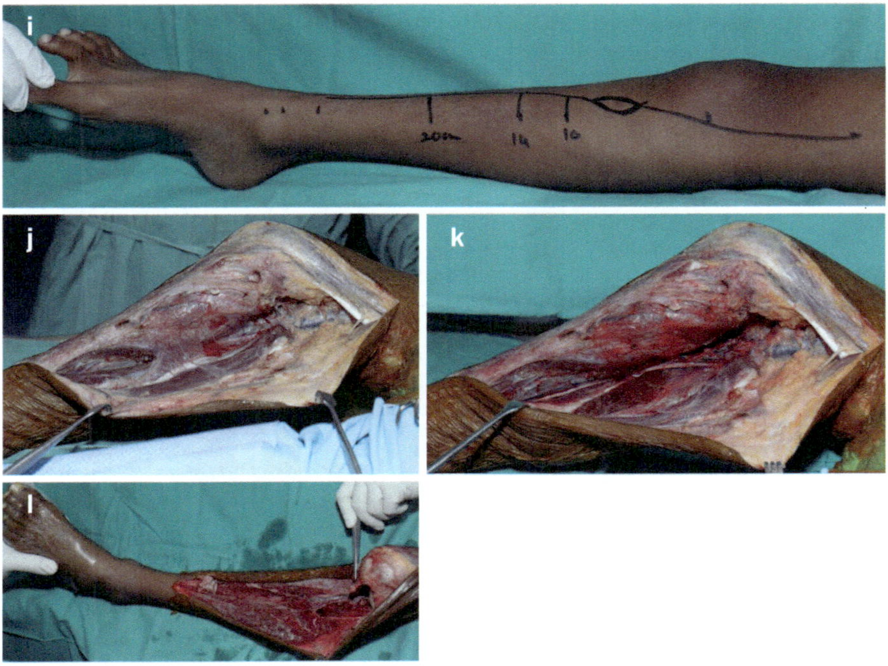

Exploration of the popliteal vessels and its trifurcation showed that the anterior tibial artery need not be sacrificed (Fig. 5i–n).

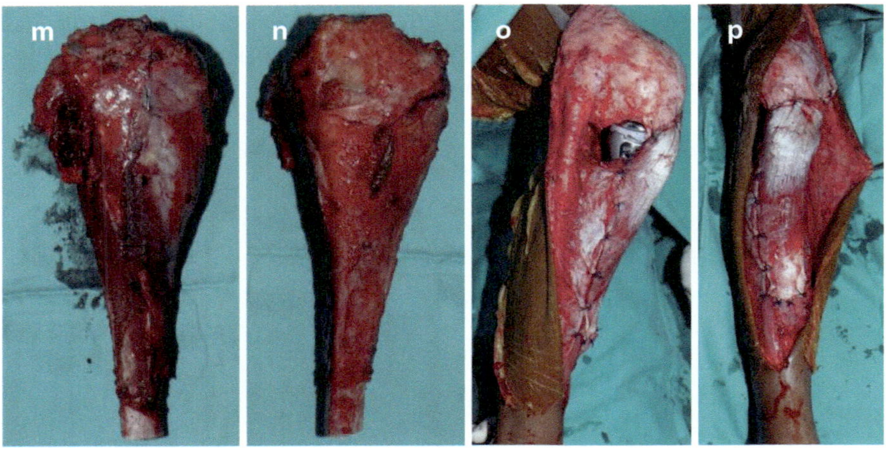

The entire prosthesis could be covered with the medial gastrocnemius muscle, and the extensor mechanism of the patella was reconstructed for better function (Fig. 5o, p).

Sarcoma with Anterior Muscle Involvement and Patella Tendon Involvement

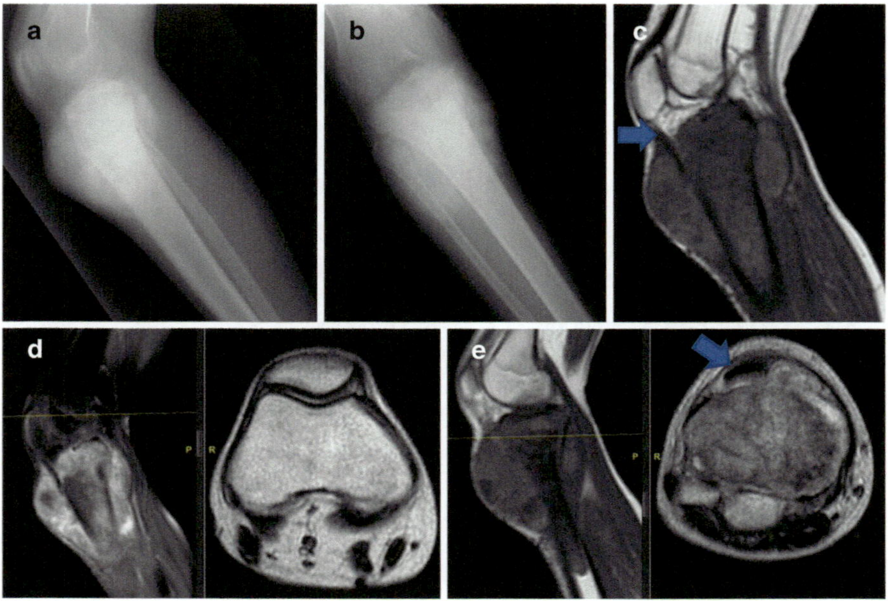

This osteosarcoma with anterior and posterior tumour extension responded well to chemotherapy. The superior part of the tumour involved the patella tubercle and left a short patella tendon for reconstruction. The posterior neurovascular structures were intact; however, the deep posterior muscle origin was involved and had to be included in the surgical margin (Fig. 6a–e).

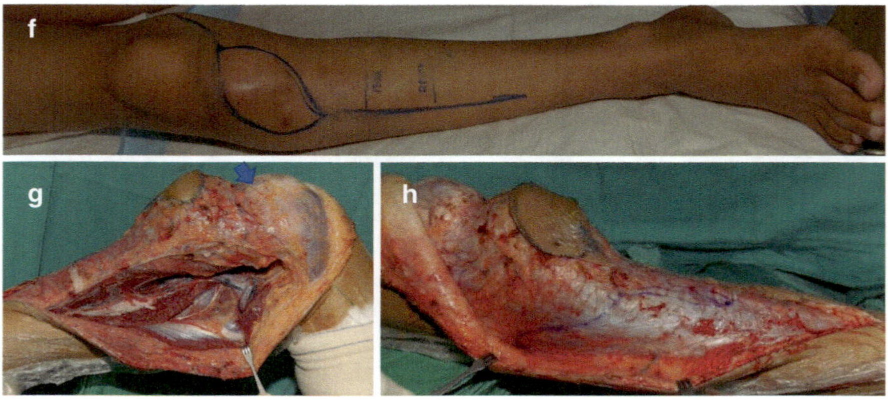

Arrow—anterior extension of tumour infiltrated and pushed the patella tendon

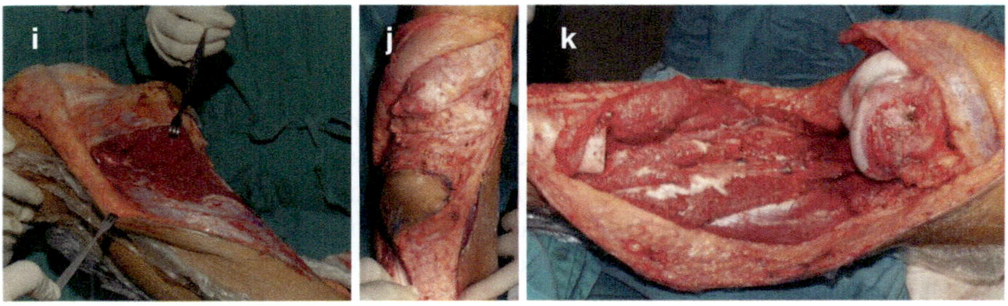

Resection of the anterior compartment muscle with half of the patella tendon and all structures attached to the proximal tibia including the iliotibial band at Gerdy's tubercle left a short patella tendon for reconstruction (Fig. 6f–m).

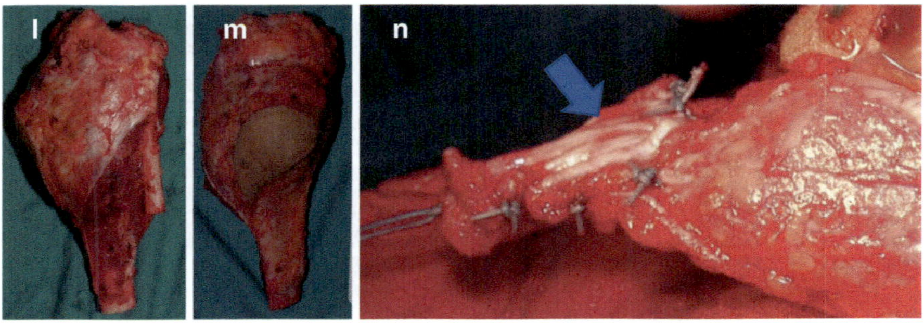

The patella tendon stump was reinforced with the remnants of the hamstring tendon and reattached to the prosthesis. The entire prosthesis was covered with the medial gastrocnemius muscle flap, and the extensor knee mechanism was maintained (Fig. 6n–p).

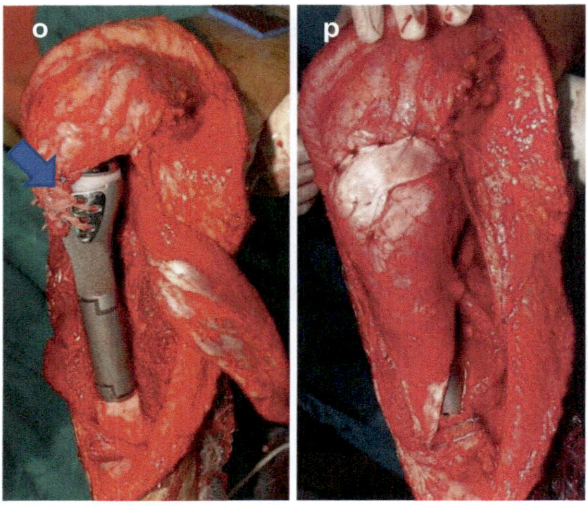

Arrow—patella tendon reconstruction with hamstring muscle and reattachment with Dacron tape.

Sarcoma with Extensive Tissue Involvement and Free Latissimus Dorsi Flap Cover

In tumours with massive anterior muscle compartment involvement, foot drop and loss of ankle dorsiflexion is to be expected. Resection of the entire extensor compartment for limb salvage is possible, provided the posterior compartment is intact with neurovascular structures for sensation and functional flexors of the foot and ankle. Remnants of the peroneal nerve can be used for motorized transfer of a free muscle flap.

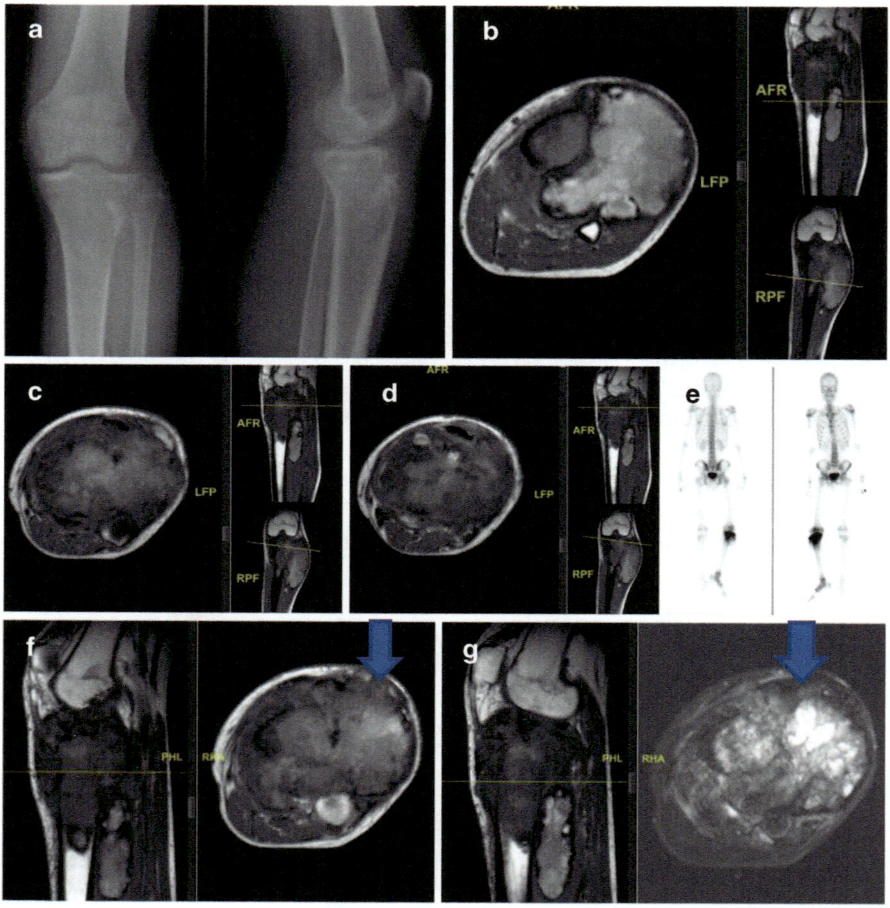

A case of proximal tibial osteosarcoma with poor response to chemotherapy with the entire extensor compartment of leg involved (Fig. 7a–i).

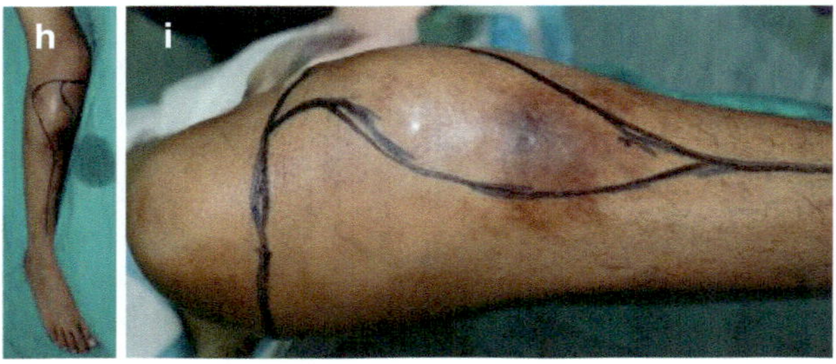

Arrow—skin infiltration on MRI, which was included in the resection margin for oncological clearance

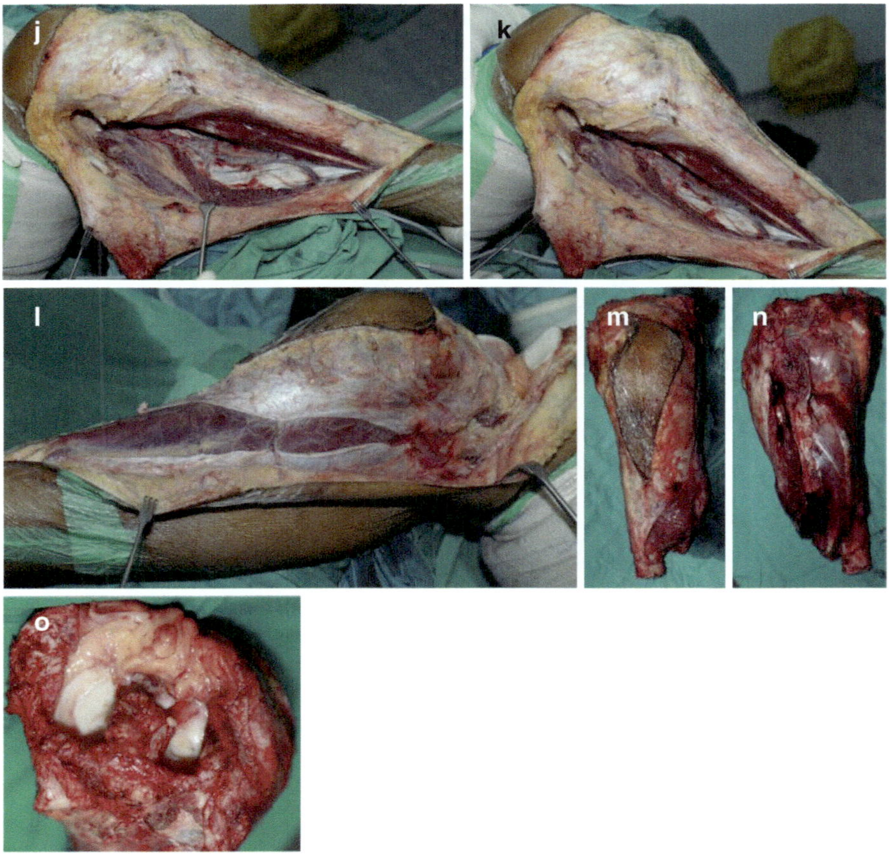

The entire anterior compartment with the peroneal nerve was resected to achieve oncological margins. Reconstruction was achieved with a latissimus dorsi motorized flap for prosthesis cover and ankle dorsiflexion function (Fig. 7j–o).

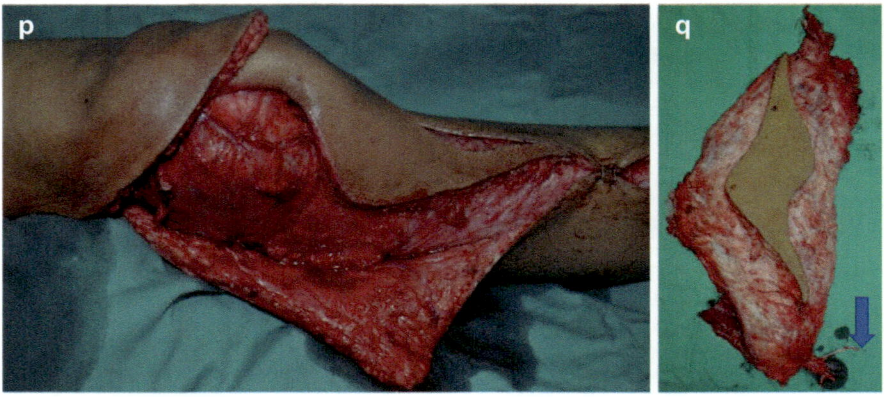

The latissimus dorsi was harvested together with thoraco-dorsal nerve for motorized transfer to the remnant of the peroneal nerve for ankle dorsiflexion function (Fig. 7p, q).

Proximal Tibial Osteosarcoma with Lesion in the Distal Femur

A case of proximal tibial osteosarcoma with skip lesion to the femoral condyle and medullary skip lesion at the distal femur. The knee joint was spared, and there was no local infiltration (Fig. 8a–d).

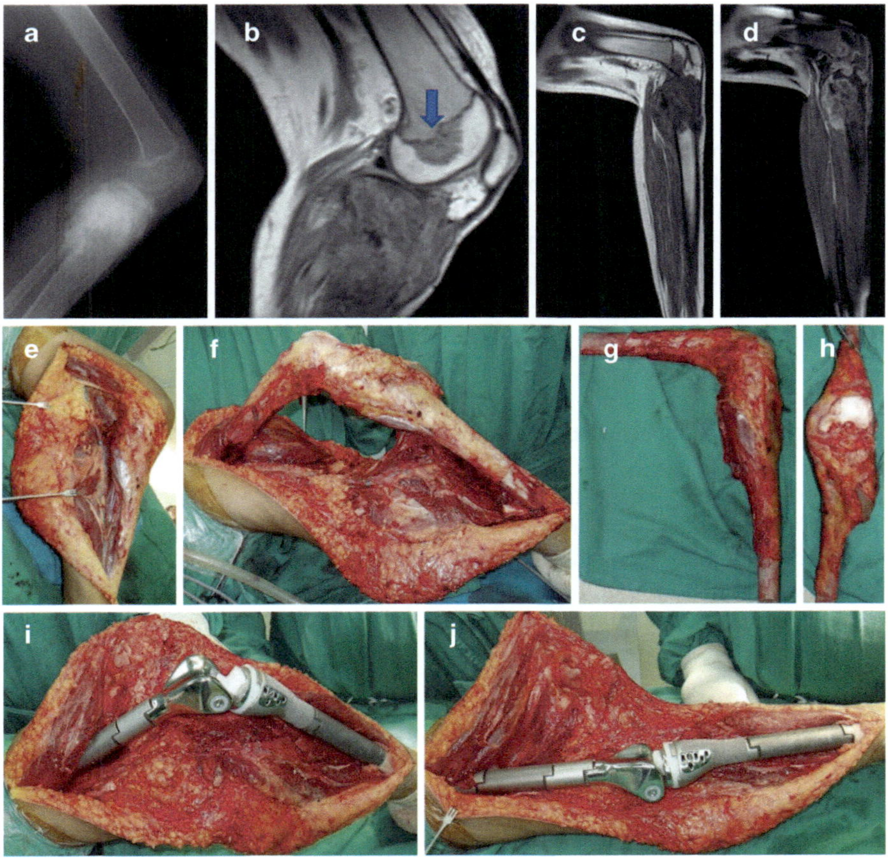

A combined resection of the distal femur and proximal tibial was accomplished. This reconstruction has an inferior functional outcome even though the reconstruction is stable and permits early rehabilitation and weight bearing (Fig. 8e–k).

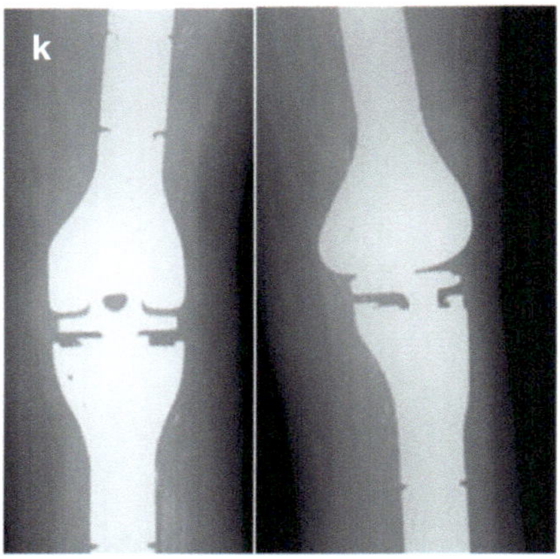

Options for Bone Reconstruction Other than Prosthesis

The following are some other options for reconstruction:

- Recycled tumour bone using extracorporeal radiation using single 60 Gy after removal of all soft tissue extension and intramedullary reaming of the tumour
  - Simple osteoarticular
  - Combined with constrained knee prosthesis
- Osteoarticular allograft in children
- Physeal preservation resection in children and intercalary allograft reconstruction

Extracorporeal Irradiation and Recycled Bone Reimplantation

Recycling the bone with extracorporeal irradiation of the primary sarcoma is an established method for bony reconstruction in children. The soft tissue extension of the resected tumour is cleared before radiation. The patella tendon is reattached, and circumferential suturing of the capsule is necessary for knee stability (Fig. 9a–h).

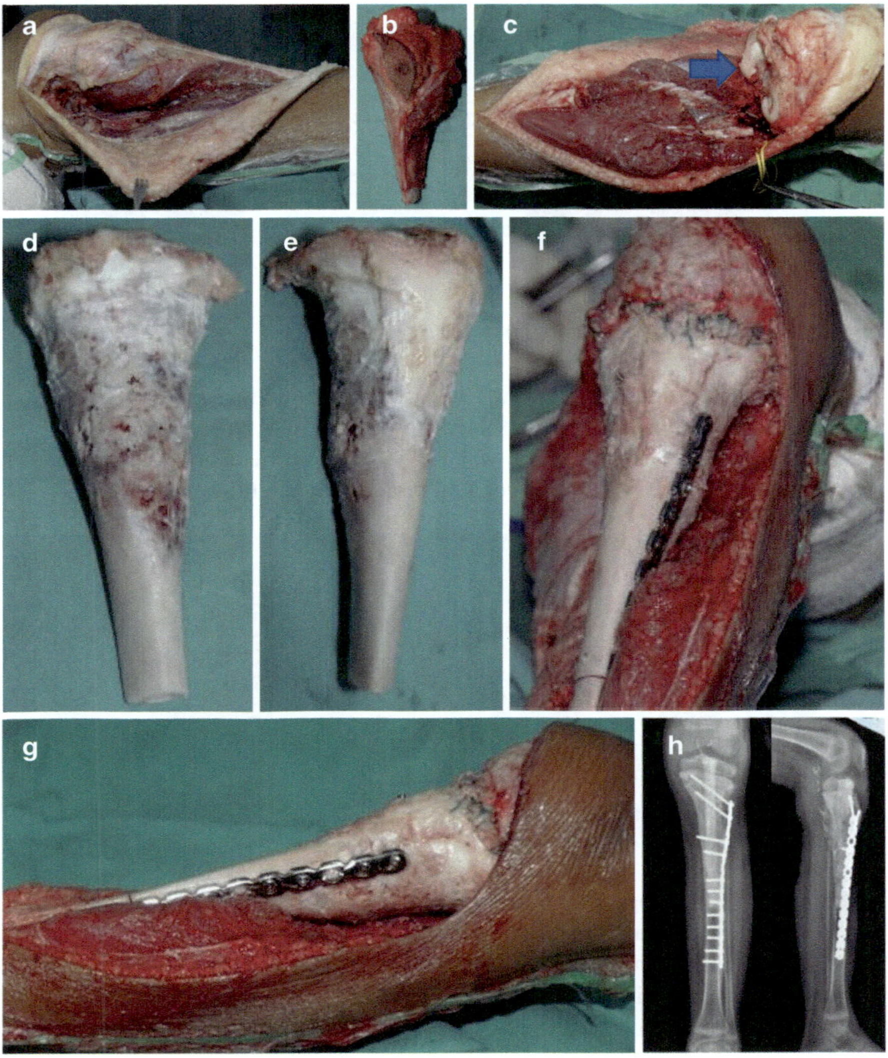

The meniscus is retained in the distal femur provided the margin is good. It will contribute towards knee stability and protect the irradiated cartilage over the tibial side (Fig. 9c).

Allograft Prosthesis Composites

Long segment proximal tibial resection also can be reconstructed with a combination of allograft and prosthesis replacement. A long intramedullary stem or intramedullary cement provides additional mechanical support against early failure (Fig. 9i, j).

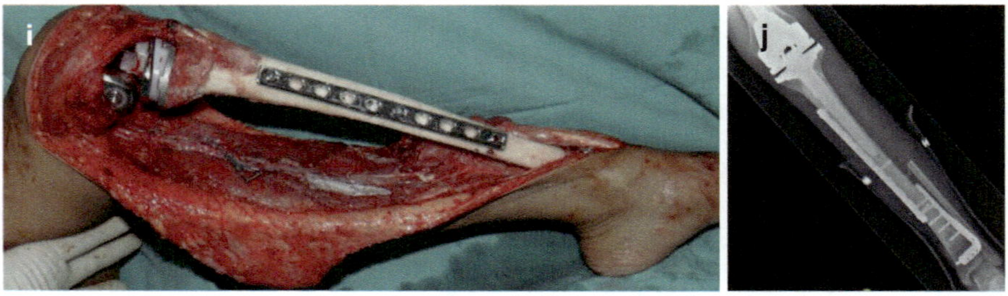

Osteoarticular Allograft Reconstruction

A proximal tibia osteosarcoma in a 13-year-old girl was managed with proximal tibial osteoarticular allograft (Fig. 9k, l). An advantage of this reconstruction was that the distal femur physeal plate was not violated for reconstruction. However, size matched allograft is a major problem, particularly in children.

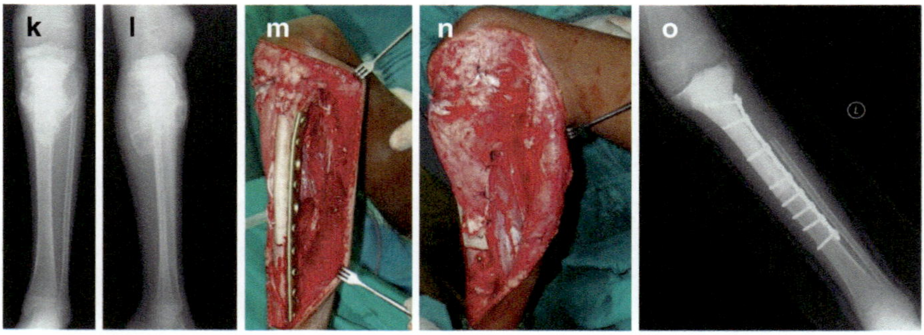

Remnant of the allograft capsule was sutured and reinforced to the distal femur. The posterior capsule and posterior cruciate ligament were tightened in flexion and tested for full extension. The patella tendon was attached to the tibial tuberosity and the medial gastrocnemius flap used to maintain the extensor mechanism. The entire intramedullary portion of the allograft was cemented to maintain strength (Fig. 9m–o).

Direct Medial Approach for Proximal Tibia Resection

Muhamad Naseh Sajadi Budi, Muhammad Phetrus Johan, and Istan Irmansyah Irsan

We describes surgical technique of direct medial approach for proximal tibial resection and how to excise the proximal tibio-fibular joint as part of margin, mobilization as well as preservation of common peroneal nerve for function.

It offers a reliable method for proximal tibial resection with several additional advantages:

- Small skin and subcutaneous flap with less skin edge necrosis and reduced risk of secondary surgical site infection
- Direct approach to neurovascular structures for better visualization and safe preservation of the peroneal nerve during dissection
- Similar exposure for medical gastrocnemius muscle flap, beneficial in cases with anterior or medial tumour extension at the tibia
- Allows for the exploration and if needed, intra-articular or extra-articular resection of the proximal tibio-fibular joint

Special Consideration for Direct Medial Approach Proximal Tibia Resection

- The fibula can be reached directly through a medial approach following the traditional medial approach by dislocating the knee joint, externally rotating the tibia, and freely mobilizing the popliteal vessels bundles.
- The common peroneal nerve and its branches are important structures that must be considered in proximal tibial resection. It follows a unique path, being easily exposed in some locations while difficult to identify in others, especially after it crosses fibula neck. Direct exploration the tibial nerve below the knee joint and trace proximally for common peroneal and tibial nerves branch is an option in this approach.

Seventeen-year-old male with osteosarcoma well responded to neo-adjuvant chemotherapy. Radiograph showed a mixed lytic and blastic bony lesion with an unclear boundary and broad transitional zone.

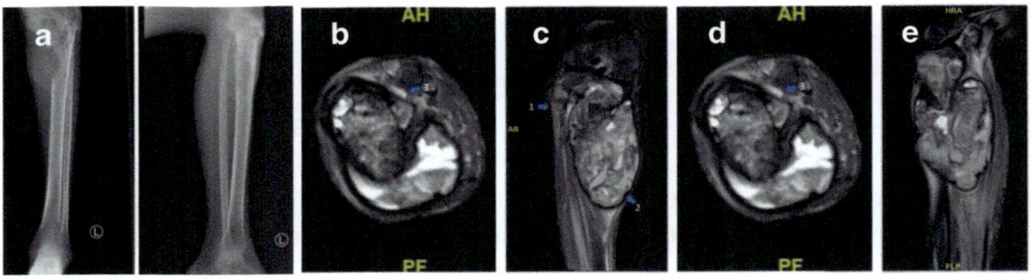

MRI reveals an extra compartment expansion of the tumour, with intact posterior neurovascular structures protected by popliteus muscle (Fig. 10a–e).

- Involvement of proximal tibio-fibular joint; extra-articular resection will be carried out.
- Medial soft tissue and periosteum involved up to 16 cm, with 14 cm marrow extension.
- Contamination of anserine bursa of and its tendon attachments.

1. Fibula
2. Pseudocapsule
3. Tibiofibular joint contaminated by tumour

Surgical Approach
A successful proximal tibia tumour resection was achieved by careful placement of the incision, ensuring the preservation of popliteal vessels and nerves. The incision's length is determined by the size of the tumour in the proximal tibia but usually ends at the point between the middle and distal third of the leg. Anteromedial approach provides a clear view of medial gastrocnemius muscle, arteries, veins, nerves and fibula.

- Biopsy scars include in the resection margin.
- Thick flaps of skin and subcutaneous tissue including fascia are raised medially and laterally to prevent flap ischemia which may result in skin necrosis (Fig. 10f).
- The insertion of the medial hamstrings on the proximal tibia is excised at the 2–3 cm proximal to their insertion to expose the popliteal fossa.
- Medial gastrocnemius muscle is mobilized posteriorly, and the soleus is detached from soleal line with cuff of normal tissue for popliteal neurovascular exploration.

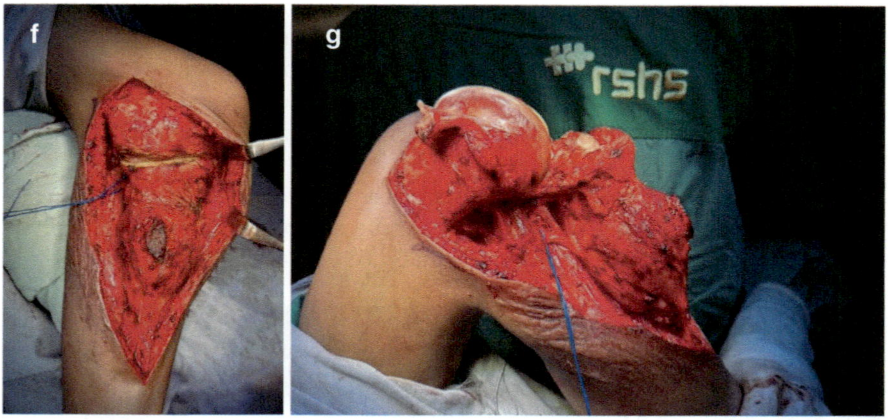

- After medial exploration of popliteal and trifurcation is completed, medial capsulotomy and dissection of collateral and cruciate ligaments are done to achieve more visualization of the tibial posterior compartment (Fig. 10g).

- The presence of a significant posterior soft tissue component frequently leads to the tethering of the blood vessels and may require careful separation to ensure that the posterior tibial arteries are completely freed from the tumour.
- The anterior tibial artery is not tied off in this case since it is not involved with the tumour. However, If the anterior tibial artery were to be ligated, the surgeon must ensure uninterrupted blood flow in the posterior tibial vessels and avoid distal vascular compromise.

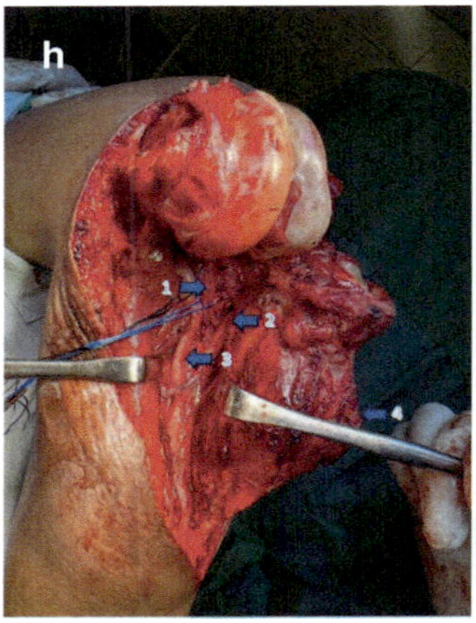

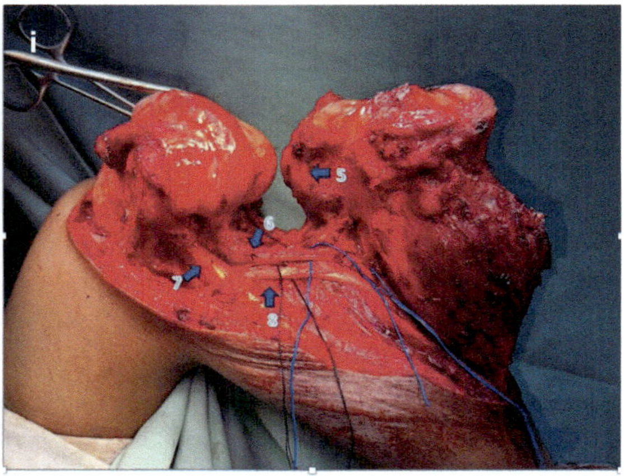

- Identification of the tibial nerve and popliteal bundle proximally is the important step in identifying the beginning of the common peroneal nerve from the medial side (Fig. 10h).
- Common peroneal nerve, head of fibula and the biceps femoris tendon are visualized by externally rotating the tibia and transecting the posterior joint capsule (Fig. 10i).
- The lateral collateral ligament and lateral capsule are transected to improve rotation for visualization of fibula head or neck.

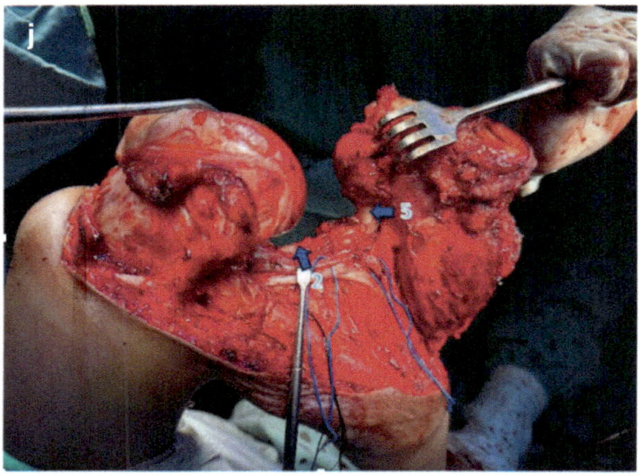

1. Popliteal bundle

2. Common peroneal nerve
3. Tibial nerve
4. Externally rotated tibia
5. Fibula head
6. Popliteal artery
7. Medial gastrocnemius muscle
8. Soleus muscle

The lateral flap is developed to mobilize anterior compartment muscle from tibia and expose the entire fibula head (Fig. 10i)

- The biceps tendon insertion is released and the previously explore peroneal nerve is mobilize with the motor unit of the anterior leg compartment from lateral border of tibia and interosseous ligament (Fig. 10k).
- Distal fibula osteotomy is prepared by mobilizing peroneal nerve distally with anterior compartment muscle.

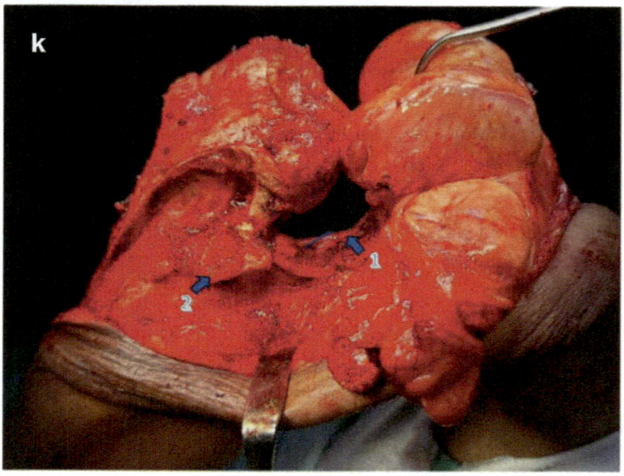

1. Common peroneal nerve

2. Peroneal muscles

Proximal Tibia Resection with Extensor Mechanism Preserving Surgery

Vivek Ajit Singh, Azura Mansor, Nor Faissal Yasin, and Wan Faisham Nu'man Bin Wan Ismail

The gastrocnemius flap is widely regarded as the gold standard in extensor mechanism reconstruction following proximal tibia resections. This flap provides robust biological reconstruction and offers essential soft tissue coverage for the implant, which has been shown to reduce the risk of postoperative infections significantly. Despite these advantages, using a gastrocnemius flap is often associated with extensor lag, primarily due to the elongation and stretching of the extensor mechanism, which can compromise knee function.

We describe a surgical technique to preserve the continuity of the extensor mechanism, eliminating the need for a gastrocnemius flap.

- It involves the subperiosteal dissection of the patella ligament in continuity with the lateral tibial compartment fascia and underlying muscles.
- It is only for selected cases in which the tumour does not involve the patella tubercle, lateral border of the tibia and lateral muscular compartment.

A Case of Osteosarcoma of the Right Proximal Tibia

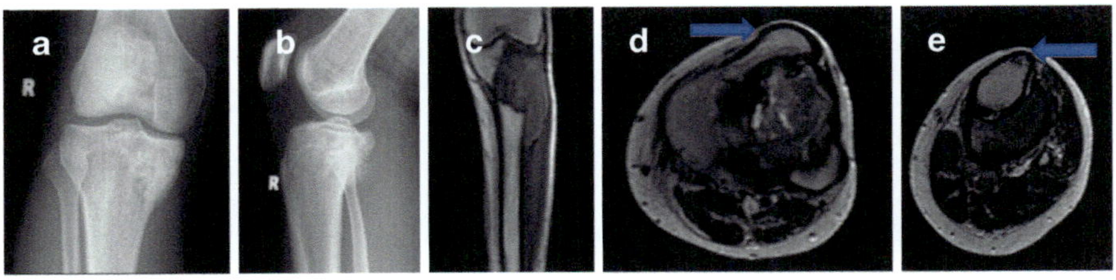

The plain radiograph shows an osteoblastic lesion over the medial tibial plateau with a sunburst periosteal reaction. MRI shows the tumour spares the tibial tuberosity and the lateral muscular compartment (Fig. 11a–e).

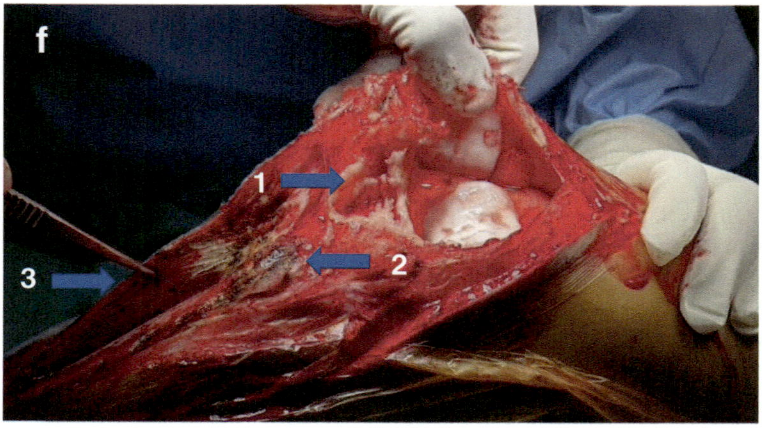

1. Patella ligament
2. Tibial tubercle
3. Lateral tibial compartment fascia

Surgical photo preservation continuity of knee extensor mechanism (Fig. 11f)

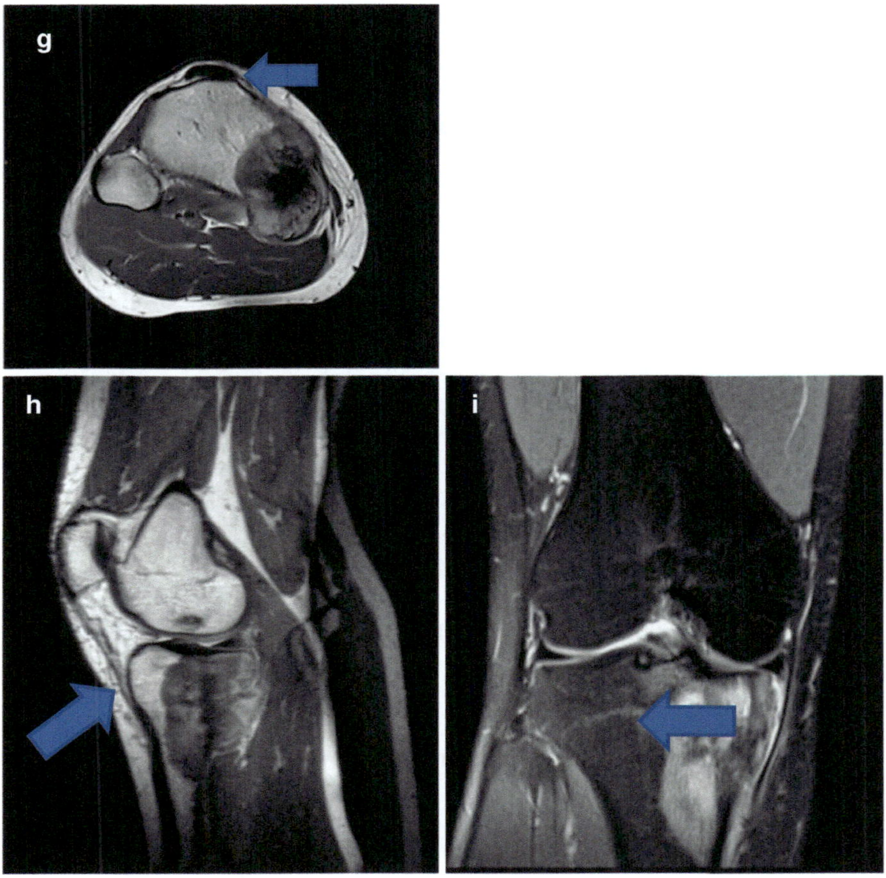

A case of osteosarcoma of the right tibia well responded to chemotherapy. MRI shows the involvement of the medial tibial plateau and preservation of lateral plateu and tibial tubercle (Fig. 11g–i).

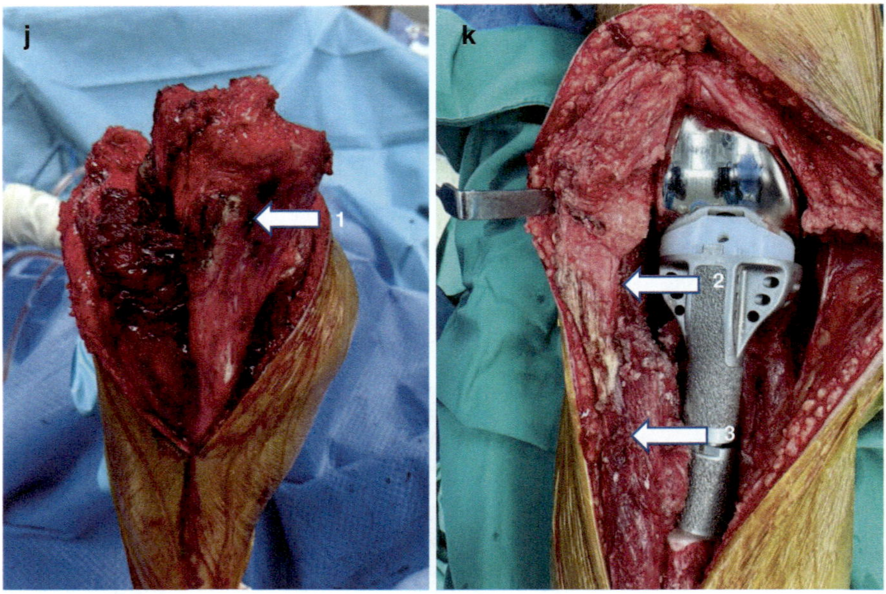

Extensor preservation surgery and method of reconstruction (Fig. 11j, k)

1. Tibial tubercle
2. Patella ligament
3. Lateral tibial compartment fascia and muscles

A case of giant cell tumour proximal tibia with cortical break and soft tissue extension medial tibial plateau. The lateral condyle, tibial tubercle and extensor muscle are not involved and suitable for preservation of continuity of knee extensor mechanism.

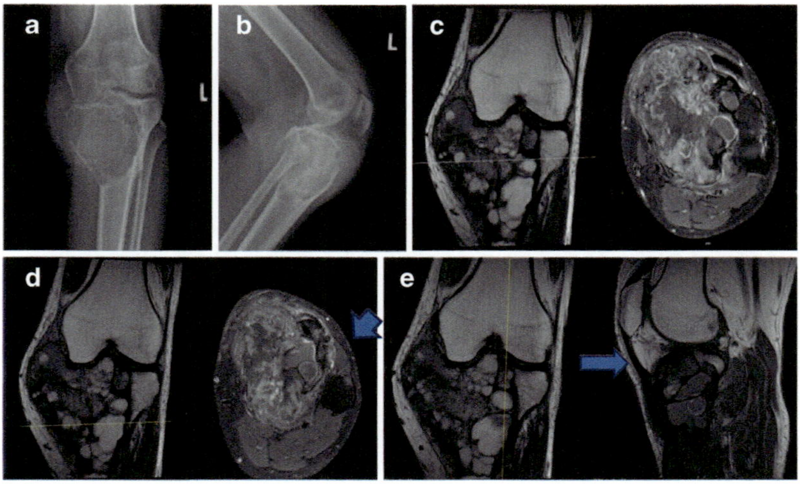

The plain radiograph shows an expansible lytic lesion with loss of medial cortex and soft tissue extension. MRI shows the tumour spares the tibial tuberosity and the lateral muscular compartment (Fig. 12a–e).

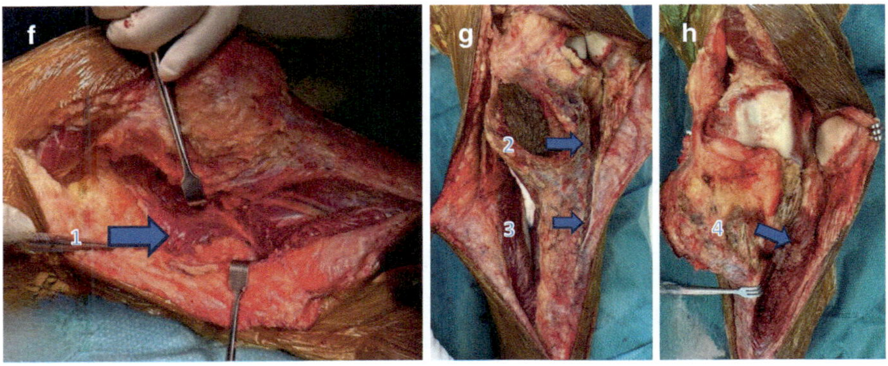

1. Gastrocnemius muscle with vascular supply
2. Tibial tubercle
3. Extensor compartment fascia
4. Tibialis anterior muscle

Technique for reservation of continuity knee extensor mechanism (Fig. 12f–h)

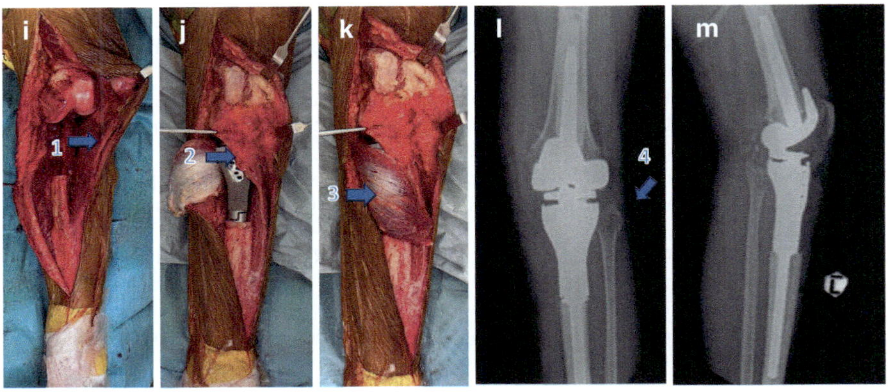

Following final resection and reconstruction, gastrocnemius muscle was used to cover the medial prosthesis and reinforce the extensor mechanism. All lateral compartment including fibula head and its muscle attachment remained intact for better knee flexion function (Fig. 12i–m).

Arrows

1. Patella tendon in continuity with extensor fascia and muscle
2. Patella tendon sutured to the prosthesis with good tension
3. Medial gastrocnemius flap
4. Fibula head

Suggested Reading

1. Abdel Rahman M, Nasser S, Safe I. The medial head gastrocnemius muscle transposition flap for coverage and functional restoration in limb-salvage surgery of bone tumors in the proximal tibia. Ain Shams J Surg. 2011;4(1):177–86.
2. Adler Z, Quinn RH. Proximal tibial resection and prosthetic reconstruction. Tech Orthop. 2007;22(2):88–98.
3. Bickels J, Wittig JC, Kollender Y, Neff RS, Kellar-Graney K, Meller I, Malawer MM. Reconstruction of the extensor mechanism after proximal tibia endoprosthetic replacement. Arthroplasty. 2001;16(7):856–62.
4. Pruksakorn D, Kongthavonskul J, Teeyakasem P, Phanphaisarn A, Chaiyawat P, Klangjorhor J, Arpornchayanon O. Surgical outcomes of extracorporeal irradiation and re-implantation in extremities for high grade osteosarcoma: a retrospective cohort study and a systematic review of the literature. J Bone Oncol. 2019;14:100210.
5. Ebeid WA, Hasan MHAE. Functional outcome following proximal tibial osteosarcoma resection and reconstruction by modular endoprosthesis. Ann Surg Oncol. 2023;30:1914–25.
6. Funovics PT. Implant reconstruction of the proximal tibia: modular prosthesis and rotational gastrocnemius flap. In: Orthopedic surgical oncology for bone tumors: a case study. Atlas; 2022. p. 299–310.
7. Bickels J, Malawer MM. Proximal tibia resection with endoprosthetic reconstruction. In: Operative technique in orthopaedic surgical oncology. Lippincott Williams & Wilkins, A Wolters Kluwer; 2012. p. 259–70.
8. Mercuri M, Errani C. Surgical technique of proximal tibia megaprosthesis. In: Master techniques in orthopaedic surgery orthopaedic oncology and complex reconstruction. Lippincott Williams & Wilkins, A Wolters Kluwer; 2011.
9. Matthias B, Zeifang F, Bernd L. Medial gastrocnemius muscle flap in limb-sparing surgery of malignant bone tumors of the proximal tibia: mid-term results in 25 patients. Ann Plast Surg. 2003;51(3):266–72.
10. Myers GJ, Abudu AT, Carter SR, Tillman RM, Grimer RJ. The long-term results of endoprosthetic replacement of the proximal tibia for bone tumours. J Bone Joint Surg Br. 2007;89(12):1632–7.
11. Ng VY, Louie P, Punt S, Conrad EU. Allograft reconstruction for sarcomas of the Tibia. Open Orthop J. 2017;11:189–94.
12. Philipp T. Funovics implant reconstruction of the proximal tibia: modular prosthesis and rotational gastrocnemius flap. In: Orthopedic surgical oncology for bone tumors. Switzerland: Springer Nature; 2022. p. 299–313.
13. Wittig JC, Villalobos CE, Hayden BL, Choi I, Silverman AM, Malawer M. Osteosarcoma of the proximal tibia: limb-sparing resection and reconstruction with a modular segmental proximal tibia tumor prosthesis. Ann Surg Oncol. 2010;17(11):3021.

Distal Tibia Resection and Reconstruction

Wan Faisham Nu'man Bin Wan Ismail,
Arman Zaharil Mat Saad, Wan Azman Wan Sulaiman,
Zulmi Wan, and Ahmad Sukari Halim

Introduction

The distal tibia is a rare site for primary sarcomas. A below-knee amputation is often an acceptable option owing to the challenges of salvaging the limb and retaining good functional outcomes. The subcutaneous position of the tibia, lack of coverage of stable soft tissue cover, narrow surgical margin with respect to the major neurovascular bundle, and a small talus for prosthesis fixation pose difficulties in reconstructive options.

Surgical Anatomy

The distal tibia is subcutaneous along the anterior part of the ankle joint. The anatomical barriers potentially infiltrated by the tumour include the following:

W. F. N. B. W. Ismail (✉)
Prince Court Medical Center, Kuala Lumpur, Malaysia

Orthopaedic Oncology Reconstructive Unit, Universiti Sains Malaysia, Kubang Kerian, Kelantan, Malaysia

A. Z. M. Saad
Plastic Reconstructive and Microsurgery, MSU Medical Centre, Management and Science University of Malaysia, Shah Alam, Malaysia

W. A. W. Sulaiman · A. S. Halim
Reconstructive Sciences Department, School of Medical Sciences, Universiti Sains Malaysia, Kubang Kerian, Kelantan, Malaysia

Z. Wan
Prince Court Medical Center, Kuala Lumpur, Malaysia

A. Puri, W. F. N. B. W. Ismail (eds.), *Atlas of Orthopedic Oncology Volume 2*,
https://doi.org/10.1007/978-981-95-8962-3_6

- In the subcutaneous layer anteriorly, the anterior part above the ankle is covered by the superior and inferior extensor retinaculum where all the anterior compartment tendons cross the ankle.
- The extensor hallucis and tibialis anterior tendon are closely related to the distal tibia along with the anterior tibial artery, which runs between the muscle tendons.
- Posteriorly, the distal tibial is covered by the muscle belly of the flexor hallucis longus and medially by the tendon of the tibialis posterior tendon where the posterior tibial nerve and artery are present.

Posterior tibial nerve is a key structure for sensation over the plantar foot and motor function of small muscles to the toe. A below-knee amputation should be suggested in cases where the posterior tibial nerve is involved. Attempts at limb salvage carry a risk of recurrent neuropathic ulcers.

Assessment

Resection and reconstruction of the distal tibia poses difficulty due to its subcutaneous location and proximity to the neurovascular bundle. Achieving a wide margin surgery is difficult, and such surgeries should be limited to sarcomas with a good response to chemotherapy or aggressive giant cell tumours. A wider oncological margin can be achieved by resecting areas of the involved skin, muscles, and tendons attached to the tumour, which includes the tibialis anterior, posterior and flexor hallucis longus muscles, and distal tibia-fibula joint.

Important structures to be critically evaluated before resection include the following:

- Subcutaneous region and skin over the anterior compartment
- Ankle joint and tibia fibula joint, including the ligaments attached to the joint
- Ligaments attached to the tibia: deltoid ligament, extensor retinaculum, and tibia fibula ligament

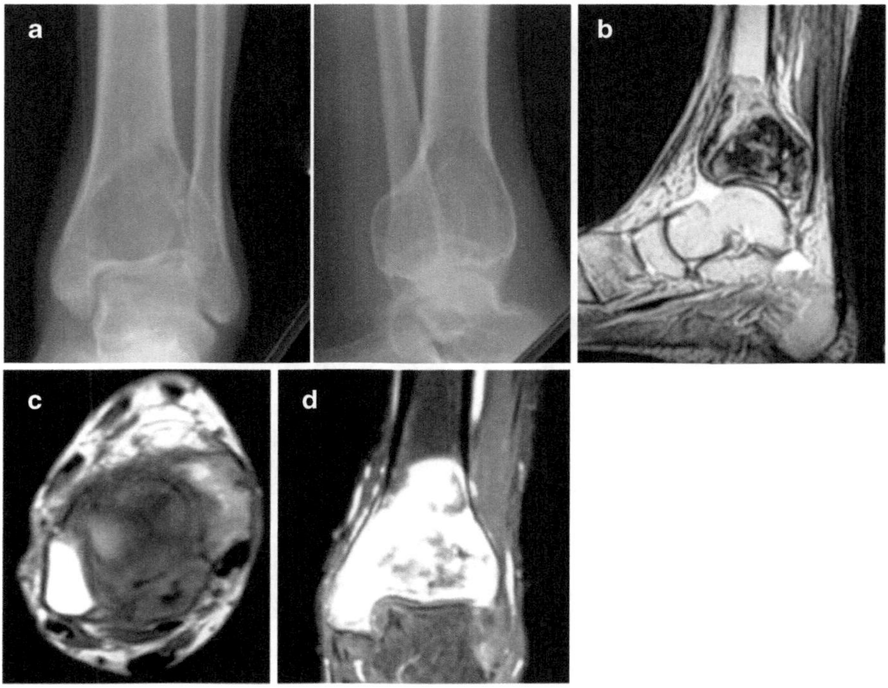

This is a case of intraosseous GCT with expansile lesion on the posterior aspect. There is no cortical breach and soft tissue extension. Considering its benign aggressive nature, a marginal margin surgery was planned (Fig. 1a–d).

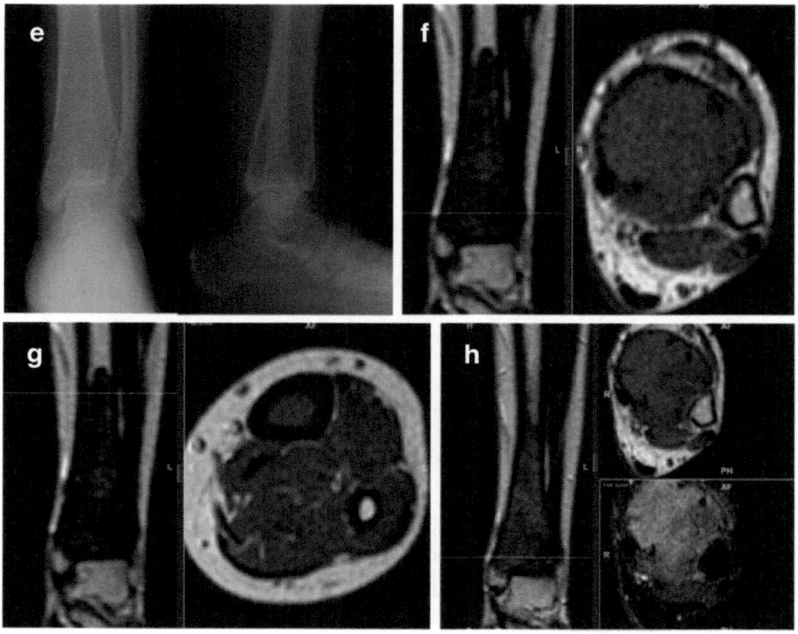

Low-grade osteosarcoma, fibrocystic variant mainly an intraosseous lesion. There is posterior extension above the ankle joint, which infiltrated the flexor hallucis longus muscle and tibialis posterior tendon. The anterior compartment structures and subcutaneous tissue were spared (Fig. 1e–h).

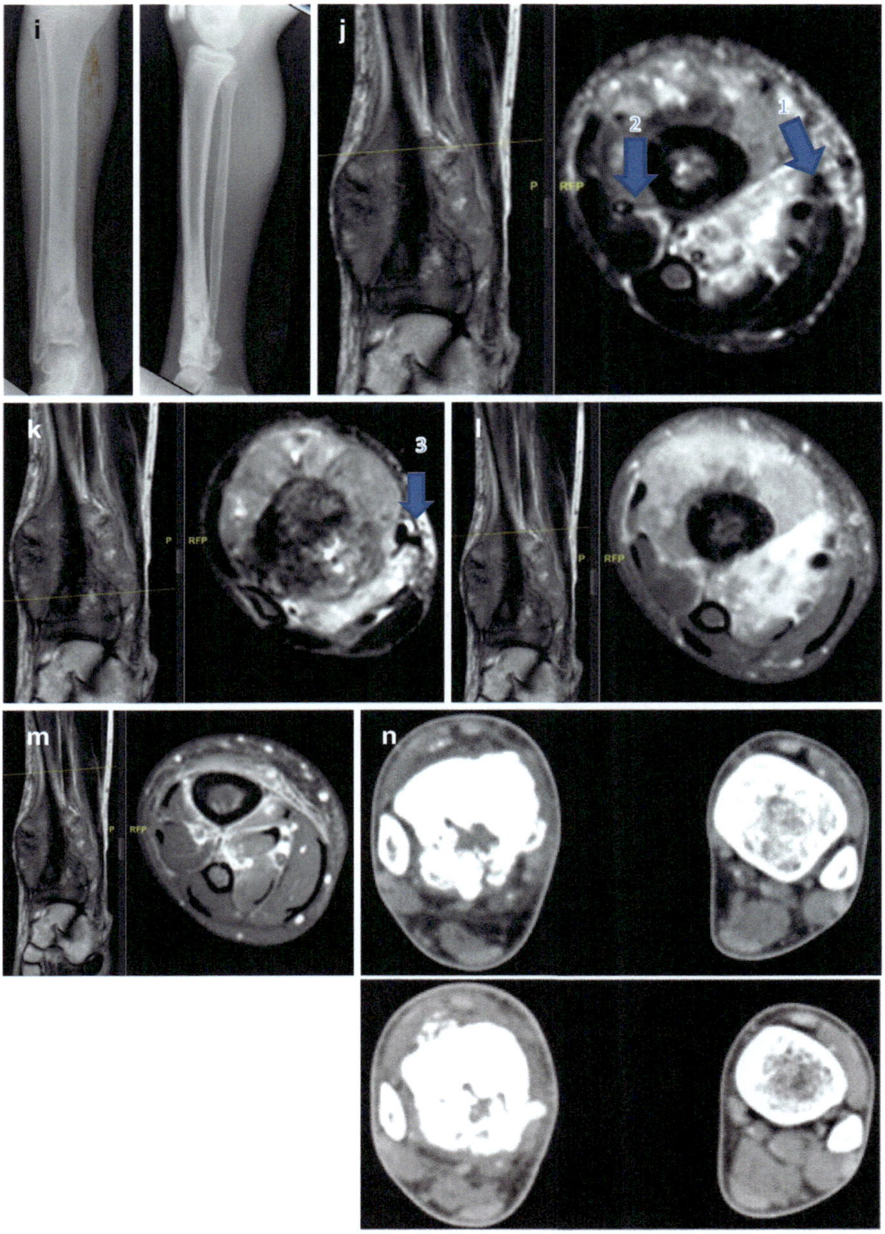

1. Posterior tibial
2. Anterior tibial vessels
3. Posterior tibial nerve

Osteosarcoma of the distal tibia with extensive circumferential soft tissue extension involving all the tendons and muscles, both anterior and posterior. The distal tibia fibula joint was closely approximated to the tumour; however, the ankle joint was spared. The neurovascular structures are best traced with contrast-enhanced MRI or contrast CT for evaluation and were within the tumour mass. The tibial nerve was within the tumour mass and potentially contaminated during exploration (Fig. 1i–n). A below-knee amputation was done as the posterior tibial nerve which is important to maintain sensations of the foot needed sacrifice.

Surgical Steps

Distal tibial resection surgical steps:

- Extensive mobilisation of the fasciocutaneous flap exposing the medial neurovascular structures and tibia fibula joint. The long saphenous vein must be mobilised together with the flap to prevent congestion and maintain its vascularity.
- Medial exploration and mobilisation of the posterior tibial artery and nerve and mobilisation of the uninvolved tendons.
- Exploration of the anterior tibial vessels and mobilisation of the tendons.
- Resection of the distal tibia fibula joint based on involvement as per the MRI.
- Proximal osteotomy and intraarticular ankle joint resection and complete mobilisation of the distal tibia.

Osteosarcoma with Extraosseous Soft Tissue Extension

Osteosarcoma in the distal tibia with significant soft tissue extension responded to chemotherapy. The tumour was abutting the fibula above the mortise and tibia-fibula joint was involved. Tibialis anterior, tibialis posterior, and flexor hallucis longus that circumferentially covered the distal tibia together with a segment of the fibula were removed to achieve adequate oncological margin.

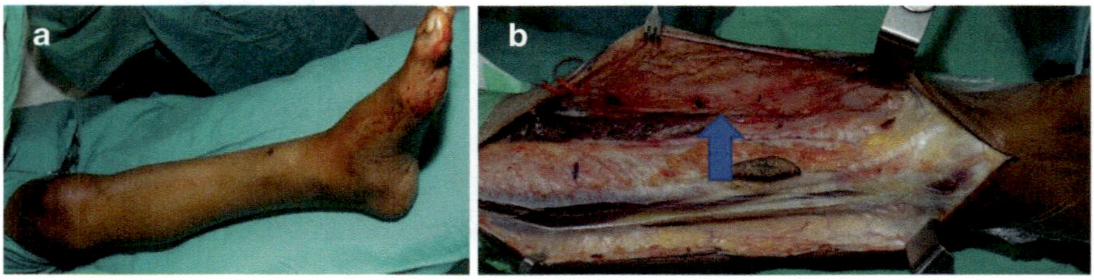

Mobilisation of the fasciocutaneous flap above the periosteum as a surgical margin is a crucial part of surgery to prevent skin necrosis (Fig. 2a, b).

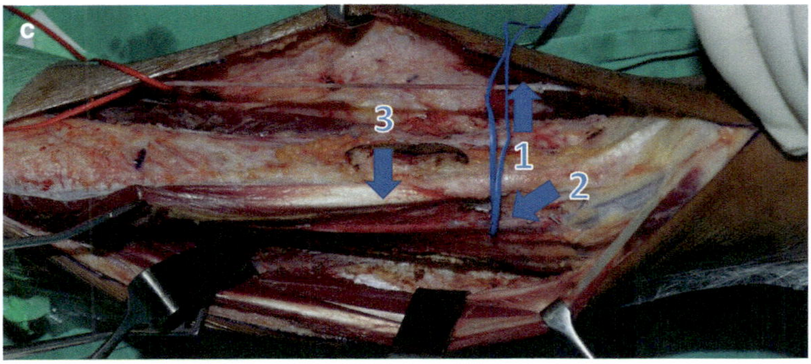

1. Medial fasciocutaneous flap with intact subcutaneous tissue and superficial vein to minimise the risk of flap necrosis
2. Anterior tibial artery and vein
3. Tibialis anterior tendon and muscle as margin

The procedure involved mobilisation of the medial fasciocutaneous flap while retaining the intact medial periosteum covering the distal tibia and elevation of the anterior compartment tendons from the tibia. The tendon and muscle of the tibialis anterior is left attached to the distal tibia for the oncological margin. The lateral inter-muscular septum and distal fibula are approached by elevating the tendon (Fig. 2c, d).

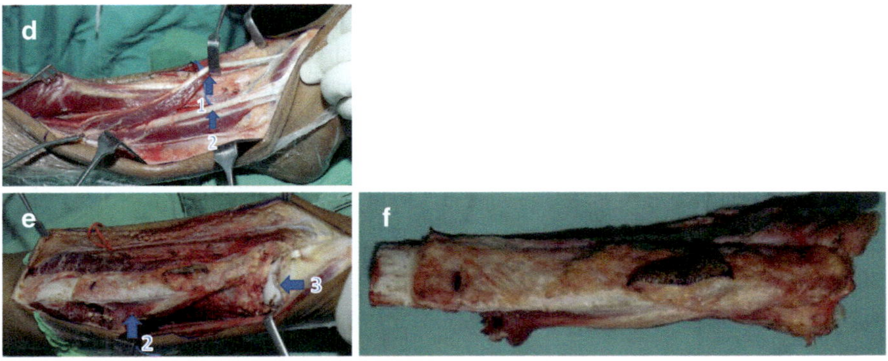

1. Mobilisation of extensor hallucis longus and extensor digitorum longus from the tibia after elevation of the extensor retinaculum
2. The tibialis anterior tendon and muscle was included as part of surgical margin
3. Capsulotomy and medial deltoid release for intraarticular ankle joint resection

Osteotomy of the proximal tibia is performed after the medial and lateral soft tissue is cleared and released. The anterior capsule and deltoid ligament are resected to mobilise the segment medially, and the medial border of the fibula is cut to elevate the entire distal tibia (Fig. 2e–g).

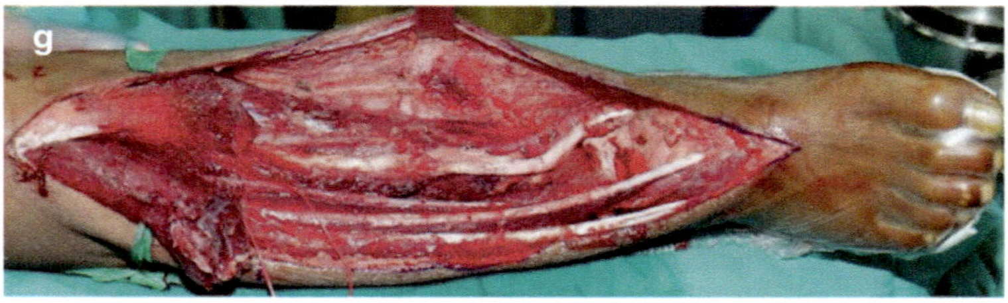

Options for Bone Reconstruction

Options for reconstruction of the osseous defect for distal tibia include the following:

- Endoprosthesis
- Recycle using extracorporeal radiation using single 60 Gy or cryotherapy with liquid nitrogen
- Osteoarticular allograft/allograft arthrodesis
- Vascularised fibula graft
- Medial transposition of fibula

Bone allograft-vascularised fibula composite with ankle arthrodesis is our preferred method as allograft provides immediate stability and vascularised fibula facilitates better incorporation and long-term biological incorporation and viability of the bone. Skin paddle from the flaps adds an additional advantage for soft tissue reconstruction and prevent skin dehiscence and failure. Ankle joint is arthrodesed, and the subtalar joint is spared to allow minimal mobility and improve gait (Fig. 2h–j).

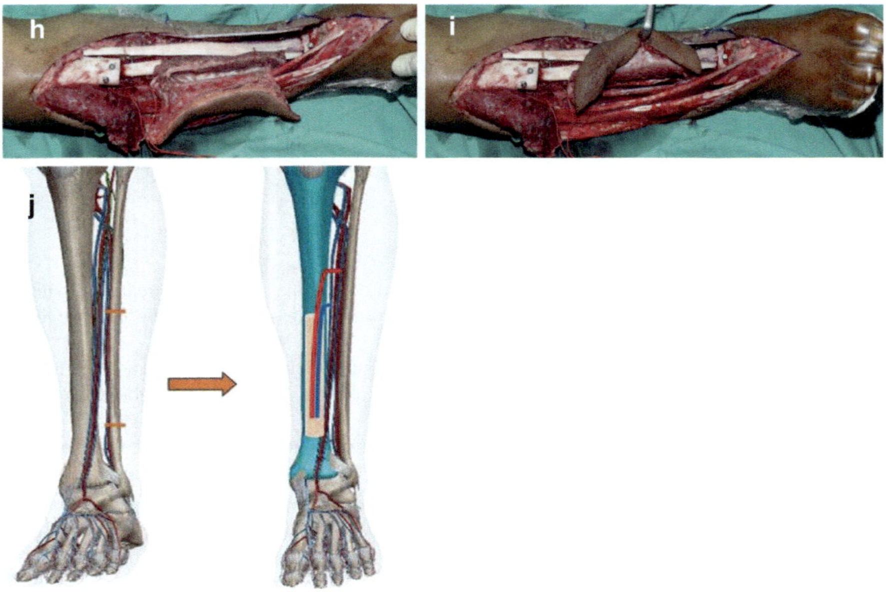

The free vascularised fibula is inserted in the intramedullary defect. It is sandwiched alongside the allograft and stabilised with plate and/or screws. The cortical allograft is trimmed to three-fourths of the diameter for comfortable placement of the vascularised fibula. Distally, cancellous allograft is placed to provide better union and stability. The entire reconstruction is stabilised with screws at the proximal tibia and at the talus.

Subsequently, the entire construct is protected by simple external fixator (one pin each at the proximal tibia and third metatarsal) for postoperative protection, flap care, and ease of dressing. Once the wound is healed and flap stabilised, a patella tendon bearing cast is applied for 2 months until junctional union. The construct is protected with a protective thermoplastic brace for 6 months until radiographs show the fibula graft and allograft was fully incorporated. The patient was allowed partial weight bearing on protective brace after 6 weeks and graduated to full weight bearing after junctional union on radiograph. Full weight bearing without the protective brace was allowed at 6 months.

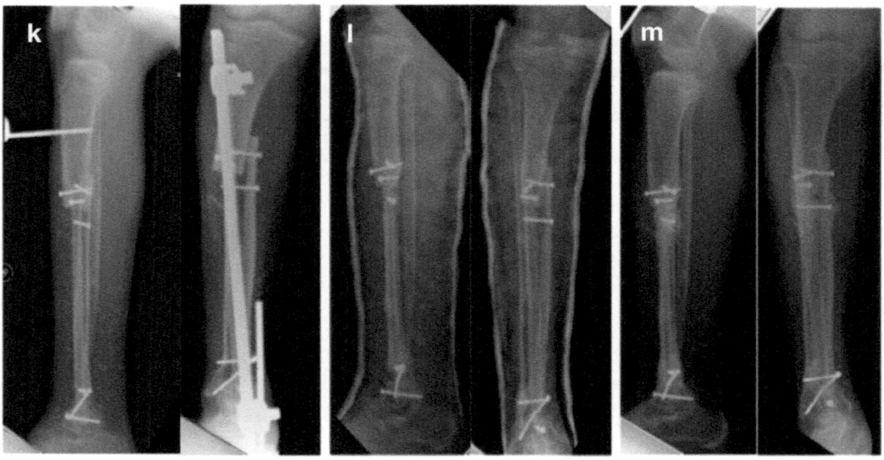

Allograft fibula composite is generally completely incorporated within 2 years. Ankle arthrodesis with mobile subtalar joint allows compensatory movement with reasonable gait and activities of daily living (Fig. 2k–m).

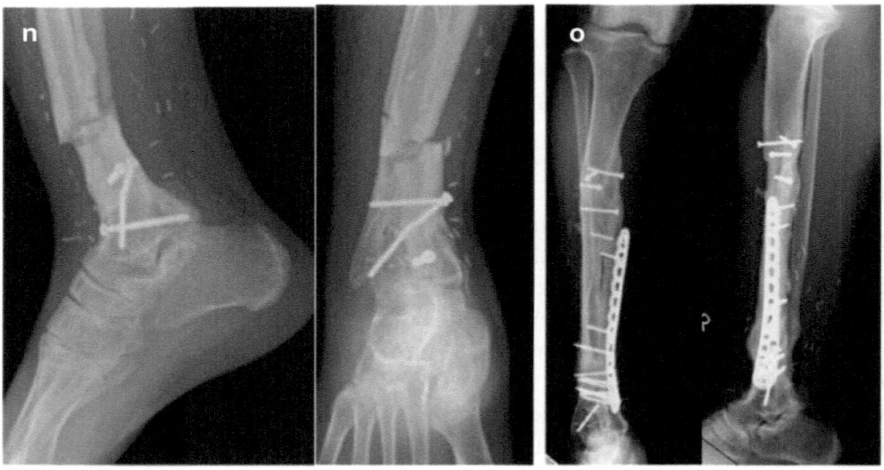

A young active patient is at risk for major injuries and fracture. Simple osteosynthesis through minimally invasive techniques is adequate for healing the fully vascularised allograft fibula composites (Fig. 2n, o).

Intraosseous Giant Cell Tumour of Distal Tibia

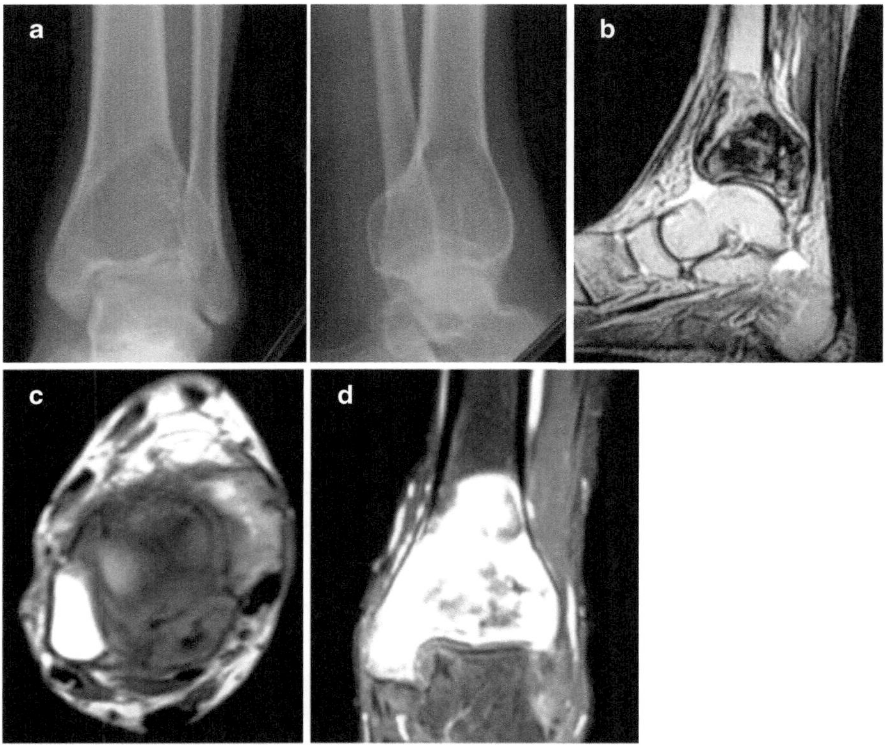

A case of intraosseous GCT presented with an expansile lesion on the posterior aspect. There is no cortical breach and soft tissue extension (Fig. 3a–d). Considering its benign aggressive nature, a marginal margin surgery was planned (Fig. 3e–h).

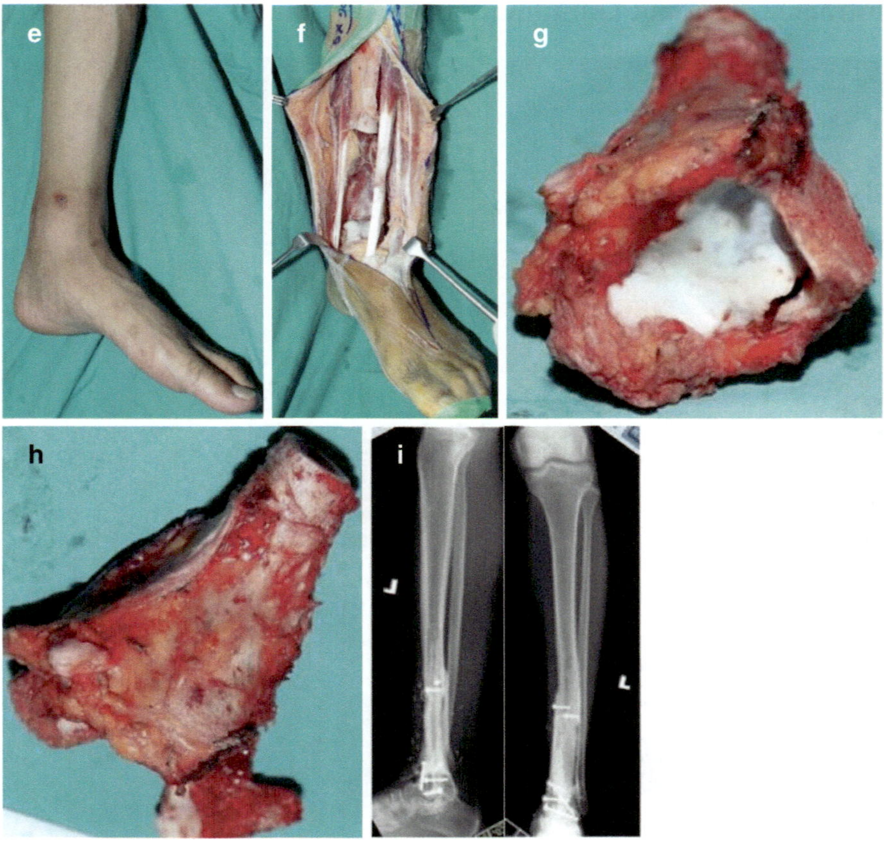

As the osseous resection length was short, anterior fasciocutaneous flap was thick and all the tendons and fascia around the ankle were maintained. An allograft was used for reconstruction. After a long-term follow-up of 15 years, a plain radiograph showed evidence of complete vascularisation of the allograft after the reconstruction (Fig. 3i).

Low-Grade Fibrocystic Type Intraosseous Osteosarcoma

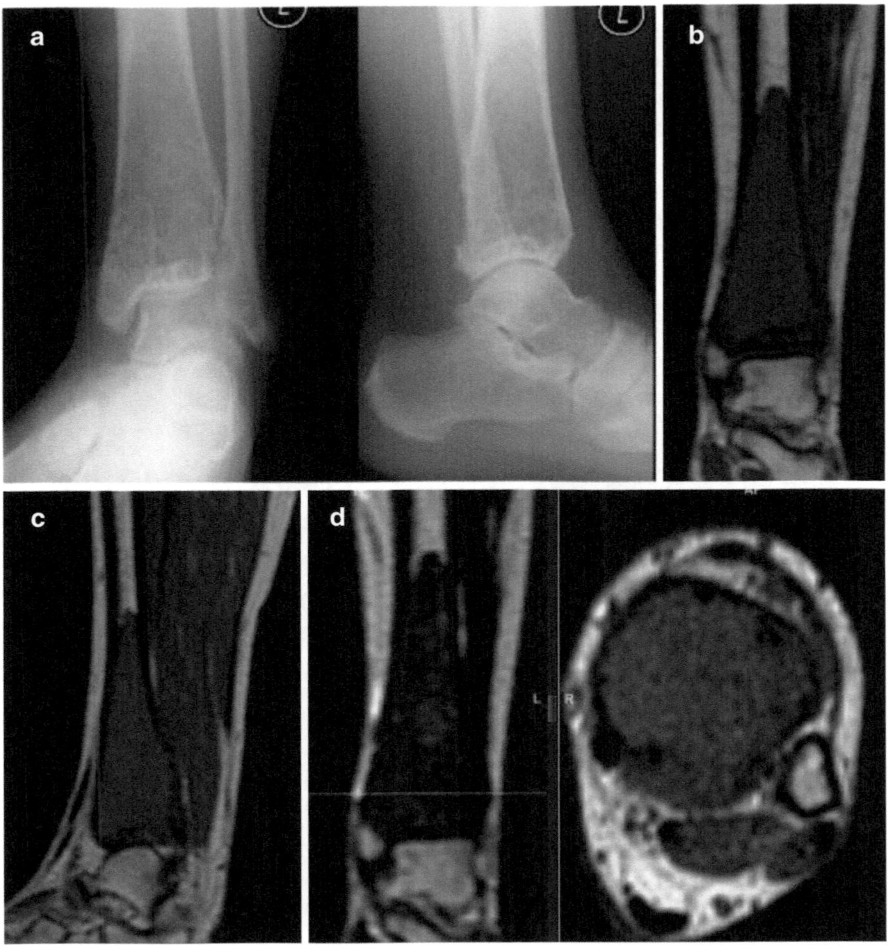

An intraosseous fibrocystic osteosarcoma was identified, where the tumour mass was confined to the bone with no extraosseous extension (Fig. 4a–d). Hence, it was suitable for limb salvage surgery. Mobilisation of the medial fasciocutaneous flaps with intact saphenous vein and nerve. The entire anterior compartment muscles and tendons were mobilised together with the anterior tibial vessels. Part of the fibula over the tibia fibula joint and syndesmotic was included in the margin prior to the tibial osteotomy and ankle joint disarticulation for final posterior exploration and distal tibia resection (Fig. 4e–j).

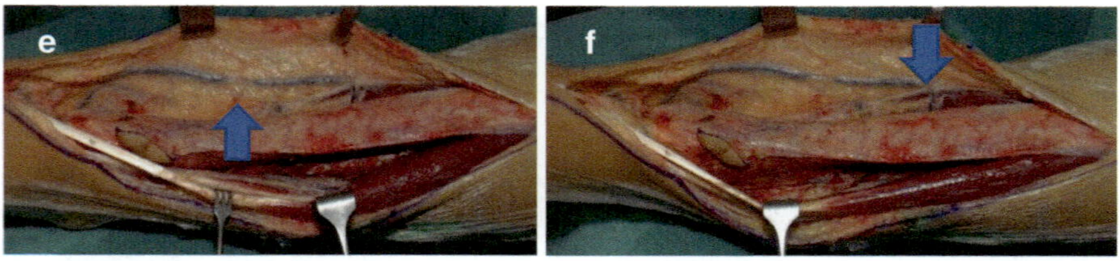

Mobilisation of the fasciocutaneous flap above the periosteum as a surgical margin is a crucial part of surgery to prevent skin necrosis. The long saphenous vein and nerve must be mobilised together to maintain venous plexus integrity and sensation.

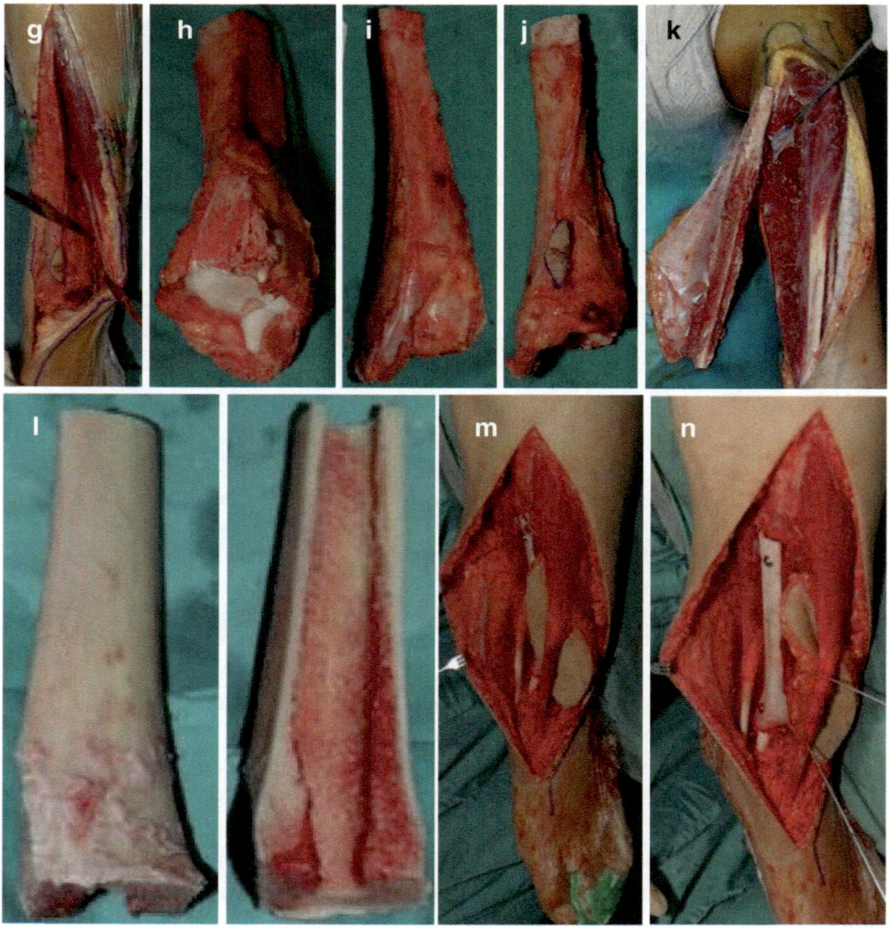

The entire distal tibia was resected with part of distal tibia fibula joint and reconstructed with an allograft vascularised fibula composite flap 'Modified Capanna

Technique'. It was fully incorporated after 3 years, and the patient remains disease free at 15 years (Fig. 4k–n).

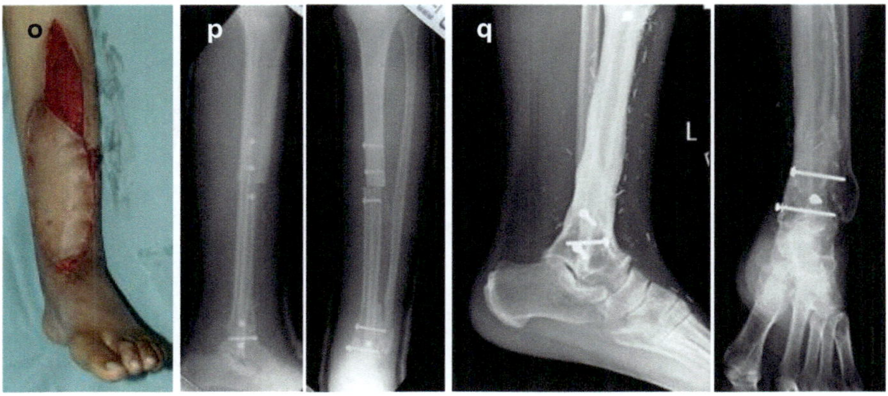

The final reconstruction was achieved with composite allograft-vascularised fibula with good soft tissue cover at the anterior shin. Subsequent hypertrophy occurred, with incorporation and vascularisation of the allograft fibula (Fig. 4o–q).

Osteosarcoma in the Distal Tibia with Extensive Soft Tissue Involvement

Osteosarcoma in the distal tibia with extensive soft tissue and fibula extension is an option for below-knee amputation and prosthesis fitting. If the posterior tibial nerve is spared and circulation of the foot is maintained, limb salvage surgery is possible. Protective sensory over the foot plantar and minimal toe tendon function is adequate for ambulation in an arthrodesis ankle (Fig. 5a–d).

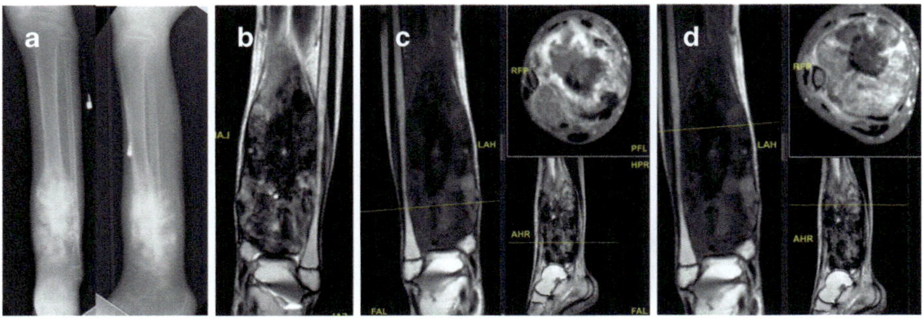

The entire anterior compartment muscle is removed and only the flexor digitorum longus and hallucis longus are maintained with the posterior neurovascular bundle (Fig. 5e–h). Extensor hallucis longus, extensor digitorum longus, and flexor hallucis longus were reconstructed using an allograft tendon for function. Simple external stabilisation was applied for easy flap monitoring, wound care, and tendon protection prior to a complete below-knee cast (Fig. 5i–k).

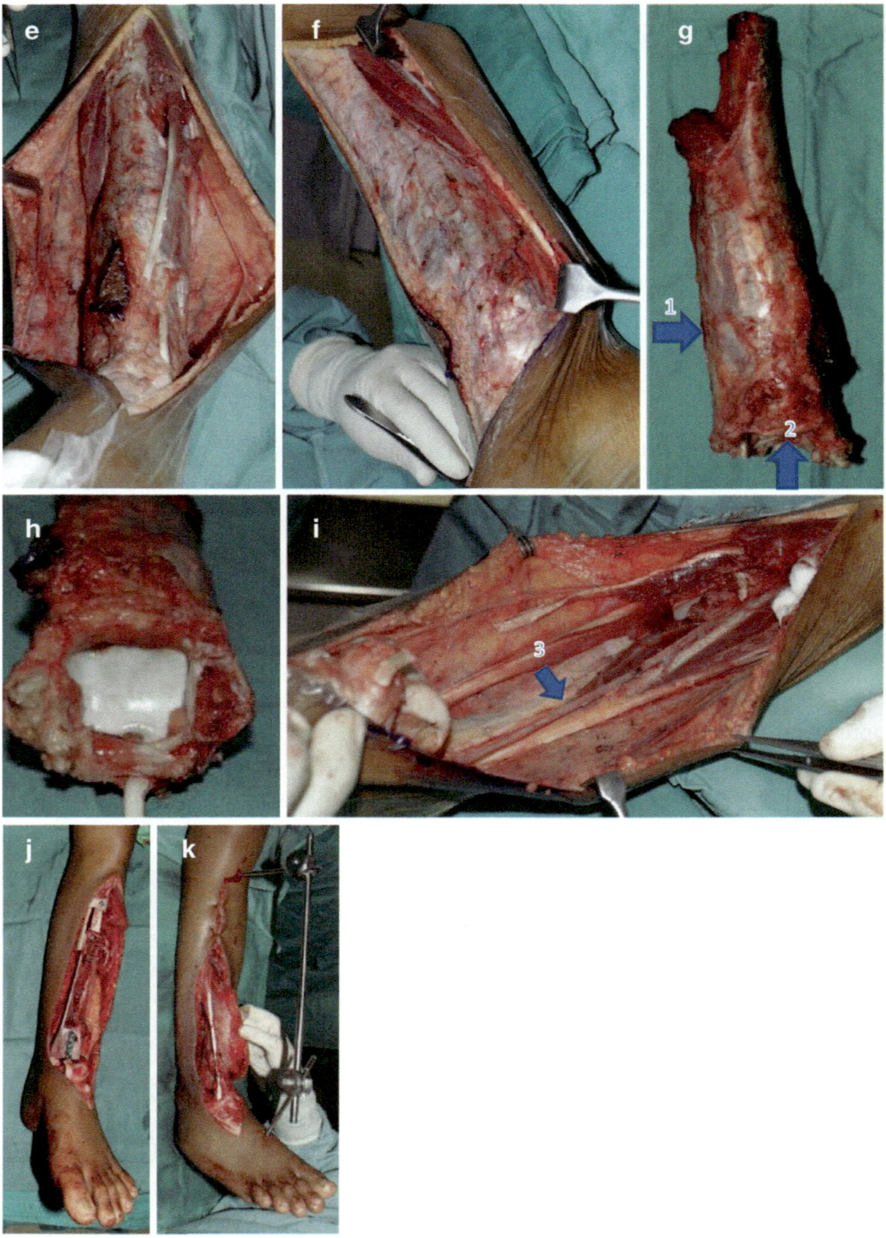

1. Entire extensor compartment
2. Flexor hallucis longus tendon
3. Posterior neurovascular bundle—posterior tibial vessels and posterior tibial nerve

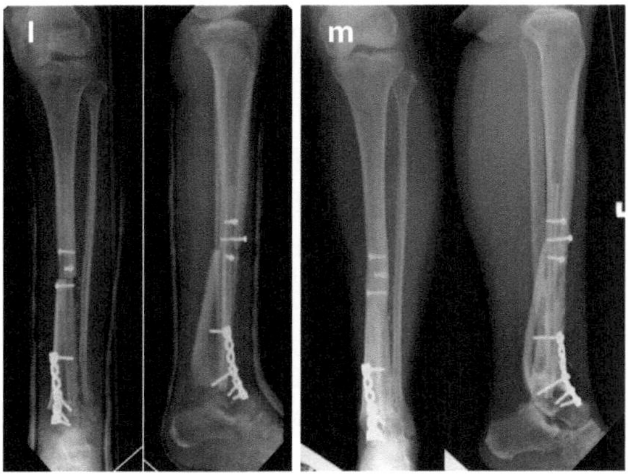

The vascularised fibula graft was slotted in the intramedullary proximal tibia and the centre of the talus dome distally. The allograft with a widened trimmed gutter to fit the fibula graft is used to reinforce the construct. The proximal part was stabilised with three screws and lower construct was stabilised with a contoured reconstruction plate. Further stabilisation with external fixation till wound healing was followed by a patella tendon bearing cast until union at both ends. Additional protection with removable brace was continued for further 6 months (Fig. 51, m).

Suggested Reading

1. Halim AS, Chai SC, Faisham WI, Azman WSW, Saad AZM, Wan Z. Long-term outcome of free fibula osteocutaneous flap and massive allograft in the reconstruction of long bone defect. J Plast Reconstr Aesthet Surg. 2015;68:1755–62.
2. Fuchs B, Ossendorf C, Leerapun T, Sim FH. Intercalary segmental reconstruction after bone tumor resection. Eur J Surg Oncol. 2008;34:1271–6.
3. Capanna R, Bufalini C, Campanacci M. A new technique for reconstructions of large metadiaphyseal bone defects: a combined graft (allograft shell plus vascularized fibula). Orthop Traumatol. 1993;2(3):159–77.
4. Scaglioni MFC, Arzi RY, Gur E, Amotz OB, Barnea Y, Kollender Y, Meller I, Bickels J, Dadia S, Zaretski A. Free fibula reconstruction of distal tibial defects after sarcoma surgery. Ann Plast Surg. 2015;74(6):680–3.
5. Capanna R, Campanacci DA, Belot N, Beltrami G, Manfrini M, Innocenti M, Ceruso M. A new reconstructive technique for intercalary defects of long bones: the association of massive allograft with vascularized fibular autograft. Long-term results and comparison with alternative techniques. Orthop Clin North Am. 2007;38:51–60.

6. Innocenti M, Abed YY, Beltrami G, et al. Biological reconstruction after resection of bone tumors of proximal tibia using allograft shell and intramedullary free vascularized fibular graft: long term results. Microsurgery. 2009;29(5):361–72.
7. Choong PF. Ankle—general consideration. In: Master techniques in orthopaedic surgery orthopaedic oncology and complex reconstruction. Lippincott Williams & Wilkins, A Wolters Kluwer; 2011. p. 273–83.
8. Colangeli S, Andreani L, D'Arienzo A, Mani O, Restuccia G, Capanna R. Biological reconstruction of the tibial diaphysis and ankle—III: arthrodesis with massive allograft. In: Orthopaedic surgical oncology for bone tumors. Springer Nature Switzerland AG; 2022. p. 333–45.

Distal Tibia Resection and Endoprosthesis Reconstruction

Vivek Ajit Singh

Introduction

Tumours in the distal tibia are uncommon. Benign aggressive bone lesions and primary bone tumours such as giant cell tumours and osteosarcoma typically affect the distal femur and proximal tibia, with the distal tibia and ankle being less frequently involved. The tibia ranks as the second most common site for osteosarcoma, with only a minority (20%) affecting the distal tibia. In contrast, giant cell tumours of the bone rarely impact the distal tibia, with less than 4% of cases occurring there. Current research indicates that osteosarcoma is the most prevalent pathological diagnosis among primary bone tumours in the distal tibia (75.1%), followed by Ewing's sarcoma (7.4%) and giant cell tumours (6.8%).

Historically, amputation was the standard treatment approach for primary bone tumours in the distal lower limb. However, with advances in surgical procedures, imaging technologies, and improved chemotherapy, limb-sparing surgeries have become the preferred method for treating distal lower limb tumours. Among the different types of limb-sparing surgeries, endoprosthesis reconstruction (EPR) in the distal tibia has been debated due to its rarity and the limited data available from most studies.

Prosthesis

The prosthesis we use is custom-made by Eagle Osteon Technologies in Chennai, India. Roentgenograms are used to measure the length of the resection segment, the size and length of the tibial stem, and the dimensions of the talar articulating

V. A. Singh (✉)
Department of Orthopaedic Surgery, Faculty of Medicine, University Malaya, Kuala Lumpur, Malaysia

A. Puri, W. F. N. B. W. Ismail (eds.), *Atlas of Orthopedic Oncology Volume 2*,
https://doi.org/10.1007/978-981-95-8962-3_7

segment. The implant will be designed based on these measurements. The prosthesis is made from a titanium alloy and consists of two components that are connected by screws and a central peg. The distal articulating segment is a saddle joint that rests on the talus dome and is secured with cementation and screws. This saddle joint includes a bar lined with a polyethene liner that moves within an oblong hole at the prosthesis's superior aspect of the talus end. The proximal component features a cylindrical stem cemented into the proximal tibia. The articular surfaces are lined with ultra-high-molecular-weight polyethene. Unlike a simple hinge movement, the ankle movement with this prosthesis replicates a saddle joint movement, aiming better to simulate the mechanics of a natural ankle joint.

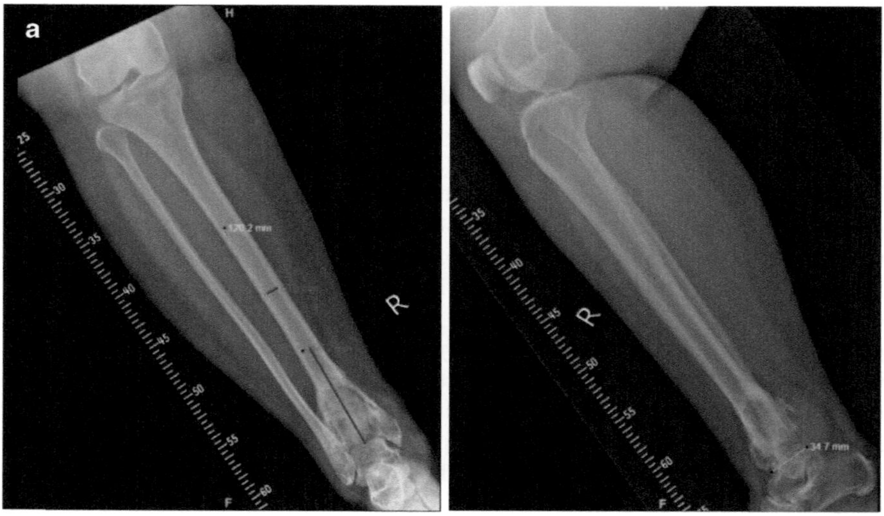

This shows the measured roentgenograms taken during the presentation. Resection measurements are taken based on the tumour extent on the MRI (Fig. 1a).

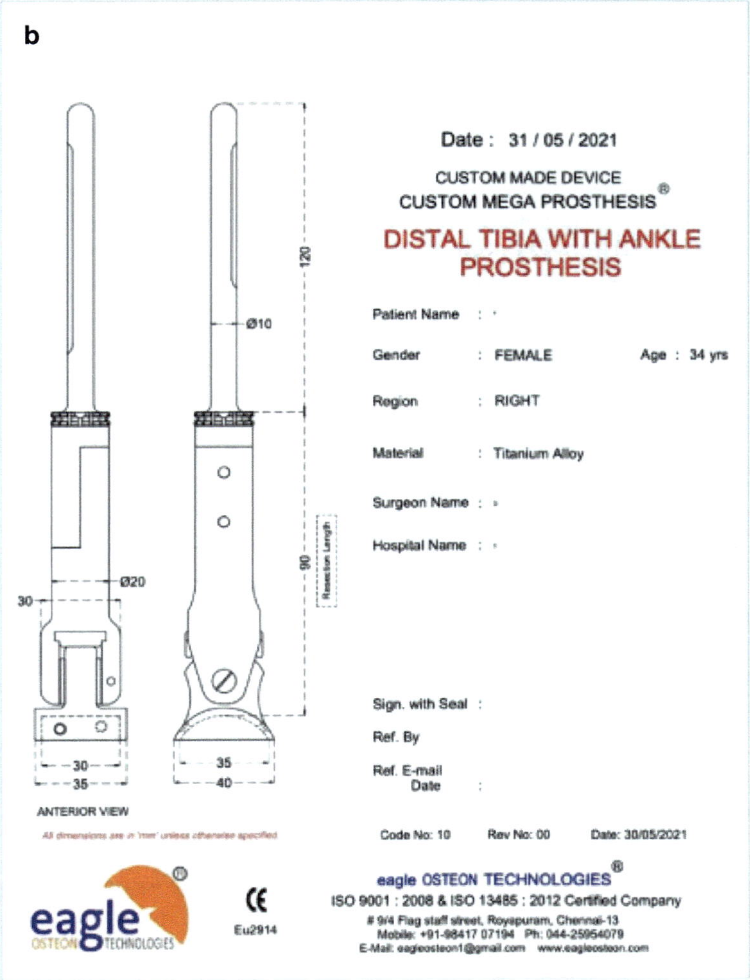

This shows the implant design for the custom-made prosthesis. This is based on the measured radiographs (Fig. 1b).

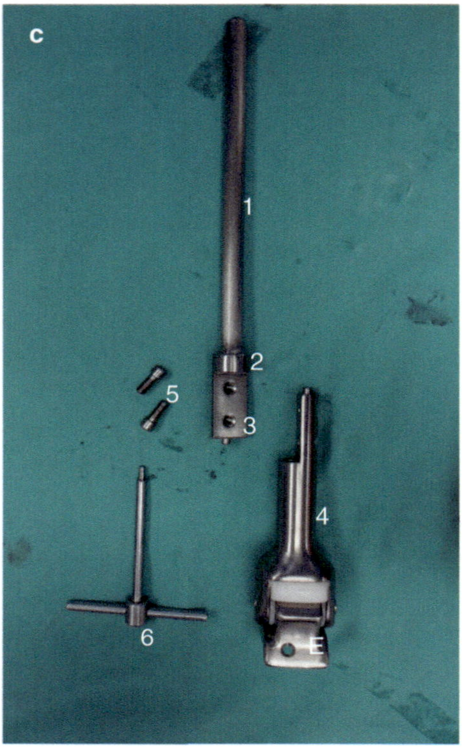

This shows the implant dismantled with the distal and proximal components (Fig. 1c). Both components interlock with each other with a peg and secured by screws (Fig. 1d). The components are as follows:

1. Tibial stem
2. Tibia shaft
3. Interlocking component with peg
4. Distal tibial stem
5. Talar component
6. Treaded screws to lock both components
7. Allen key

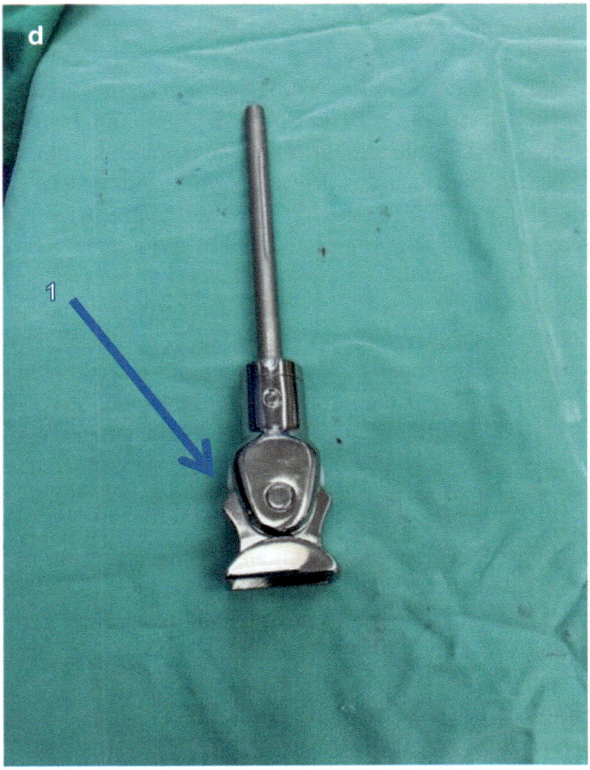

1 shows the saddle ankle joint. The talar component is oblong, allowing semicircular movement of the joint.

Operative Criteria

All patients selected for this procedure met the following criteria for limb salvage surgery:

1. There is no involvement of the neurovascular bundle, which includes the anterior tibial artery, posterior tibial artery, and posterior tibial nerve.
2. There are no skip lesions present within the same tibia.
3. There is no additional involvement of the ipsilateral talus or Calcaneum.

Operative Technique

The surgical approach involves an anterior lateral incision. The biopsy tract and the tumour are included in this incision and removed. The soft tissue dissection is similar to all other forms of resection of distal tibia tumours and reconstruction. Tumour dissection aims to achieve wide resection margins. Preservation of the anterior or posterior tibial artery, or both, along with the posterior tibial nerve, is carried out during resection. Efforts are made to spare the superficial and deep peroneal nerve branches; however, they may be removed with the tumour. Proximal tibial bone cuts are performed approximately 2 to 3 cm proximal to the tumour's proximal margin, and this resection length is integrated into the implant design. The tumour is excised at the ankle joint, separating the talus from the distal tibia fibula joint without violating the distal tibia's articular cartilage. The distal portion of the fibula with the distal tibia fibula joint is typically excised with the tibia with the distal tibia fibula joint intact to prevent potential recurrence due to tumour infiltration in that area. Hemostasis is ensured after tumour removal, followed by thorough irrigation of the wound.

Subsequently, the cartilage on the talar dome is removed using a power saw, reshaping to fit the prosthesis's cup end. Drill holes are made on the talus dome for cement anchorage. The component is then cemented onto the talus and secured with threaded cancellous screws. The remaining proximal tibia end is reamed slightly larger than the stem diameter, and the stem is cemented for fixation. A cement plug is usually unnecessary as the implant's stem is designed to be long enough to accommodate the remaining bone segment. The two implant components are then aligned, locked together with the peg, and secured by two screws.

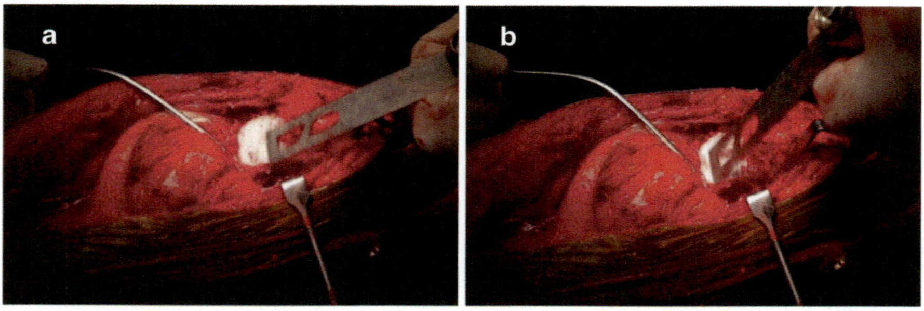

This shows the shaving of the talar articular cartilage with a power saw (Fig. 2a, b).

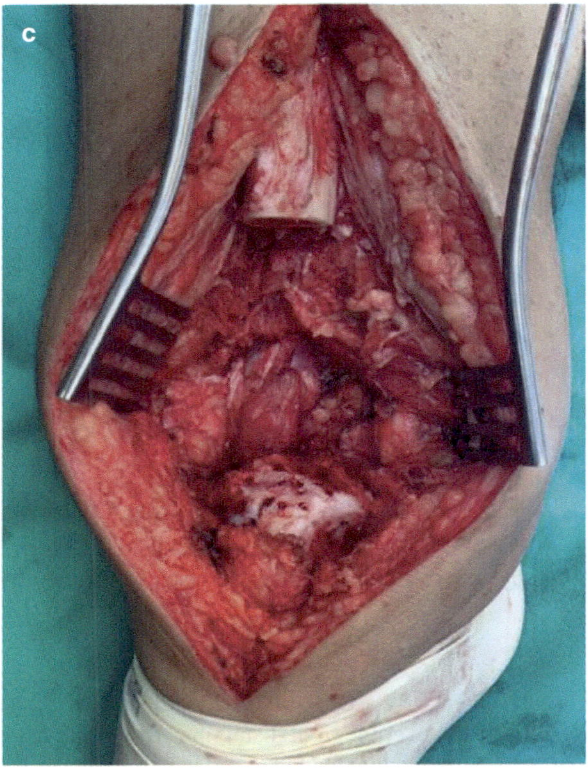

This shows multiple drill holes made into the talar dome to improve the implant's talar component's anchorage with the talus (Fig. 3c).

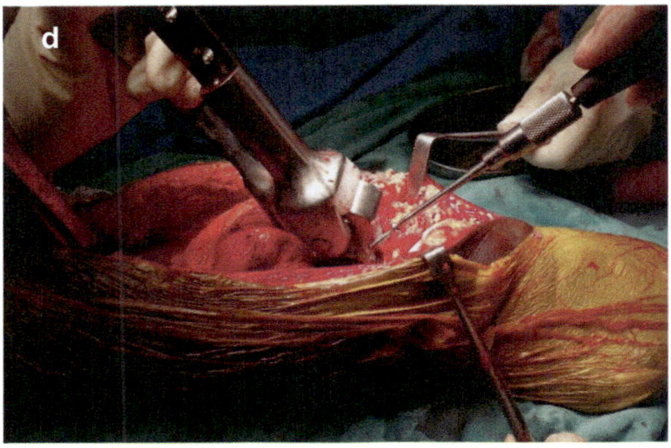

This shows the talar component is further secured with screws (Fig. 2d).

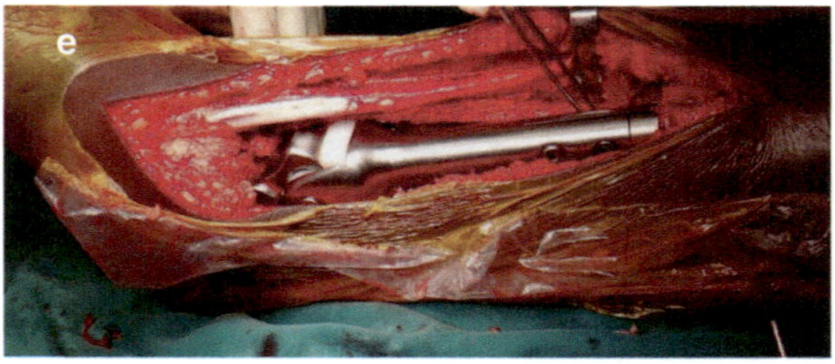

This shows both proximal and distal components reduced and locked with threaded screws (Fig. 2e).

Postoperative Rehabilitation

On day 2 postoperatively, patients are allowed full weight bearing. They are advised to use a walking aid, either a walking frame or crutches, for the first 2 weeks to attain balance while walking. At 2 weeks, the sutures are removed, and the patient is referred for formal physiotherapy, where ankle mobility exercises and stretching are started.

Case 1

This is a 33-year-old lady who presented with a GCT of the right distal tibia. The radiograph shows an expansile lytic lesion over the right distal tibia, extending from the metaphysis to the epiphysis. She underwent extended curettage and bone grafting. However, on a 1-year follow-up, recurrence was detected. She subsequently underwent a wide resection and endoprosthesis replacement. She is currently disease free and ambulating without support.

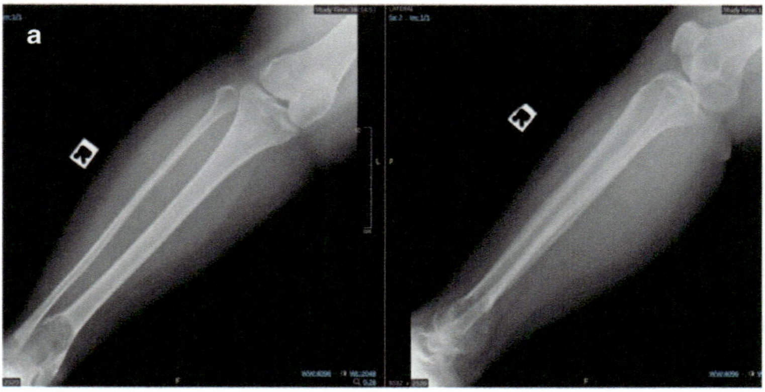

This shows an expansile lytic lesion over the right distal tibia. There is soap bubble appearance.

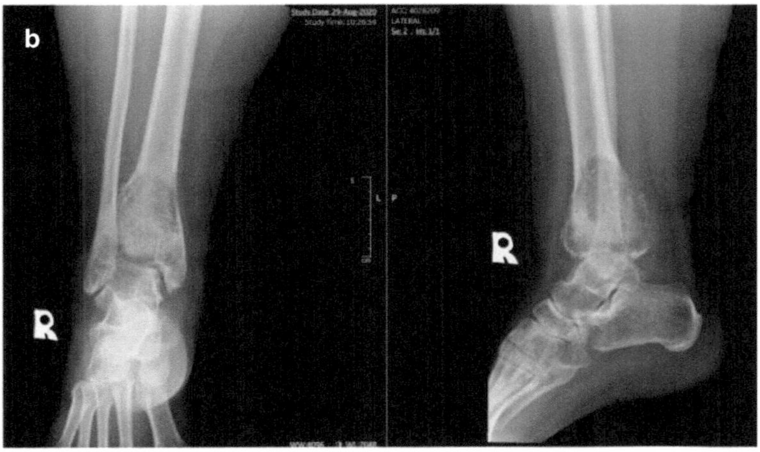

The postoperative radiograph of post-extended curettage and bone grafting. The tumour is curetted, filling the cavity with morselised bone grafts.

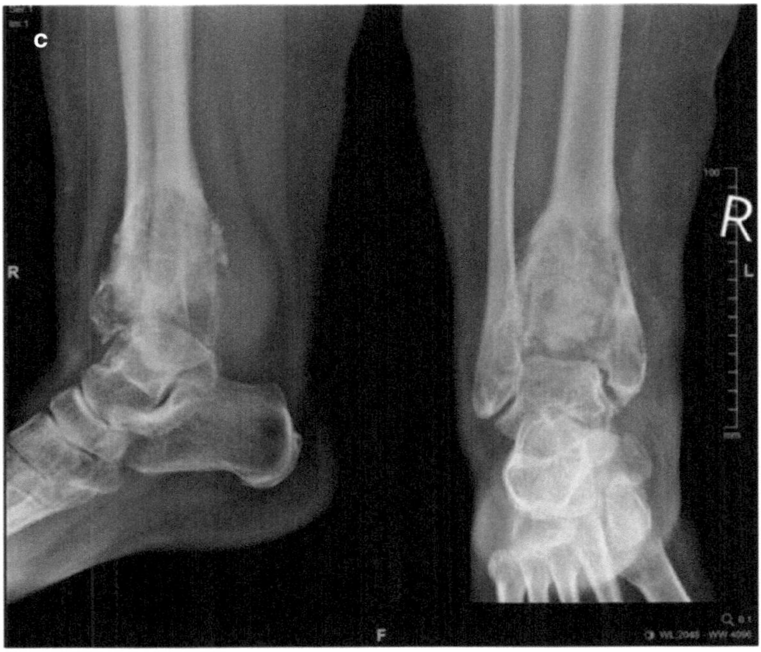

This radiograph shows the recurrence of the disease with a lytic area over the anterior right distal tibia and a break in the posterior cortex with soft tissue extension.

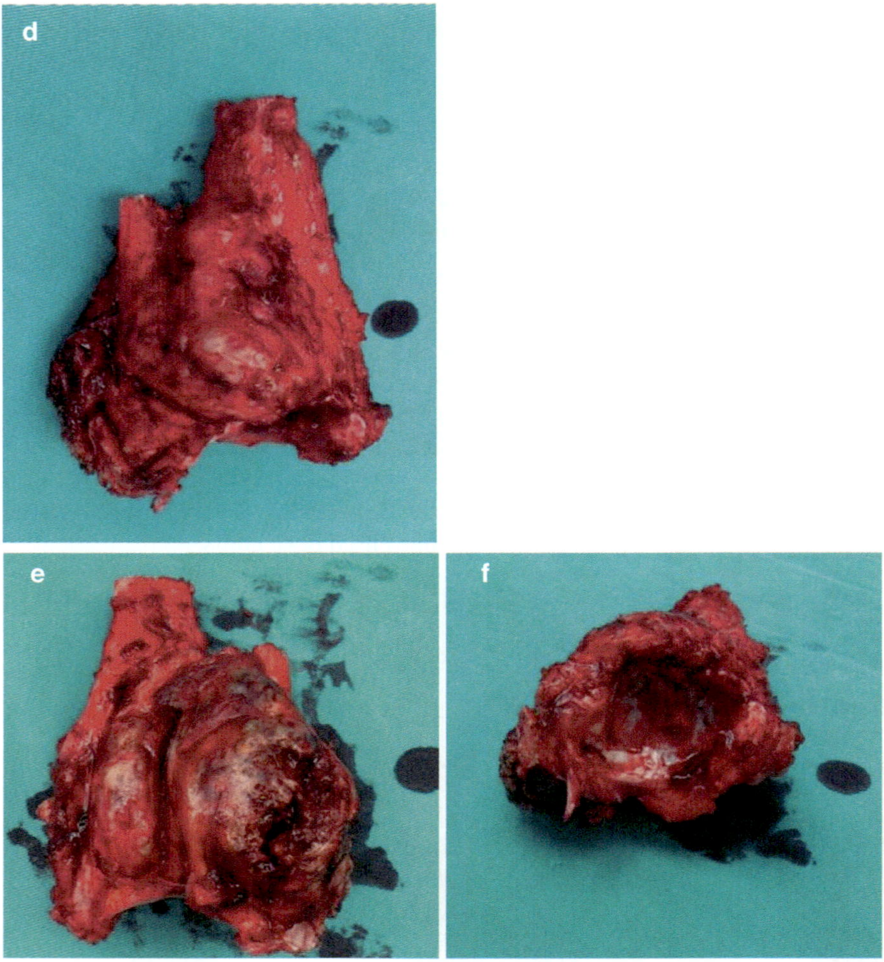

This shows the resected specimen. The distal tibia and fibula are excised. There is a soft tissue extension over the posterior distal tibia. The distal tibia articular surface is intact.

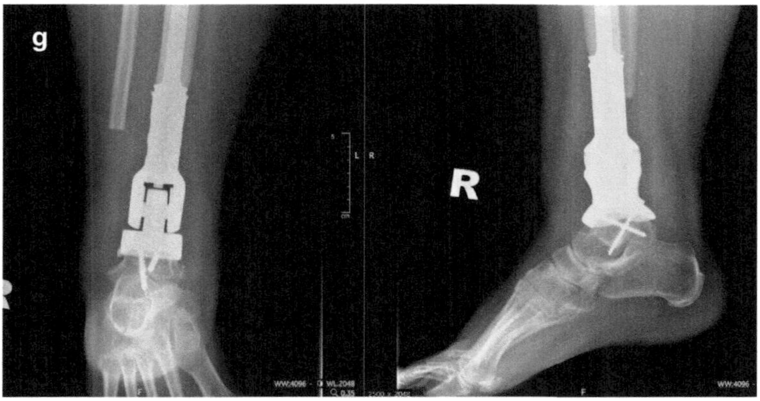

This shows the plain radiograph of the postoperative distal tibia endoprosthesis.

Case 2

This is a 12-year-old boy with osteosarcoma of the right distal tibia. The plain radiograph shows an osteoblastic lesion over the right distal tibia with Codman's triangle and sunburst appearance. The MRI showed no neurovascular involvement; therefore, limb salvage was possible. He underwent three cycles of neoadjuvant chemotherapy. After which, a wide resection and endoprosthesis replacement were carried out. Post-surgery, the patient had another three cycles of adjuvant chemotherapy. It has been 10 years since the index surgery. The patient is walking without support and has a normal gait; radiologically, there is no evidence of implant failure.

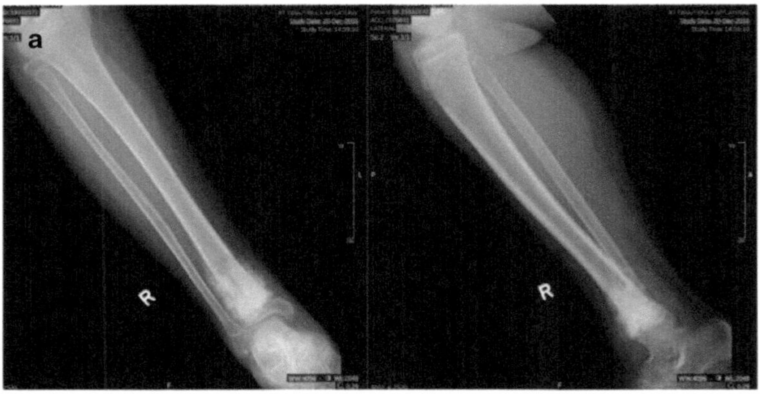

The plain radiograph shows an osteoblastic lesion over the right distal tibia metaphysis with a sunburst periosteal reaction and Codman's triangle (Fig. 4a).

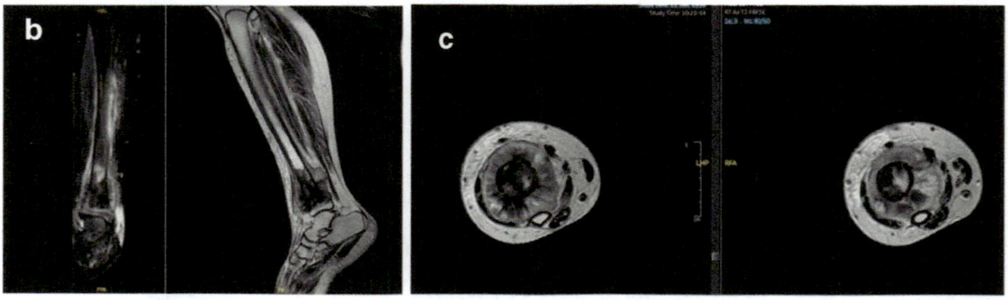

This shows the coronal, sagittal, and axial view of the MRI. The tumour is confined to the distal tibia metaphysis, the neurovascular bundles are spared, and there are no skip lesions (Fig. 4b,c).

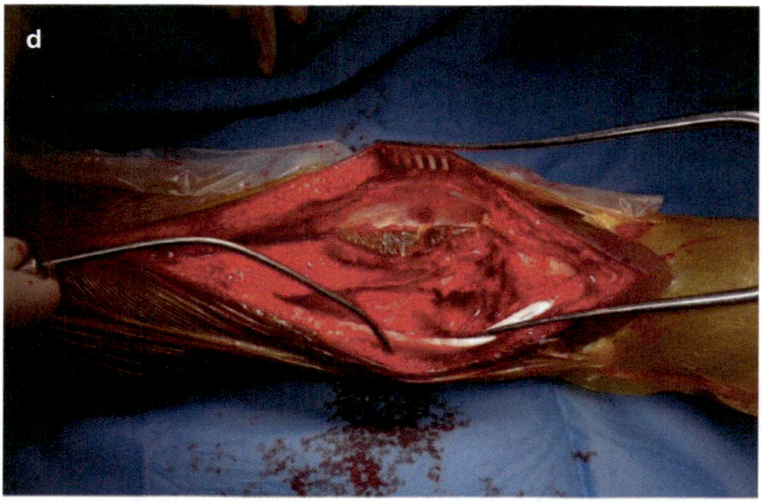

This shows the distal tibia dissected with the biopsy tract (Fig. 4d).

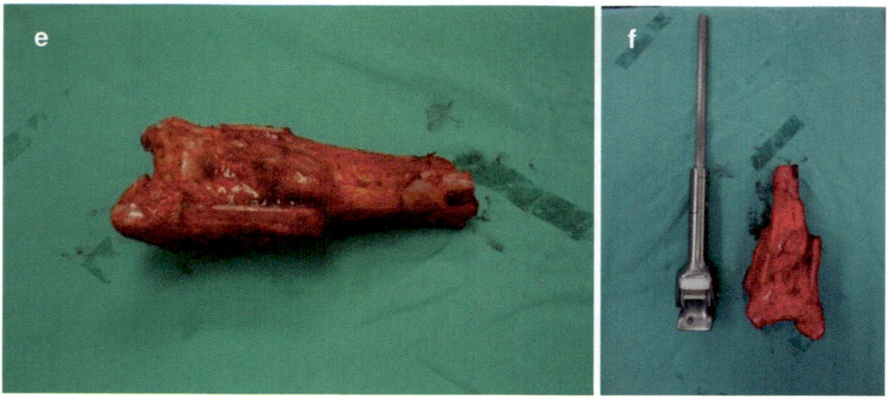

This shows the resected specimen with the custom-made endoprosthesis. The distal tibia was resected with the distal fibula, and the distal tibia fibula joint was intact (Fig. 4e,f).

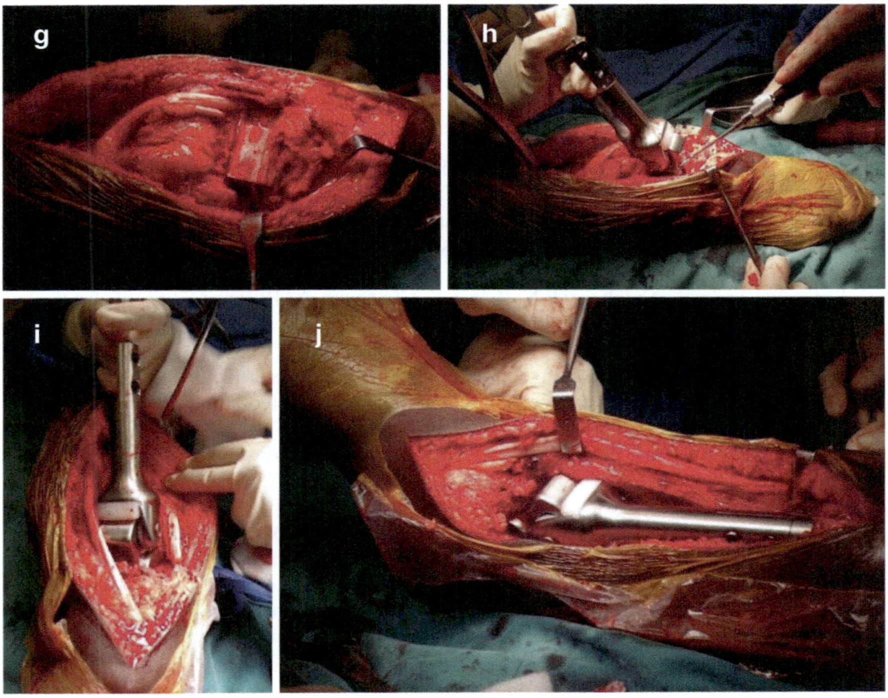

This shows the surgical procedure of inserting the endoprosthesis, where the talus cartilage is shaved off, the dome of the prosthesis is anchored to the talus with screws, and the proximal end of the prosthesis is cemented into the proximal tibia. The prosthesis is finally reduced, and the connection is secured with screws (Fig. 4g–j).

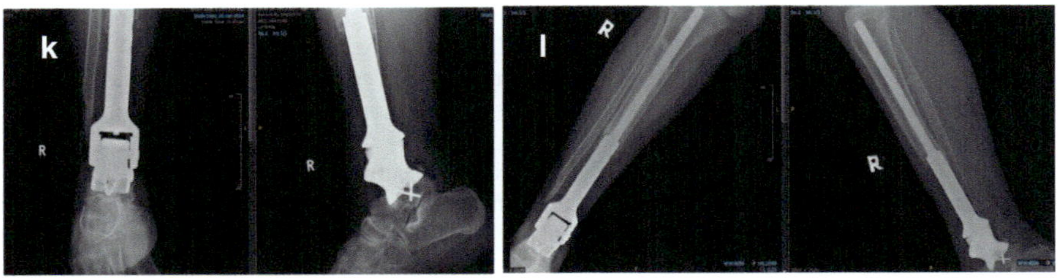

This shows a follow-up radiograph taken 10 years after the procedure. There is no evidence of implant failure (Fig. 4k–l).

Outcome

We reviewed and published the outcomes of nine cases that underwent this prosthesis with a follow-up of 39.3 months (range 12 to 112). The mean MSTS score for the nine patients during their last follow-up is 87.8% (range 73.3 to 100). The mean TESS score is 84.4% (range 69.2 to 100). There were no implant failures [21].

Suggested Reading

1. Bielack SS, Kempf-Bielack B, Delling G, Exner GU, Flege S, Helmke K, Kotz R, Salzer-Kuntschik M, Werner M, Winkelmann W, Zoubek A, Jurgens H, Winkler K. Prognostic factors in high-grade osteosarcoma of the extremities or trunk: an analysis of 1,702 patients treated on neoadjuvant cooperative osteosarcoma study group protocols. J Clin Oncol. 2002;20(3):776–90.
2. Ebeid W, Amin S, Abdelmegid A, Refaat Y, Ghoneimy A. Reconstruction of distal tibial defects following resection of malignant tumours by pedicled vascularised fibular grafts. Acta Orthop Belg. 2007;73(3):354–9.
3. Mavrogenis AF, Abati CN, Romagnoli C, Ruggieri P. Similar survival but better function for patients after limb salvage versus amputation for distal tibia osteosarcoma. Clin Orthop Relat Res. 2012;470(6):1735–48.
4. Lee SH, Kim HS, Park YB, Rhie TY, Lee HK. Prosthetic reconstruction for tumours of the distal tibia and fibula. J Bone Joint Surg (Br). 1999;81(5):803–7.
5. Natarajan MV, Annamalai K, Williams S, Selvaraj R, Rajagopal TS. Limb salvage in distal tibial osteosarcoma using a custom mega prosthesis. Int Orthop. 2000;24(5):282–4.
6. Faisham WI, Zulmi W, Halim AS, Biswal BM, Mutum SS, Ezane AM. Aggressive giant cell tumour of bone. Singapore Med J. 2006;47(8):679–83.
7. Ottaviani G, Jaffe N. The epidemiology of osteosarcoma. Cancer Treat Res. 2009;152:3–13.
8. Karpik M. Giant Cell Tumor (tumor gigantocellularis, osteoclastoma) – epidemiology, diagnosis, treatment. Ortop Traumatol Rehabil. 2010;12(3):207–15.
9. Zeytoonjian T, Mankin HJ, Gebhardt MC, Hornicek FJ. Distal lower extremity sarcomas: frequency of occurrence and patient survival rate. Foot Ankle Int. 2004;25(5):325–30.
10. Ajit Singh V, Nasirudin N, Bernatt M. Endoprosthetic reconstruction for giant cell tumors of the distal tibia: a short term review. Asia Pac J Clin Oncol. 2013;9(2):182–9.
11. Zhao Z, Yan T, Guo W, Yang R, Tang X, Wang W. Surgical options and reconstruction strategies for primary bone tumors of distal tibia: A systematic review of complications and functional outcome. J Bone Oncol. 2019;14:100209.
12. Abudu A, Grimer RJ, Tillman RM, Carter SR. Endoprosthetic replacement of the distal tibia and ankle joint for aggressive bone tumours. Int Orthop. 1999;23(5):291–4.
13. Laitinen M, Hardes J, Ahrens H, Gebert C, Leidinger B, Langer M, et al. Treatment of primary malignant bone tumours of the distal tibia. Int Orthop. 2005;29(4):255–9.
14. Yang P, Evans S, Khan Z, Abudu A, Jeys L, Grimer R. Reconstruction of the distal tibia following resection of aggressive bone tumours using a custom-made megaprosthesis. J Orthop. 2017;14(3):406–9.
15. Simon MA, Aschliman MA, Thomas N, Mankin HJ. Limb-salvage treatment versus amputation for osteosarcoma of the distal end of the femur. J Bone Joint Surg Am. 1986;68(9):1331–7.
16. Rougraff BT, Simon MA, Kneisl JS, Greenberg DB, Mankin HJ. Limb salvage compared with amputation for osteosarcoma of the distal end of the femur. A long-term oncological, functional, and quality-of-life study. J Bone Joint Surg Am. 1994;76(5):649–56.
17. Kamal AF, Widyawarman H, Husodo K, Hutagalung EU, Rajabto W. Clinical outcome and survival of osteosarcoma patients in Cipto Mangunkusumo hospital: limb salvage surgery versus amputation. Acta Med Indones. 2016;48(3):175–83.

18. Laitinen M, Hardes J, Ahrens H, Gebert C, Leidinger B, Langer M, Winkelmann W, Gosheger G. Treatment of primary malignant bone tumours of the distal tibia. Int Orthop. 2005;29(4):255–9.
19. Moore DR, Halpern JL, Schwartz HS. Allograft ankle arthrodesis: a limb salvage technique for distal tibial tumors. Clin Orthop Relat Res. 2005;440:213–21.
20. Campanacci DA, Scoccianti G, Beltrami G, Mugnaini M, Capanna R. Ankle arthrodesis with bone graft after distal tibia resection for bone tumors. Foot Ankle Int. 2008;29(10):1031–7.
21. Wei KK, Singh VA, Wen LX, Yasin NF, Mansor A. Distal tibia endoprosthesis reconstruction after resection of aggressive bone tumors: is it a reliable treatment option? World J Surg. 2023;10(2):2–7.

Fibula Resection

Wan Faisham Nu'man Bin Wan Ismail

Introduction

Tumours of the proximal fibula are rare. Resection is always challenging due to its close proximity to two major structures: the peroneal nerve and the anterior tibial artery. Malawer has previously described the two types of resections for aggressive benign and malignant tumours of the proximal fibula.

- Benign tumour—all the covering muscle and common peroneal nerve is spared during excision
- Malignant tumour—en bloc extraarticular excision, including resection of the anterior, peroneal group of muscles together with the peroneal nerve and lateral part of tibia cortex in cases proximal tibial fibula joint contaminated

Surgical Anatomy

- The fibula head is situated at the posterolateral corner of the tibia and articulates with the lateral condyle of the tibia. The biceps femoris muscle and lateral collateral ligament of the knee are directly attached to the surface of the head. The tibiofibular joint, stabilised by a strong interosseous ligament, is a true synovial joint. Anteriorly, it is covered by the origin of peroneus longus and posteriorly by the soleus origin.
- The fibula neck is a short bare region below the fibula head where the common peroneal nerve lies crossing below the biceps femoris to the anterior compart-

W. F. N. B. W. Ismail (✉)
Prince Court Medical Center, Kuala Lumpur, Malaysia

Orthopaedic Oncology Reconstructive Unit, Universiti Sains Malaysia, Kubang Kerian, Kelantan, Malaysia

A. Puri, W. F. N. B. W. Ismail (eds.), *Atlas of Orthopedic Oncology Volume 2*,
https://doi.org/10.1007/978-981-95-8962-3_8

ment of the leg. Evaluation of its involvement is important prior to surgical intervention.

- Both the flexor and extensor hallucis longus originate from the fibula together with the extensor digitorum longus and soleus and tibialis posterior. These are important structures for the surgical margin. Extensive resection of these muscles will lead to distal disability.
- The popliteal artery lies medial to the proximal fibula over the soleus muscle and branches into the trifurcation of anterior tibial artery, tibia peroneal trunk, and fibula artery. All these structures are at risk in a large malignant proximal fibula tumour. Exploration and identification prior to resection are mandatory to minimise vascular complication.

The peroneal nerve is divided into the deep and superficial peroneal nerves: branches of the anterior branch are articular branch of the tibia fibula joint, followed by the motor branch to the tibialis anterior. The deep peroneal follows the course of the anterior tibial artery after piercing the anterior compartment. Exploration and identification at the neck fibula neck is required to examine where the first articular branch can be sacrificed for fibula resection (Fig. 1a, b).

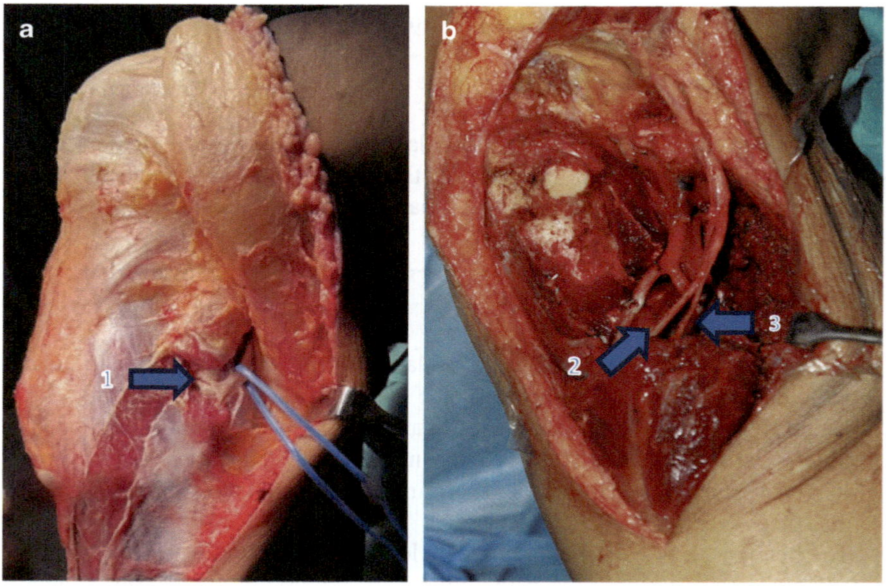

1. Articular branch
2. Deep peroneal
3. Superficial peroneal

Assessment

Anatomical boundaries around the fibula are an important part of the assessment to achieve a wide surgical margin for the malignant tumours:

- Proximal tibia fibula joint—involvement and infiltration to the lateral condyle of the tibia warrants extraarticular resection involving the condyle of tibia.
- Peroneal nerve—whether it should be retained or sacrificed to achieve a wide margin. Informed consent of functional morbidity is important to avoid medical litigation.
- Muscle origin and its involvement, particularly for a long segment fibula resection.
- Popliteal vessels and its branch and their correlation with the tumour.

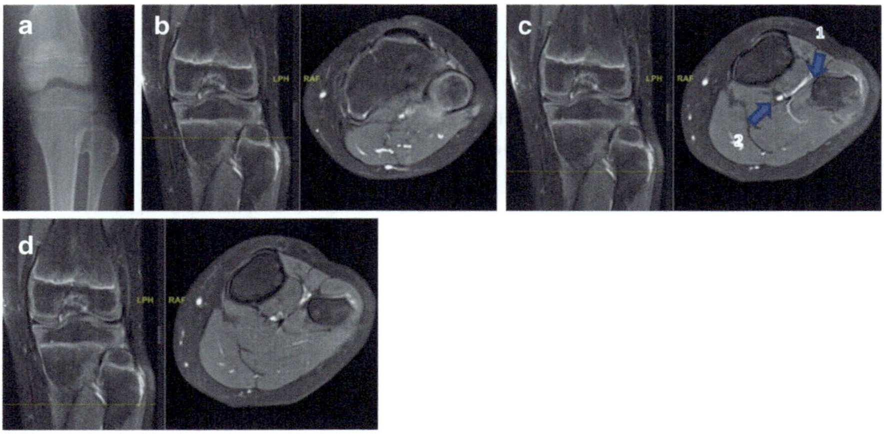

A 6-year-old girl with multiple hereditary exostosis presented with foot drop. The MRI showed a small lesion below the epiphyseal fibula plate. The popliteal vessels branched to the anterior tibial and were in close proximity to the exostoses (Fig. 2a–d).

1. Posterior tibial vessels
2. Anterior tibial vessels

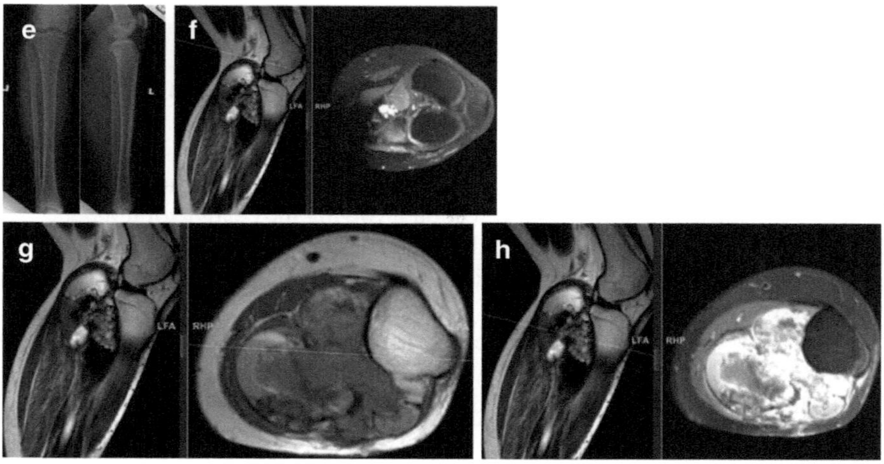

This is a case of osteosarcoma of the fibular head in a 15-year-old boy that responded poorly to chemotherapy and had a massive soft tissue extension. The popliteal vessels and its trifurcation together with the posterior tibial nerve were within the tumour, and the best option was above knee amputation (Fig. 2e–h).

Type I Resection for Benign Tumour

Surgical Steps (Fig.3a-c)

- Exploration of the common peroneal nerve below the biceps femoris tendon. The nerve is freed proximally to minimise tension during manipulation for removal of the tumour.
- The anterior compartment muscle is mobilised from the tibia with the nerve to maintain motor unit for function and minimise traction injury.
- Distal fibula osteotomy and mobilising of the proximal fibula as the common peroneal nerve is reflected anteriorly to minimised nerve stretching.
- The proximal attachment of the biceps femoris and lateral collateral ligament were detached from the fibula. The tibia fibula interosseous ligament was detached by external rotation of the fibula.

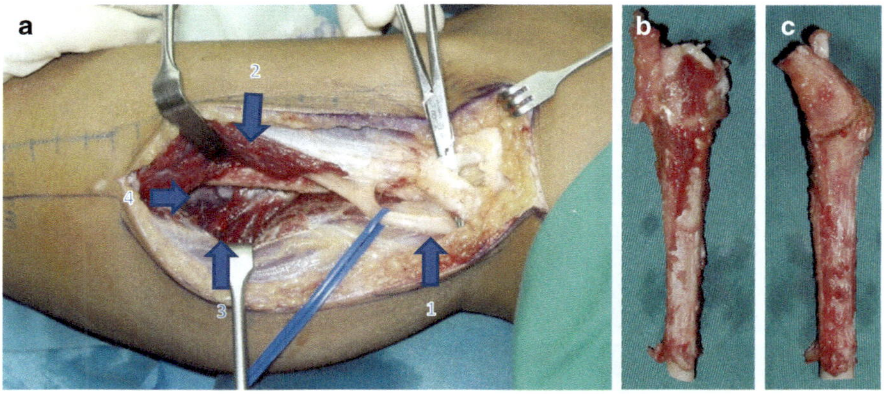

1. Peroneal nerve
2. Extensor digitorum longus
3. Peroneal longus
4. Peroneal vessels

The proximal fibula is a well-established donor for reconstruction of a distal radius tumour. A biceps femoris tendon is required and the lateral collateral ligament provides good soft tissue reconstruction for mobile and stable wrist. The peroneal nerve must be protected properly while harvesting the proximal fibula to minimise disability.

Tips and Tricks

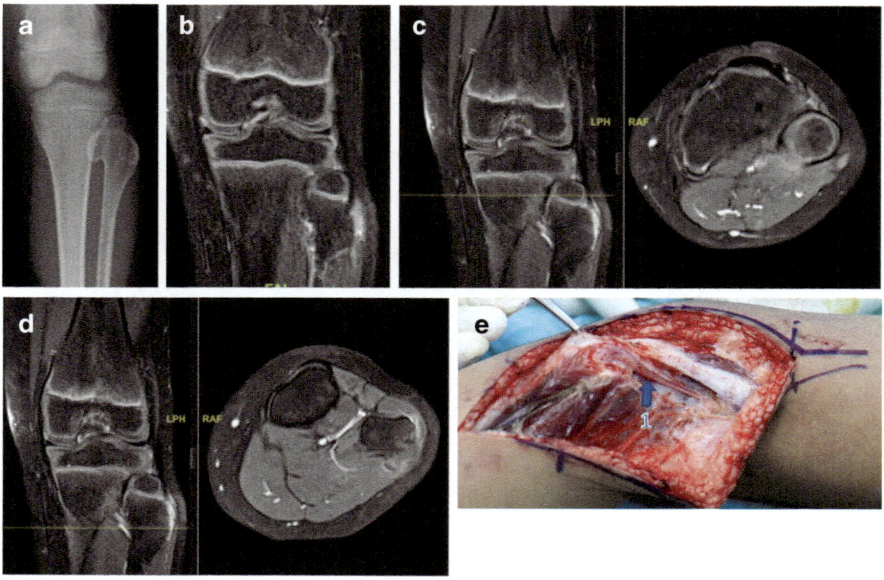

A 6-year-old girl with MHE presented with foot drop secondary to fibula exostosis (Fig. 4a–d). The first step in a surgical approach is to mobilise the peroneal nerve from the fibula neck. The proximal part is mobilised to minimise tension injury when resecting the fibula (Fig. 4e).

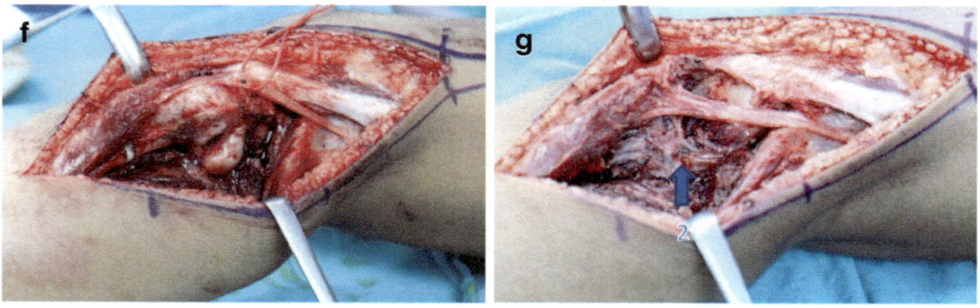

1. Compressed peroneal nerve
2. Tibia-peroneal trunk vessels

The anterior tibial vessel crosses the proximal part of the fibula and is closely attached. Careful mobilisation of the fibula is important during resection to minimise injury (Fig. 4f, g).

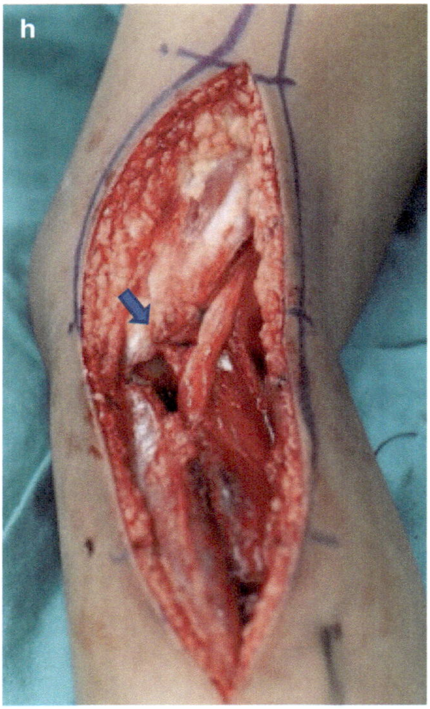

The biceps femoris tendon and lateral collateral ligament were sutured together with the peroneus longus origin and anchor sutured to the tibial condyle for lateral stability (Fig. 4h).

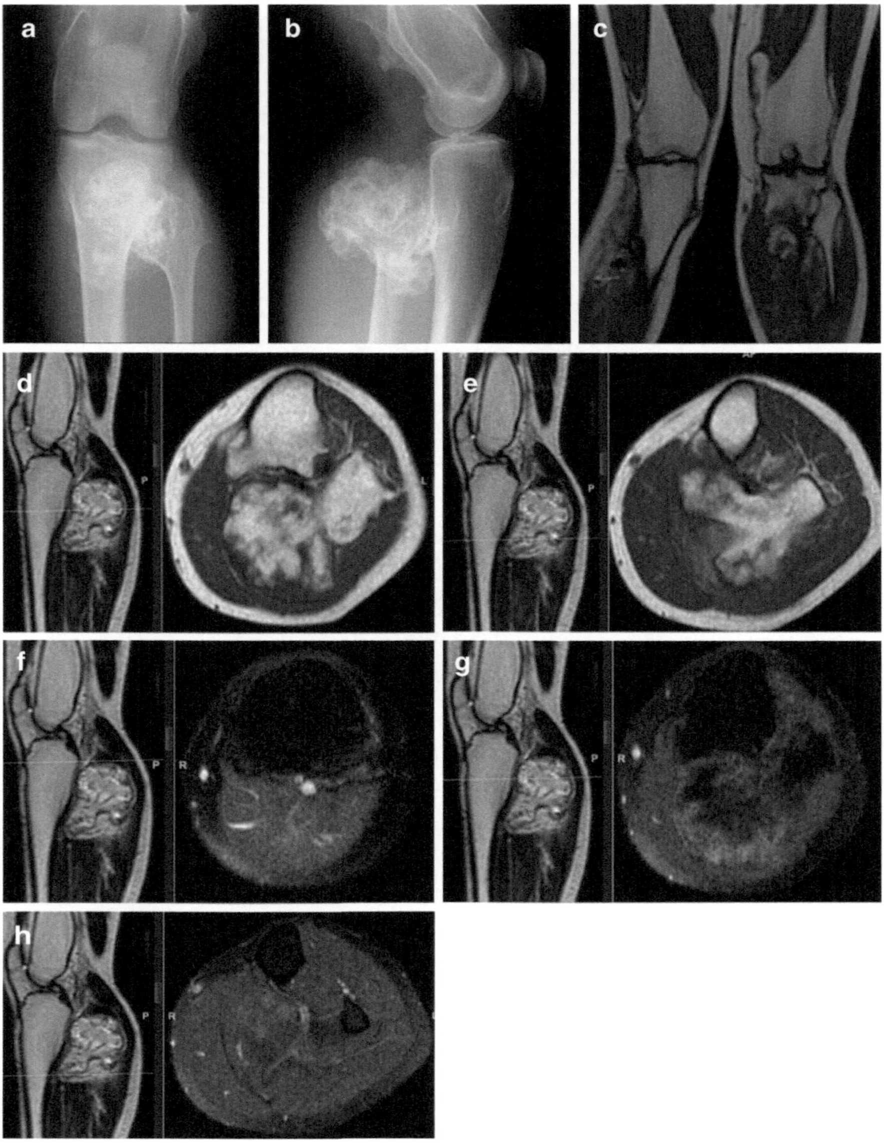

A larger exostosis displaced the popliteal vessels. The main trifurcation and posterior tibial vessels were attached to the fibula due to the proximal nature of the lesion (Fig. 5a–h).

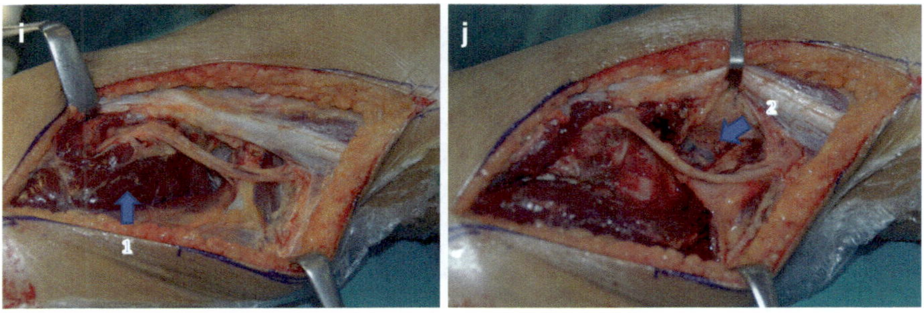

Resection of the fibula exostosis starts with exploration of the common peroneal nerve below the biceps femoris tendon. The proximal fibula exostoses is mobilised after distal osteotomy and the common peroneal nerve is reflected anteriorly to minimise nerve tension. Marginal resection of the benign mass is achieved, and all the muscles are maintained (Fig. 5l, l).

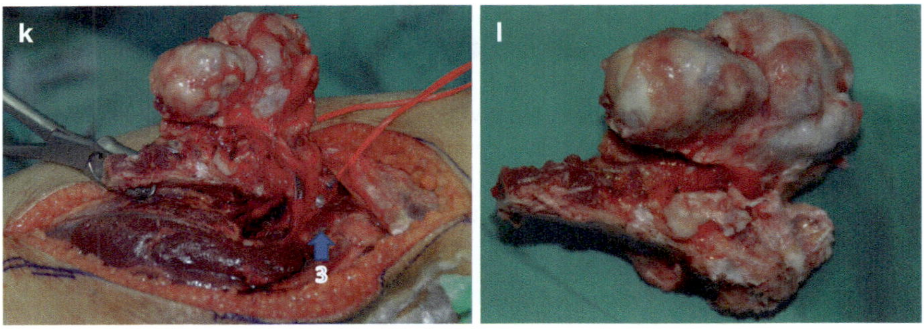

1. Soleus muscle
2. Popliteal vessels
3. Trifurcation trapped within the lobulated mass—mobilisation to clear anterior tibial vessels

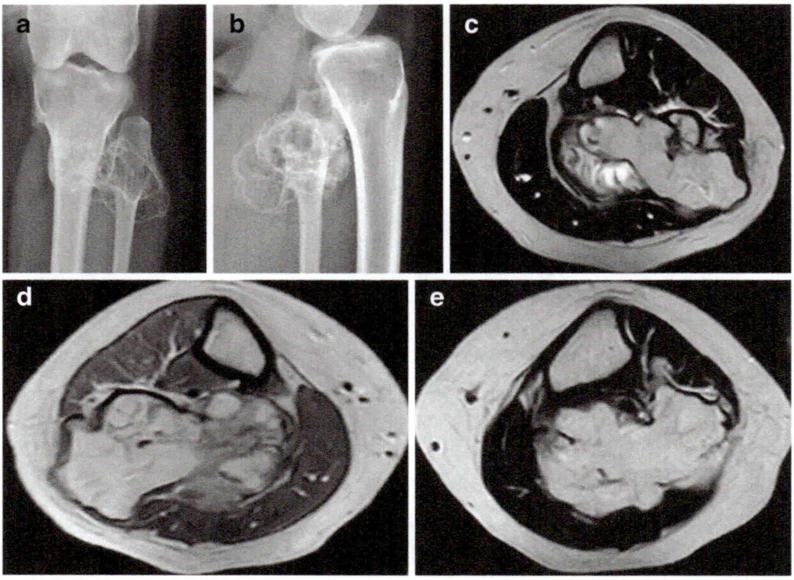

This shows a larger fibula exostoses with posterior projection compressing on the posterior tibial artery and nerve. The neurovascular structure is closely attached to the tumour and at risk during removal (Fig. 6a–e). The peroneal compartment and soleus attachment over the fibula are detached to free the vessels posteriorly prior to final resection to minimise injury to the vessels (Fig. 6f–h).

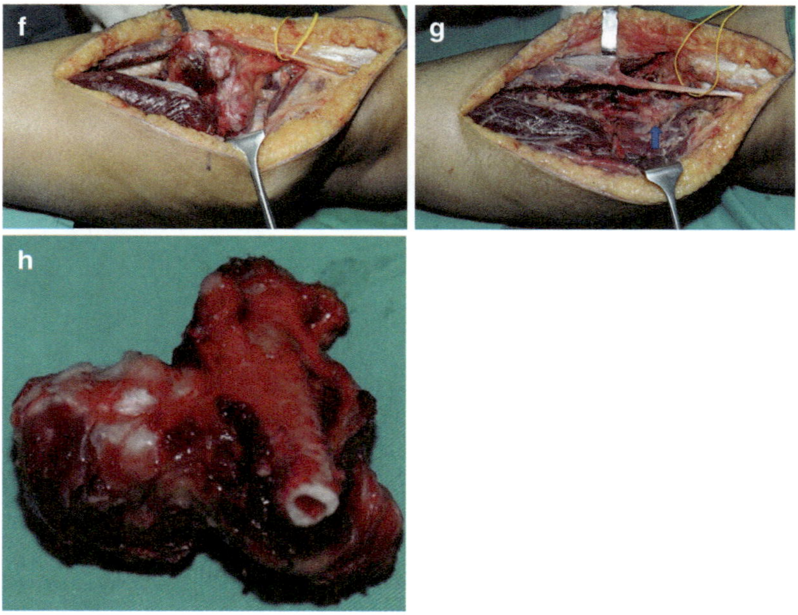

- Popliteal vessels and trifurcation branch: tibia-peroneal trunk and anterior tibia

Type II Fibula Resection

The procedure involved a wide intra-compartmental resection of the proximal fibula with 3 cm marrow margin, including the following:

- The anterior and lateral muscle compartments
- The peroneal nerve
- The anterior tibial artery
- The proximal tibiofibular joint (intra-/extraarticular)
- Gastrocnemius flap reconstruction

Surgical treatment of benign aggressive tumours is based on their grade, anatomical location, and local recurrence rate. Great care must be taken to avoid inadequate surgical margins while also trying to preserve the peroneal nerve and other important anatomical structures.

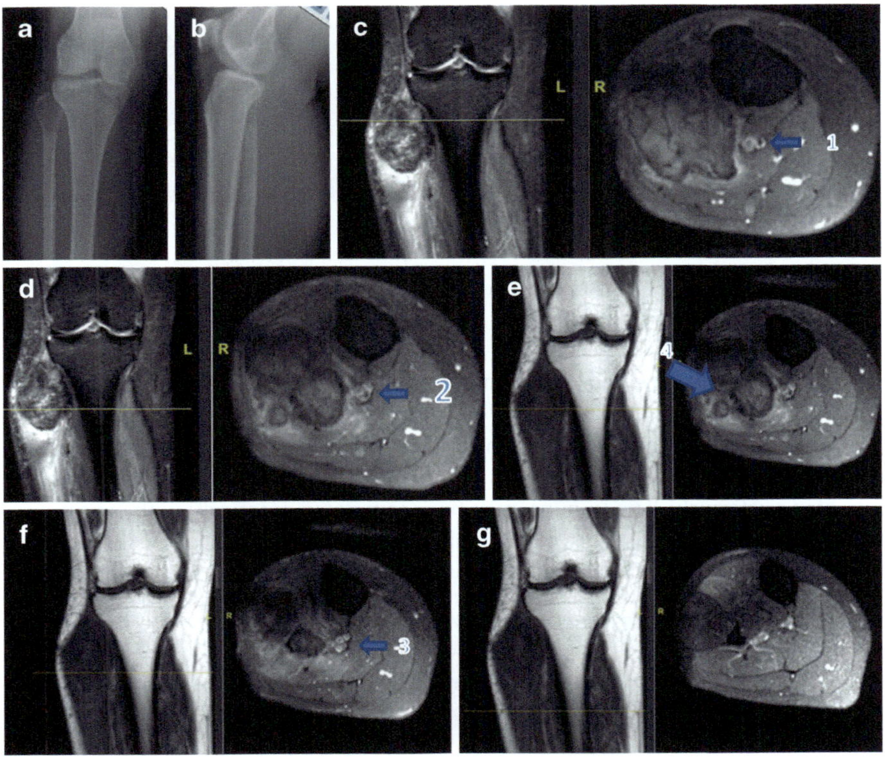

Giant cell tumour of the proximal fibula with extraosseous extension requires a wide margin with a cuff of normal soft tissue. The peroneal nerve is maintained if the motor unit to the anterior compartment muscle is preserved. The MRI revealed that the posterior tibial neurovascular structure was in close proximity to the tumour and must be explored and protected prior to resection (Fig. 7a–g).

1. Popliteal vessels
2. Knee trifurcation vessels
3. Peroneal vessels
4. Extensor digitorum longus, tibialis anterior, peroneus longus, and soleus muscle

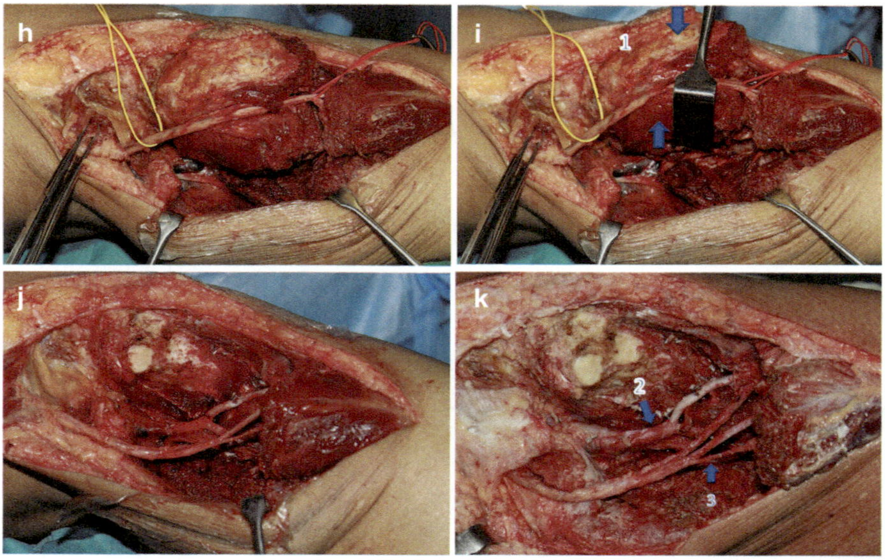

1. Soft tissue margin: extensor digitorum longus, peroneus longus, and tibialis anterior
2. Popliteal vessels branch: anterior tibial, tibia-peroneal trunk, and posterior tibial vessels
3. Peroneal nerve branch: to tibialis anterior, peroneal muscle, and superficial sensory

The peroneal nerve is reflected posteriorly with the anterior compartment muscle. To minimise tension to the motor unit, the muscle is detached from the tibia and retracted posteriorly. The tumour must be manipulated anteriorly with care to protect the anterior tibial vessels from trifurcation. The motor branch of the peroneal nerve is maintained to the anterior tibial muscle (Fig. 7h–k).

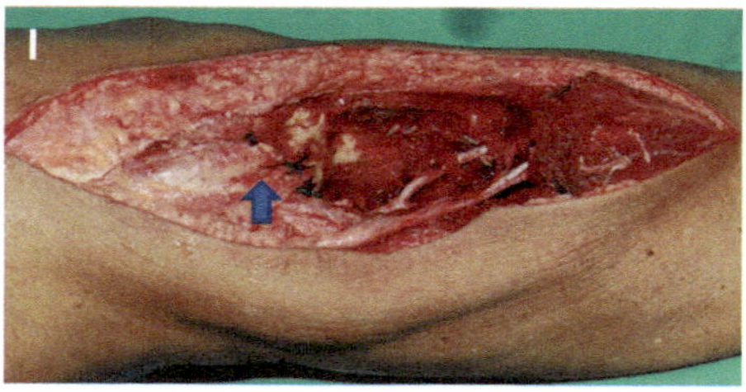

Remnants of the lateral collateral ligament and biceps femoris tendon are attached to the lateral tibia and Gerdy's tubercle to improve lateral stability (Fig. 7l).

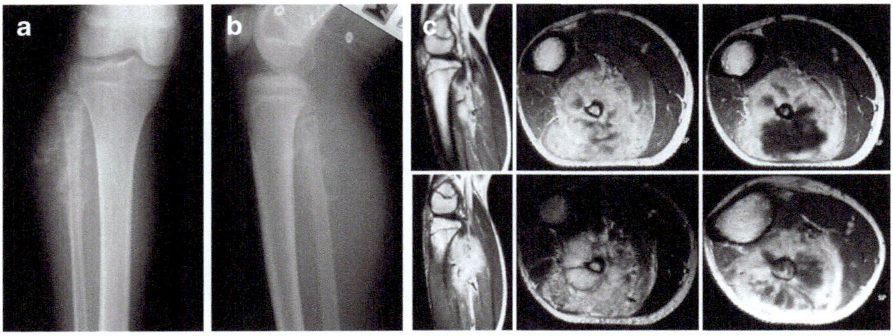

Osteosarcoma of the proximal fibula needs a wide margin for surgical resection (Fig. 8a–c). The anterior and peroneal compartments with part of the soleus must be resected. The lateral gastrocnemius muscle can be detached for wider exposure of the popliteal vessels. The soleus muscle is released with good margin for final exploration (Fig. 8d–f).

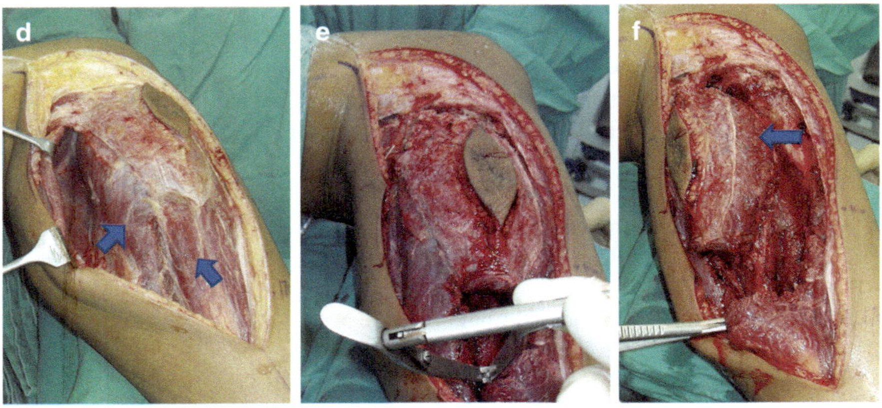

Proximal fibula with extensive tissue extension was in close proximity to proximal tibia fibula joint and removed together with the lateral tibial cortex. The posterior neurovascular structures were in close proximity to the mass; however, they were circumferentially free. The anterior compartment, lateral compartment, and part of the soleus were removed in total with the tumour (Fig. 8g–i).

- Surgical margin—soleus, peroneus longus, extensor digitorum longus, and tibialis anterior

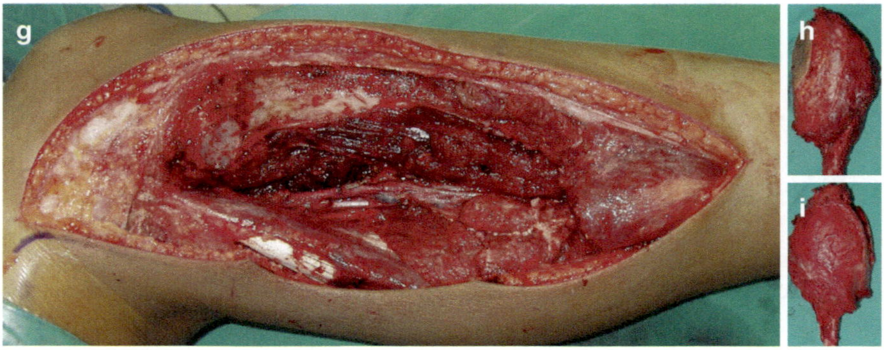

Distal Fibula Resection

Distal fibula excision poses various challenges for reconstruction, as a lateral malleolus resection can lead to lateral instability and valgus deformity of the ankle. The following reconstructive techniques can overcome this problem:

- Ankle arthrodesis
- Proximal fibula graft reconstruction
- Reinforcement of soft tissue reconstruction of the remaining lateral collateral ligament
- Size-matched allograft of distal fibula

A 23-year-old lady with Ewing's sarcoma distal fibula that responded well to chemotherapy (Fig. 9a–d). The tip of the fibula and lateral collateral ligament were not involved and retained for reconstruction. The syndesmotic joint was reconstructed with an autogenous tricortical iliac crest, which was size matched to maintain lateral stability (Fig. 9e–l).

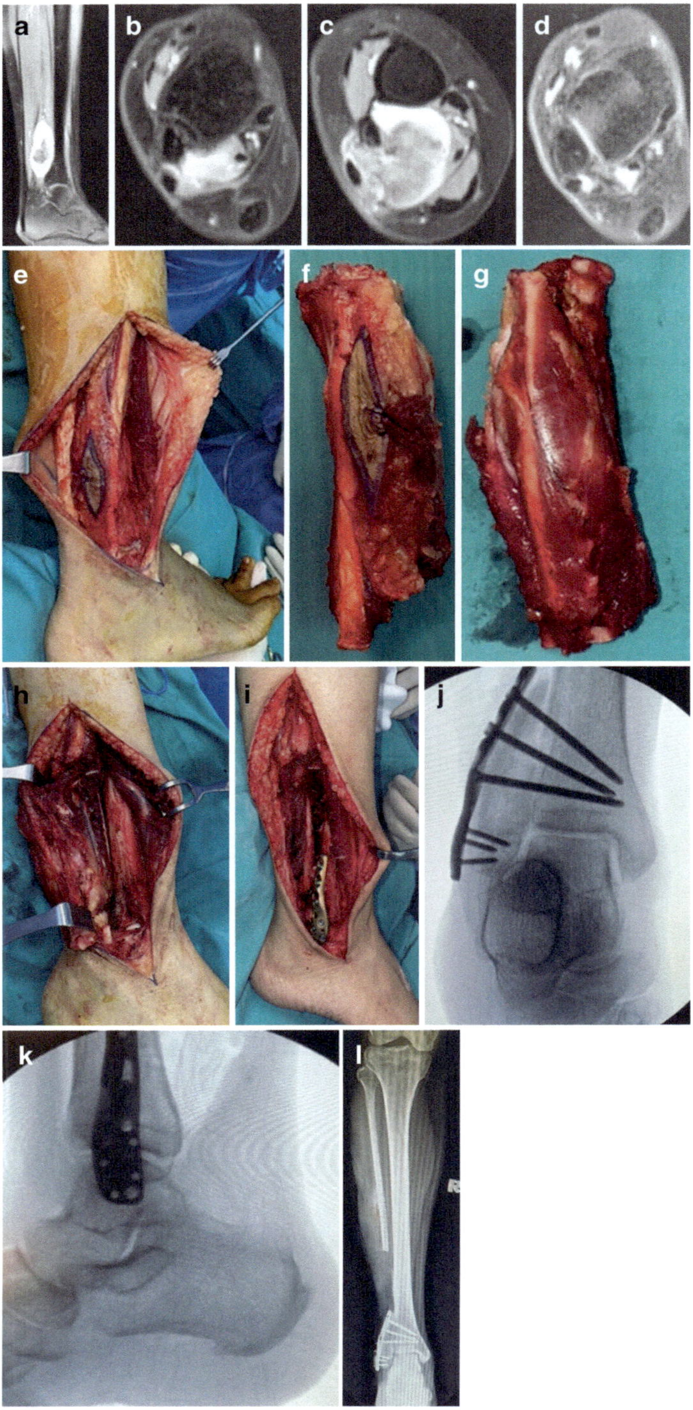
a
b
c
d
e
f
g
h
i
j
k
l

Acknowledgement The author thanks Professor Nor Hazla Muhammad Hafiah, Dr. Mohamed Hafizudin Abdullah Sani, and Dr. Levin Kesu Belani for their contributions and team members for managing the patients in this chapter.

Suggested Reading

1. Abdel MP, Papagelopoulos PJ, Morrey ME, Wenger DE, Rose PS, Sim FH. Surgical management of 121 benign proximal fibula tumors. Clin Orthop Relat Res. 2010;468(11):3056–62.
2. Bickel J, Kollender Y, Pritsch T, Meller I, Malawer MM. Knee stability after resection of the proximal fibula. Clin Orthop Relat Res. 2007;454:198–201.
3. Jamshidi K, Mazhar FN, Masdari Z. Reconstruction of distal fibula with osteoarticular allograft after tumor resection. Foot Ankle Surg. 2013;19:31–5.
4. Malawer MM. Surgical management of aggressive and malignant tumors of the proximal fibula. Clin Orthop Relat Res. 1984;186:172–81.
5. Einoder PA, Choong PFM. Tumors of the head of the fibula. Acta Orthop Scand. 2002;73(6):663–6.
6. Ozaki T, Hillmann A, Lindner N, Winkelmann W. Surgical treatment of bone sarcomas of the fibula analysis of 19 cases. Arch Orthop Trauma Surg. 1997;116:475–9.

Foot Tumour

Wan Faisham Nu'man Bin Wan Ismail

Introduction

The primary goal of surgical treatment for malignant tumours involving the foot is to achieve local control with good oncological margins and maintain a painless, stable foot for ambulation. In the foot, the anatomical boundaries are not well established. In addition, the surgical margin is narrow, and a wider margin is always complicated with poor function and disability. Below-knee amputation is preferred as the surgical option in majority of the cases.

Advances in oncologic treatment modalities and developments in axial imaging techniques have made limb salvage procedures in the ankle and foot increasingly possible. Adjuvant chemotherapy and radiotherapy provide better local control and enable wide resection. Modern reconstruction techniques include free tissue transfer of the bone and soft tissue to provide skeletal and soft tissue reconstruction, minimise wound complication, provide flexibility for rehabilitation and optimise foot function.

Surgical Anatomy

The function of the foot is to support the body weight and enable locomotion. The foot specifically acts as a platform for stance, as a shock absorber for impact during gait, and a lever to propel the body forward during gait. It is important to be maintain basic foot function when considering major oncological resection and advanced reconstruction.

W. F. N. B. W. Ismail (✉)
Prince Court Medical Center, Kuala Lumpur, Malaysia

Orthopaedic Oncology Reconstructive Unit, Universiti Sains Malaysia, Kubang Kerian, Kelantan, Malaysia

A. Puri, W. F. N. B. W. Ismail (eds.), *Atlas of Orthopedic Oncology Volume 2*, https://doi.org/10.1007/978-981-95-8962-3_9

There are nine anatomical compartments of the foot and four plantar layers of the foot. These barriers do not hold true when considering oncological anatomical barrier compartments and detailed imaging evaluation is mandatory for surgical planning.

Compartments of the foot

- Medial: abductor hallucis and flexor hallucis brevis
- Superficial: flexor digitorum longus and flexor digitorum brevis
- Lateral: abductor digiti minimi and flexor digiti minimi brevis
- Adductor: oblique head of the adductor hallucis
- Interossei: compartment includes the dorsal and plantar interosseous muscle
- Calcaneal: quadratus plantae

Plantar layer of the foot

- 1st: abductor hallucis, flexor digitorum brevis, and abductor digiti minimi
- 2nd: quadratus plantae and lumbricals
- 3rd: flexor hallucis brevis, adductor hallucis, and flexor digiti minimi brevis
- 4th: plantar and dorsal interossei

Anatomical Boundaries and Foot Compartmentalisations

The foot has compact structures and lacks true anatomical boundaries. Early tumour extension outside the compartment leads to involvement of the adjacent bone and soft tissues. There is no true compartmentalisation for wide surgical margin.

- Metatarsal and its surrounding interosseous muscle provide a good cuff of soft tissue for oncological margins in metatarsal resection and rays amputation.
- Fascial planes superficial to the metatarsal and tarsal structures, between the layers of the foot, lack sufficient integrity to resist tumour extension. Once this anatomic plane is contaminated, the entire compartment must be considered involved.
- Tendon sheaths of the extrinsic foot muscles:- posterior tibial, peroneal, and anterior compartment tendons, extend and cross the joint and should be evaluated for tumour contamination.

Foot Neurovascular Surgical Anatomy

The medial and lateral plantar arteries supply the toes through the deep plantar arch. The medial plantar artery supplies part of the hallux (big toe), and the lateral plantar artery supplies the vast majority of the foot.

The plantar arch is circulatory an anastomostic arc by deep arch plantar branch of the dorsalis pedis artery. The lateral plantar artery runs from the 5th metatarsal and extends medially to the 1st metatarsal. The dorsal metatarsal artery from the plantar arch supplies the artery to the toes. Resection of two middle metatarsals with interossei muscle poses a risk and impairs the blood supply to the toe.

The foot is innervated by five main nerves: superficial peroneal, deep peroneal, tibial, sural, and saphenous nerves. The main nerve supply for plantar sensation is the medial plantar nerve, a branch of the posterior tibial nerve. It supplies sensation to the great toe, second, third, and medial side of the fourth toe.

Understanding the arch of the foot is important for reconstruction following major foot resection. Foot arches and their flexibility facilitate weight bearing and locomotor functions.

- Medial arch is formed by the calcaneus, talus, navicular, three cuneiforms, and first, second, and third metatarsals. It plays a critical role in shock absorption and propulsion while walking.
- Lateral arch is formed by the calcaneus, cuboid, and fourth and fifth metatarsals. It is the flatter of the two longitudinal arches and lies flat on the ground in the standing position The talocalcaneal articulation and calcaneocuboid articulation have special mechanism for locking, and allow only limited movement while walking
- Transverse arch is formed by the bases of the five metatarsal heads, three cuneiforms, and cuboid in the coronal plane. The dome-shaped transverse arch is elevated medially across the tarsal bones at the tarsometatarsal joints.

Surgical Steps

The principle of surgical treatment for foot sarcomas is to achieve oncological clearance with painless preservation of ambulation. This strategy may include radiotherapy or chemotherapy on an adjuvant or neoadjuvant basis. The decision to opt for limb-sparing surgery or amputation is based on many factors, which include the compartment involved and ability to obtain R0 resection with anticipated functional outcome. Marginal resection is not suitable due to high local recurrence.

We have highlighted few cases of foot sarcoma and discussed the surgical steps of resection and reconstruction.

Aggressive Sarcoma of Dorsum Foot and Interossei Muscle

A 24-year-old lady presented with slow growing mass on the dorsum of the foot with discomfort and difficulty in wearing shoes. The lesion occupied the dorsal medial part of the foot with extension to the 1st and 2nd interossei muscle. An MRI revealed the interosseous ligament of the tarsus showed infiltrative signal intensity suggestive of involvement. There was no bony erosion on the radiograph and MRI (Fig. 1a–e).

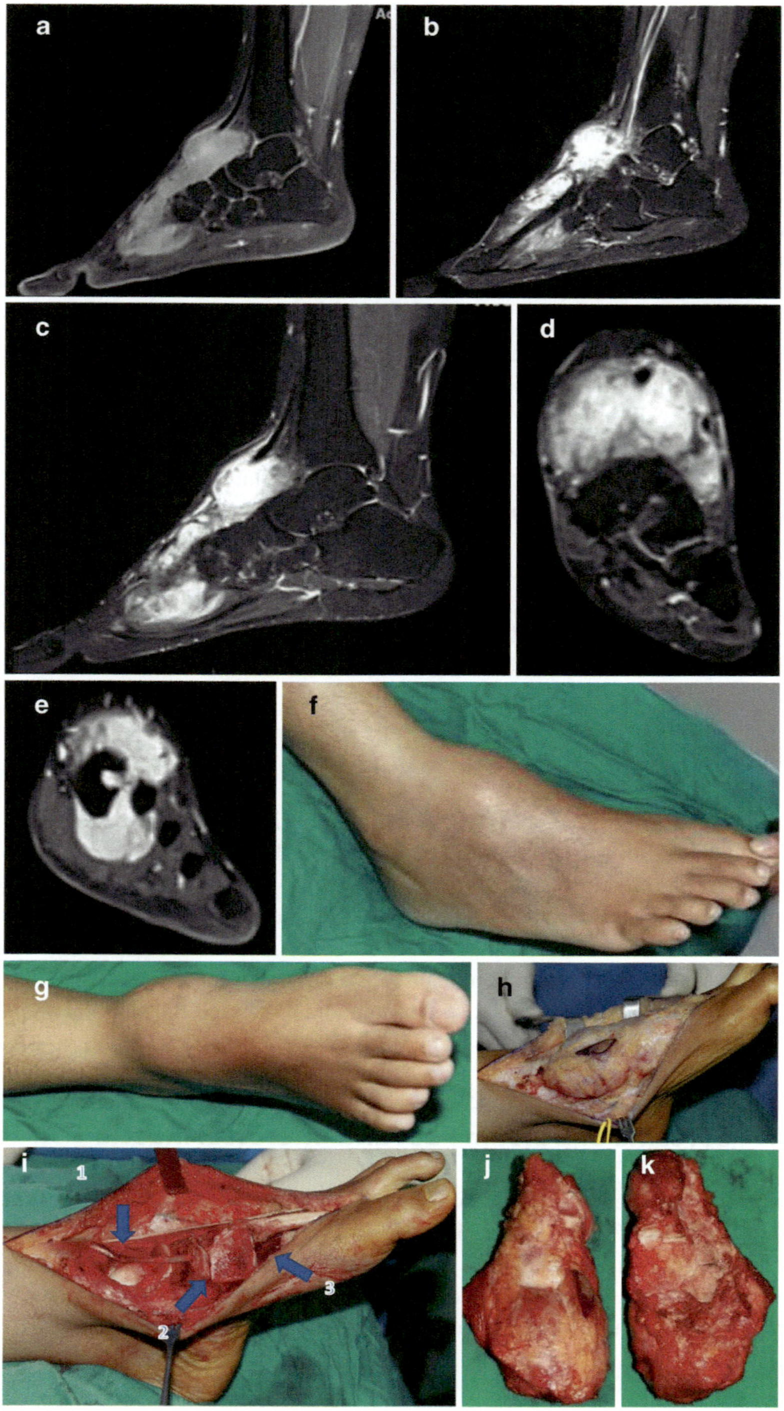
a
b
c
d
e
f
g
h
i
1
2
3
j
k

1. Extensor hallucis longus and tibialis anterior removed as margin
2. Talar head, navicular and medial cuneiform were shaved for margin
3. 1st metatarsal partially removed as margin with both the medial interossei muscles

The entire proximal part of 1st and partial 2nd metatarsals together with partial medial tarsal bone was removed for quality margins (Fig. 1f–k). Stability of the medial arch was provided by tricortical iliac graft for 1st metatarsal, and the entire construct was maintained with a reconstruction plate. The surgical bed was subjected for 60Gy radiotherapy for better local control (Fig. 1l–o).

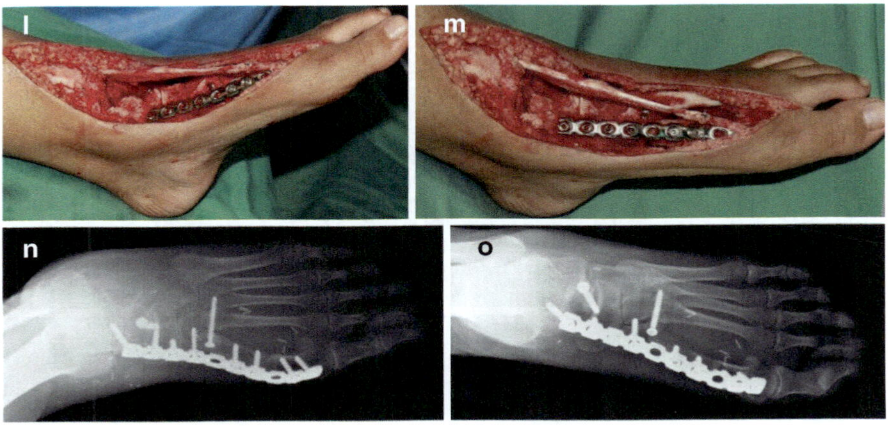

Midfoot Giant Cell Tumour—Bony Resection and Simple Bony Reconstruction

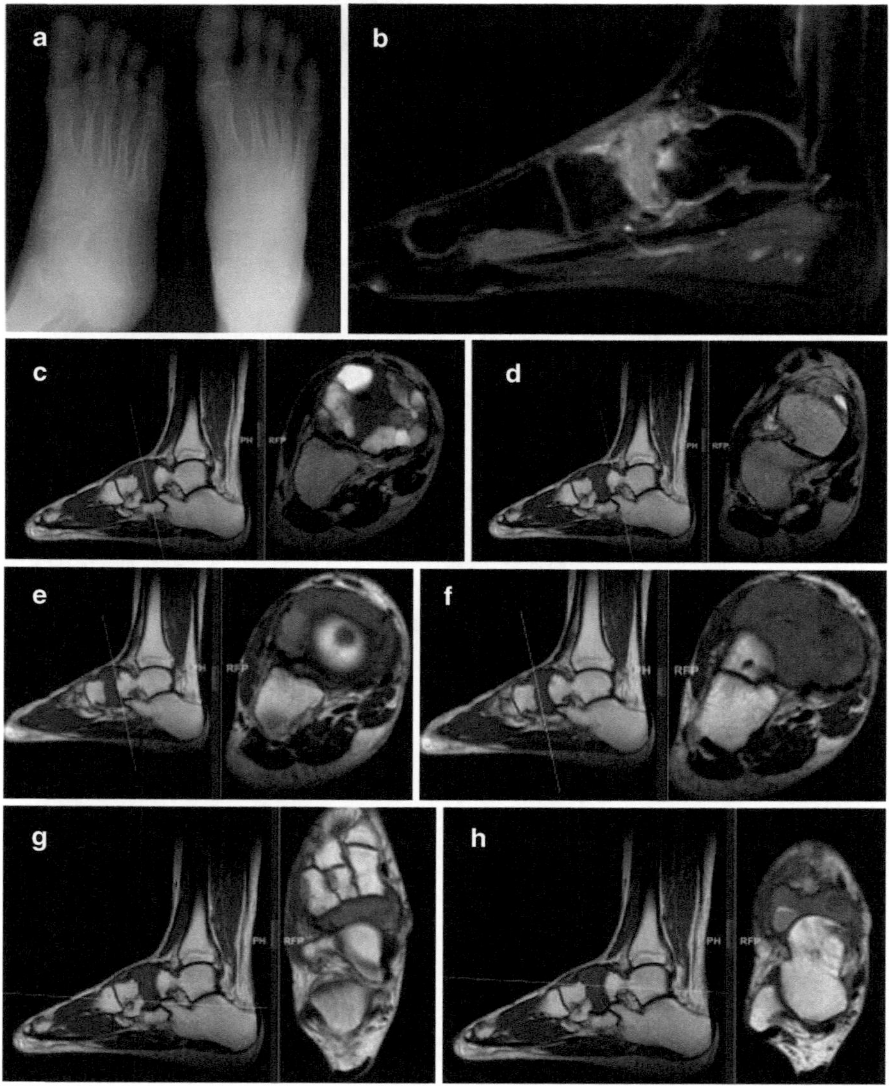

This is a case of giant cell tumour of the navicular with infiltration to cuneiform articulation (Fig. 2a–h). Shot segment bony resection with intact soft tissue was reconstructed with structural non-vascularised iliac crest graft.

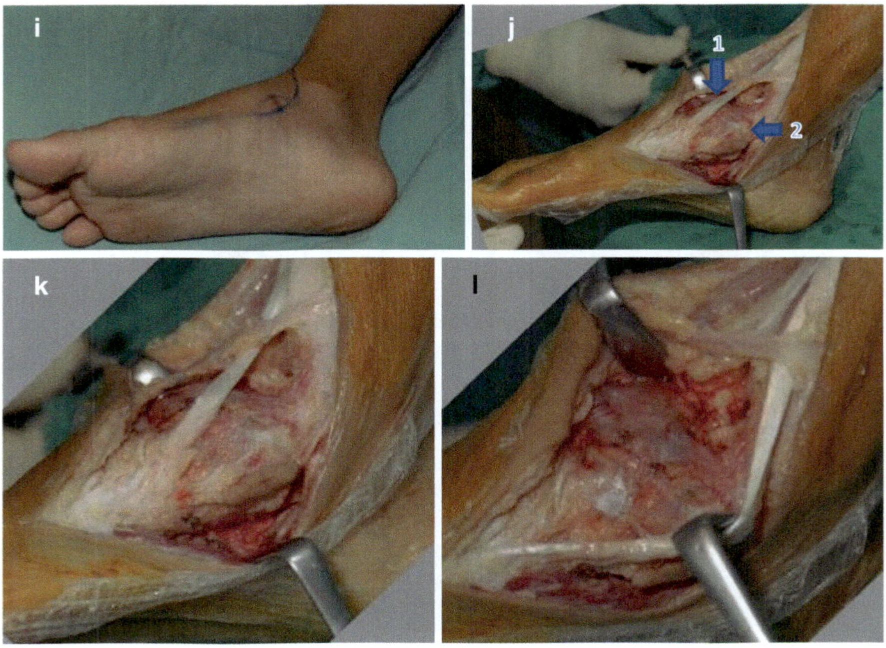

1. Tibialis anterior tendon
2. Talonavicular joint

Medial exploration was performed by mobilisation of the abductor hallucis muscle, and all the plantar tendons from the navicular. A complete resection of the navicular was carried out, including parts of the cuneiform and intraarticular talonavicular joint as part of the margin. The talonavicular joint was free from tumour extension, and evaluation of the joint was required for erosion of the talus cartilage. The plantar margin of the navicular and cuneiform was protected by malleable retractor prior to osteotomy with saw and osteotomes and intraarticular resection (Fig. 2i–p).

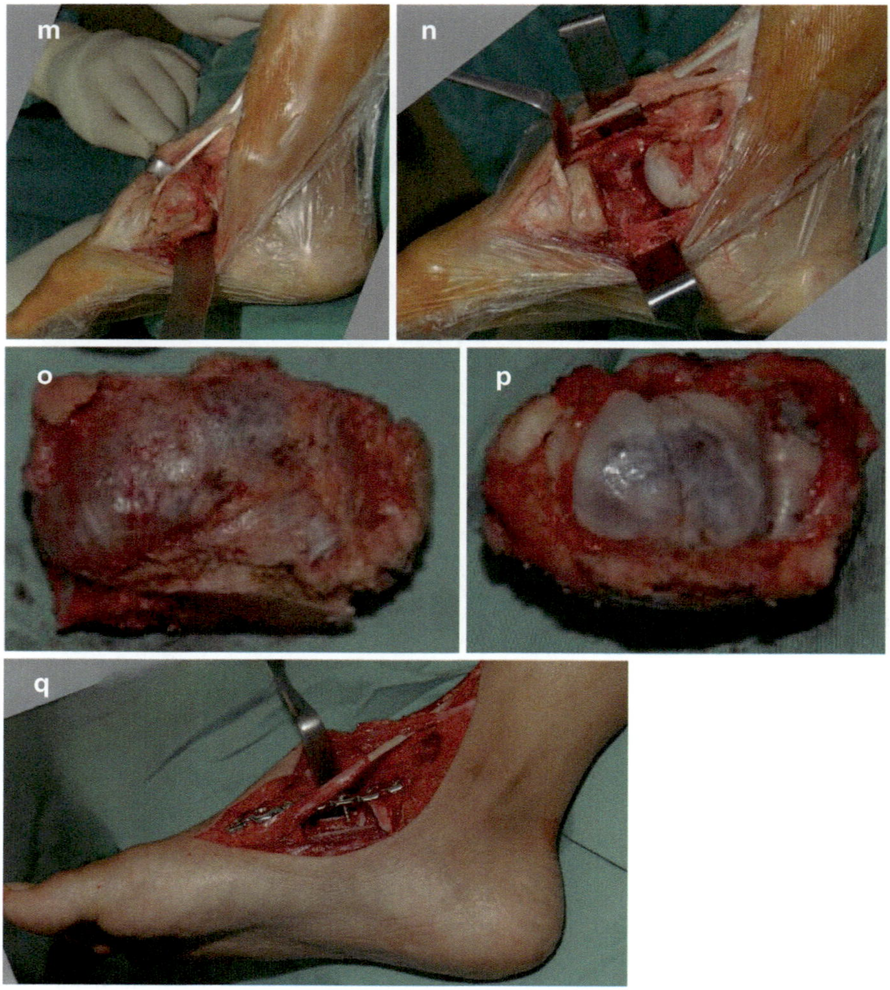

The segment defect was reconstructed with tricortical bone graft. Solid integration was observed and sustained even 10 years after surgery (Fig. 2q–w).

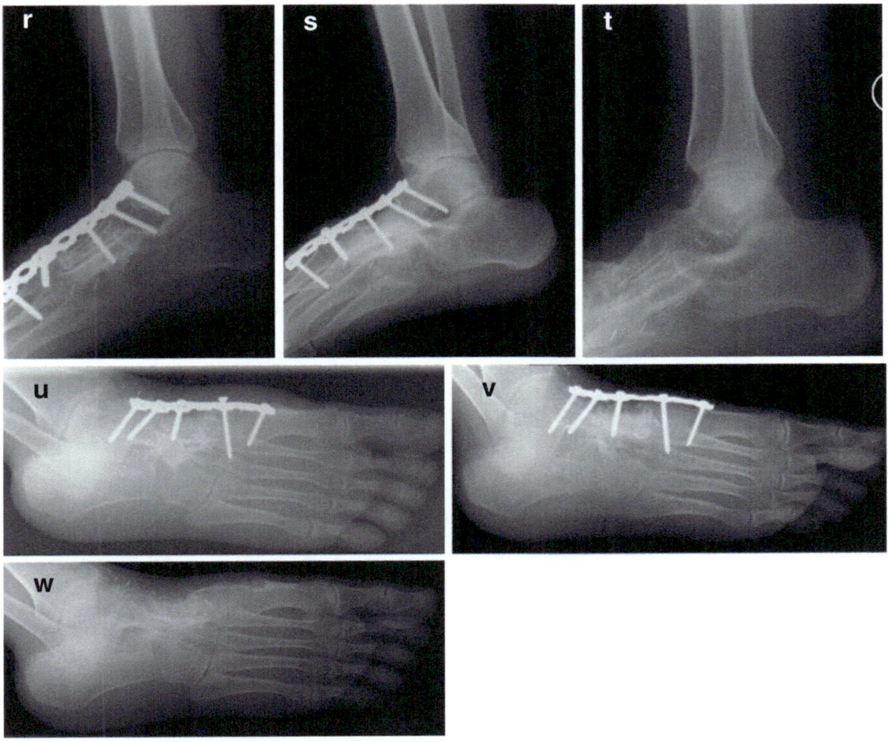

Soft Tissue Sarcoma with Bony Resection and Flap

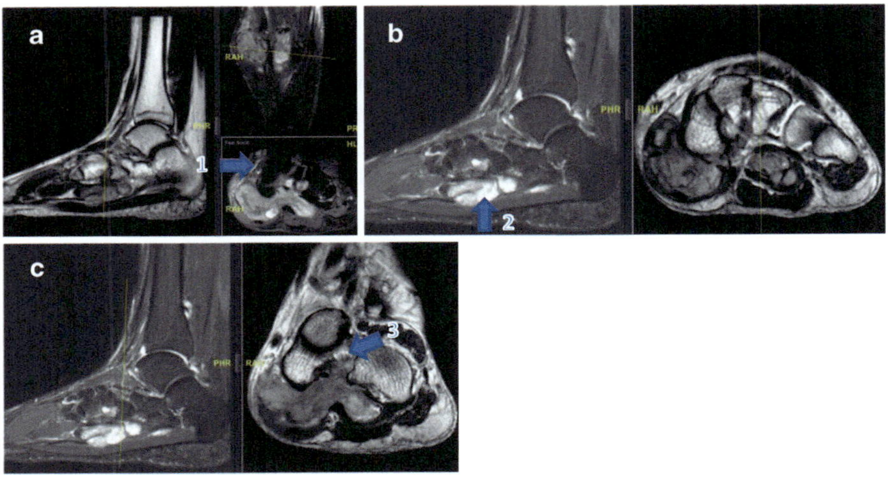

1. Medial cuneiform
2. Adductor hallucis muscle
3. Navicular bone

A 35-year-old gentleman presented with low-grade fibromyxoid sarcoma involving the adductor hallucis muscle and medial compartment of the foot. The tumour infiltrated the plantar surface of the bone and joint of the navicular, medial to lateral cuneiform and occupied the 3rd layer of the foot within the flexor tendon. The attachment of the tibialis posterior and plantar interosseus ligament was also involved. The medial skin was thin and included as resection margin (Fig. 3a–f).

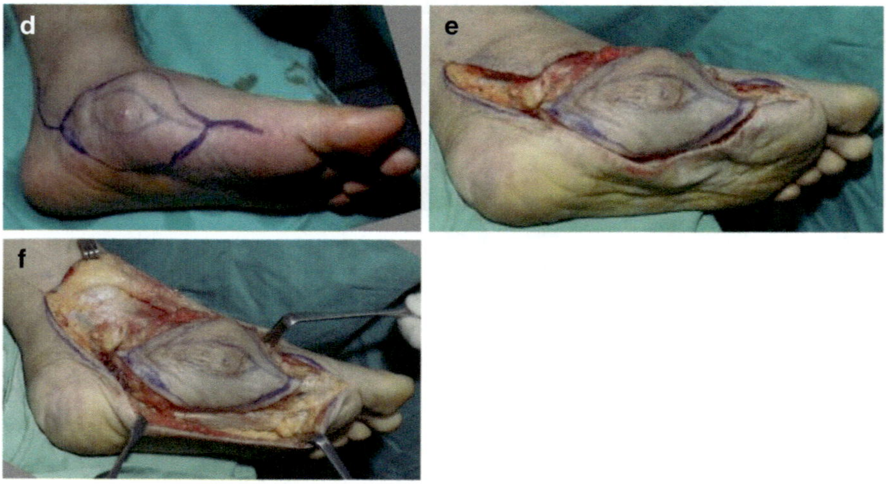

The medial arch of the foot was exposed. A plantar flap was created to identify the plantar aponeurosis to expose the 2nd and 3rd layer of the foot. The adductor hallucis muscle and its origin were included as margin. The plantar surface of the half of the talus, navicular, medial, middle, and lateral cuneiform were osteotomised and included as bony margin to achieve oncological clearance. The flexors of the hallucis longus and digitorum were sectioned and included as margin (Fig. 3g–k).

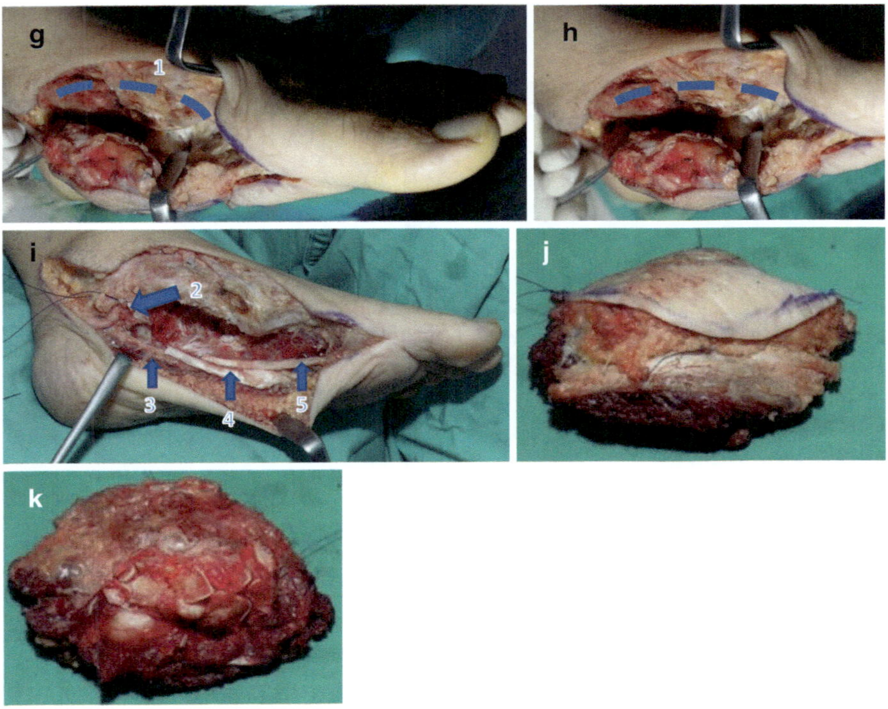

1. Midfoot osteotomy line
2. Posterior tibial nerve and lateral plantar branch
3. Medial plantar branch posterior tibial nerve
4. Flexor hallucis longus tendon
5. Flexor digitorum longus tendon
6. End to side anastomosis of the lateral femoral circumflex to posterior tibial vessels

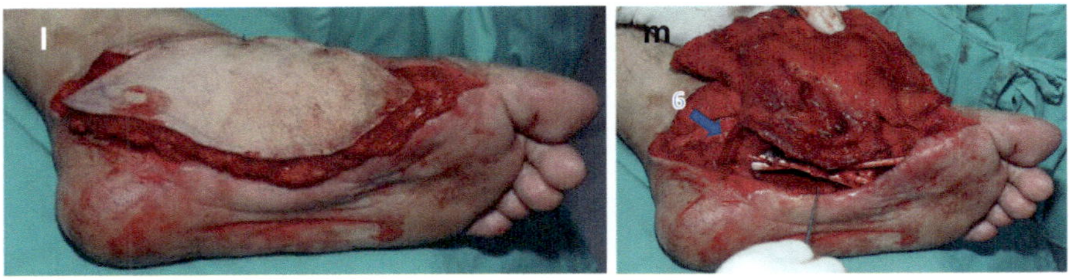

Soft tissue and skin defect were reconstructed with an anterolateral thigh flap. The fascia was used to reinforce the medial structures and remnant of the tendon were grafted for flexion of all toes. He underwent 60Gy of local radiation for local control and 5 years postoperative disease free with no local recurrence (Fig. 3l–o).

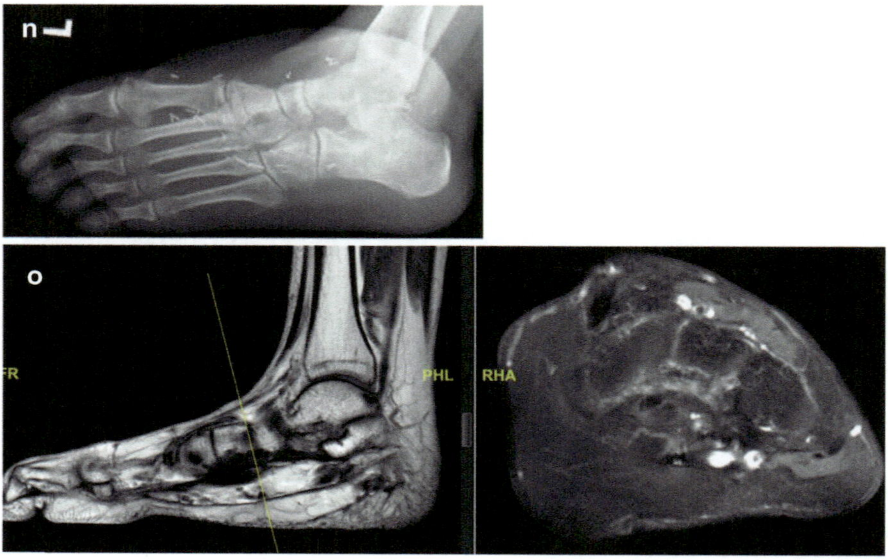

Benign Aggressive Tumour with Metatarsal Resection and Reconstruction

A case of fibromatoses presented with encasement of the entire 1st metatarsal and erosion of the 2nd metatarsal. The medial skin was thin, abductor hallucis and long flexor to big toe were involved and must be included as margin. The tumour was attached to the plantar surface of the 1st to 4th metatarsal and needed to be removed in total (Fig. 4a–g).

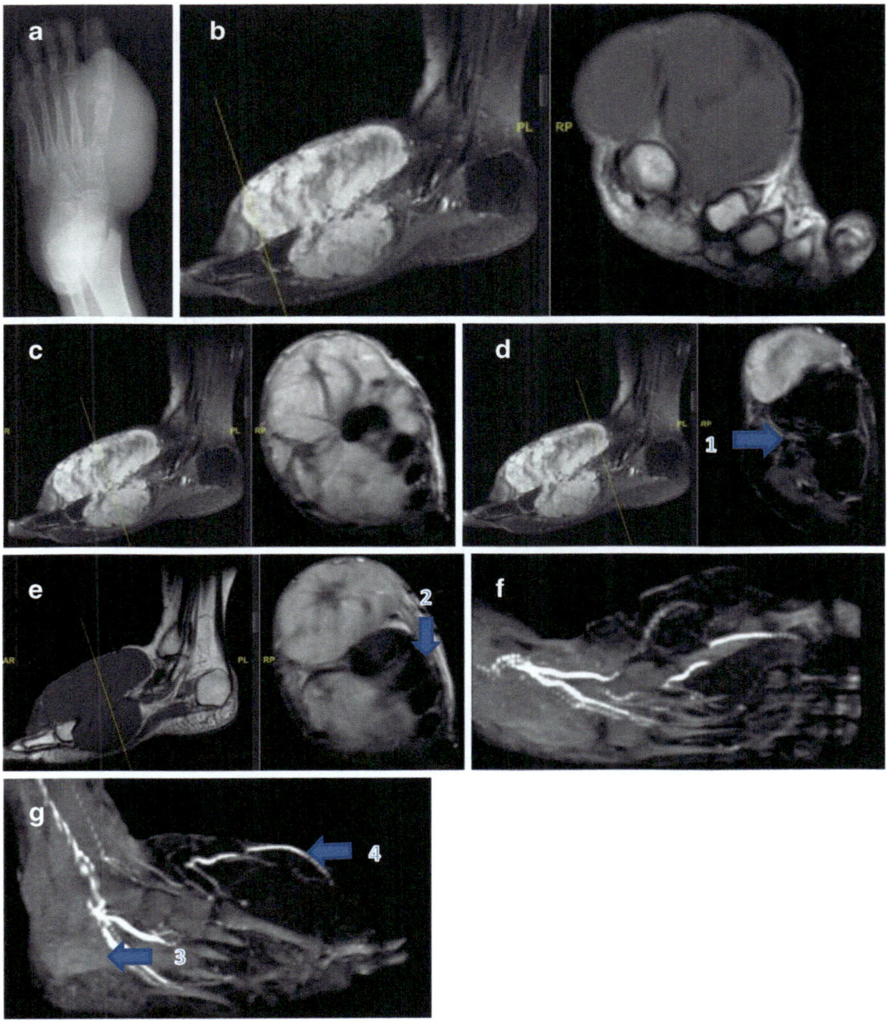

1. Common flexor tendon
2. 1st-3rd metatarsal base
3. Common plantar artery
4. Dorsalis pedis artery pushed by the tumour

The 1st and 2nd interossei muscle and entire abductor hallucis and long segment of the flexor hallucis were included as surgical margin. The second metatarsal bone was elevated at the Lisfranc joint subperiosteally for resection of the 2nd interossei muscle and entire tumour over the plantar layer of the foot (Fig. 4h–o).

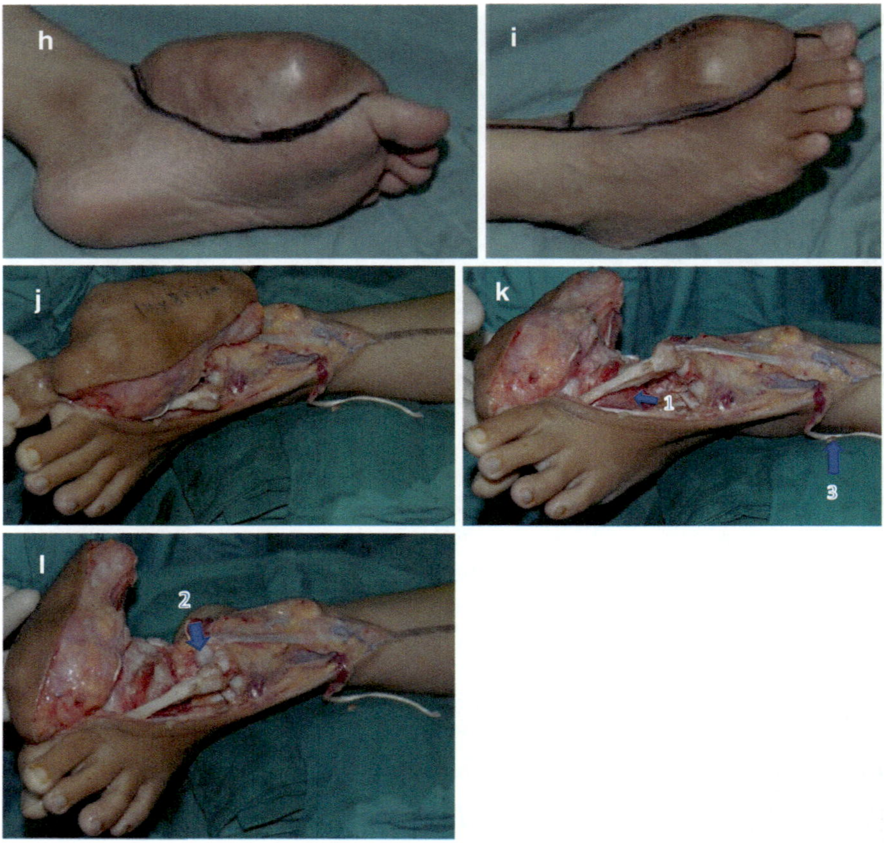

1. Mobilisation of the entire tumour and 1st metatarsal after elevation of the 2nd metatarsal
2. Lisfranc joint
3. Extensor hallucis longus and brevis resect in segment
4. Dorsalis pedis vessels for recipient vascularised for 1st metatarsal reconstruction

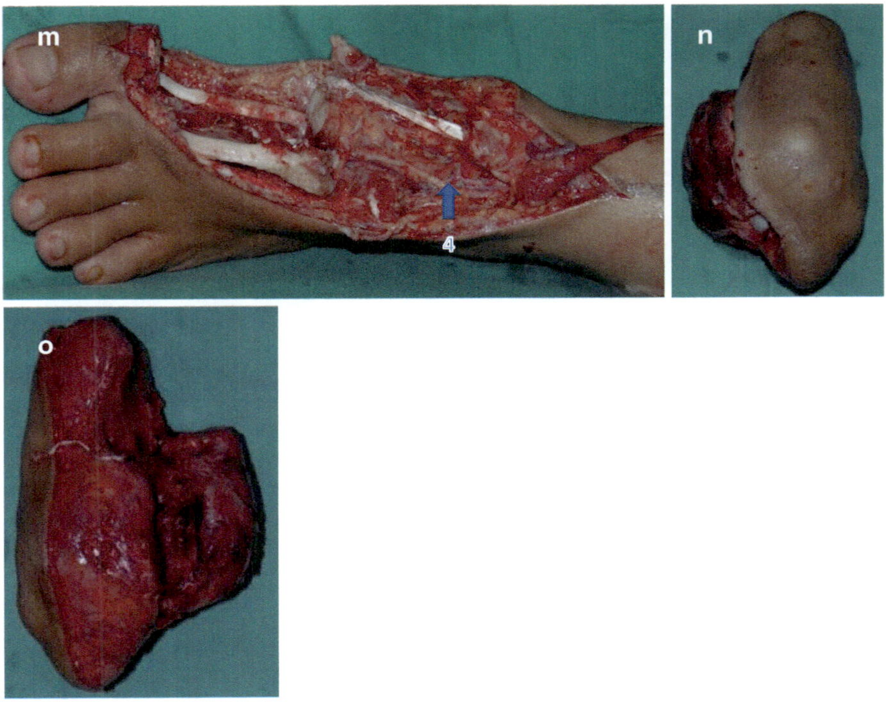

Vascularised osteocutaneous fibula graft for medial arch reconstruction and soft tissue defect coverage allows early ambulation and minimises wound complication and early adjuvant radiotherapy for local control (Fig. 4p–s).

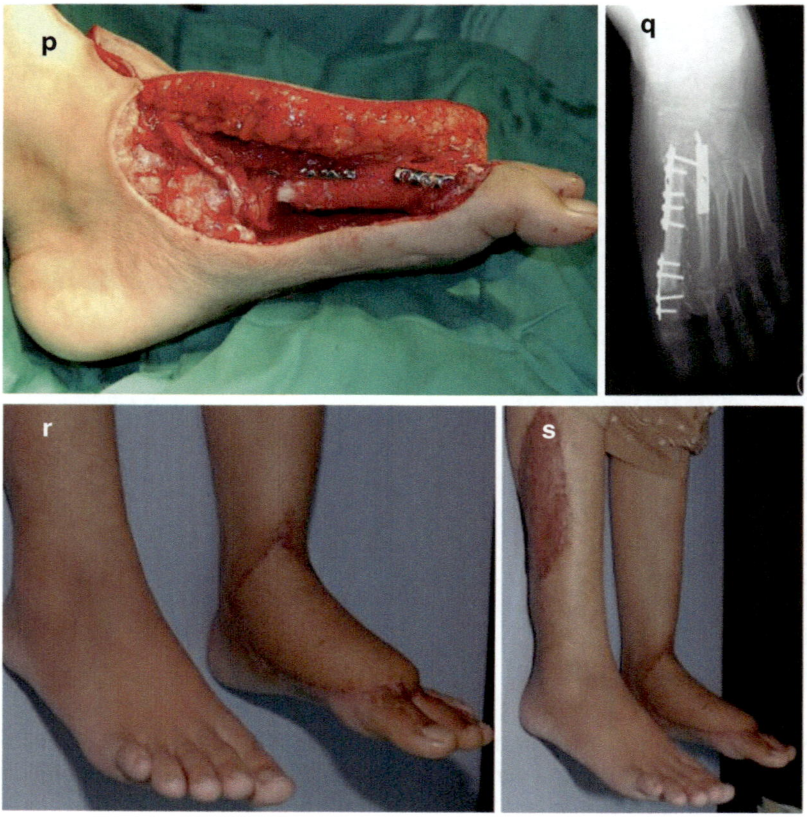

Talus Resection with Triangular Vascularised Fibula Graft Reconstruction

The talus is a complex bone that transmits weight from the body. It articulates with three joints, and it is stabilised mainly by ligaments. There is a close relationship between the talus and posterior tibial neurovascular structures. Preservation of these structures during tumour resection is vital to maintain foot vascularity and protective sensation.

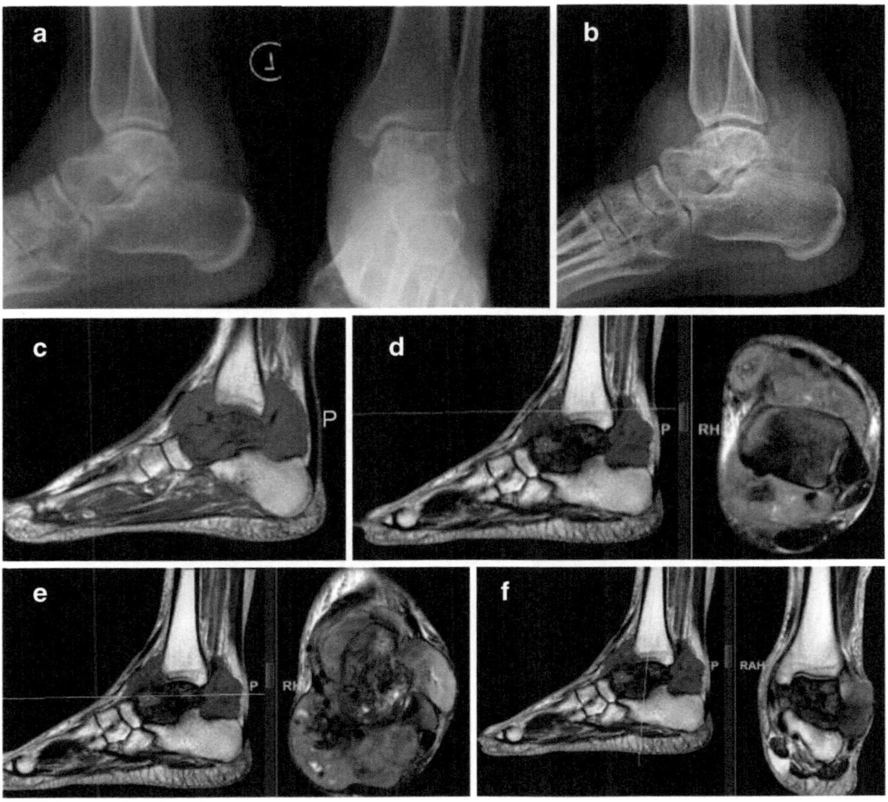

A case of GCT talus presented with extraosseous extension to the soft tissue surrounding the distal tibia, navicular, and calcaneum. The posterior tibial vessels were encased by the tumour and should be included as margin (Fig. 5a–f).

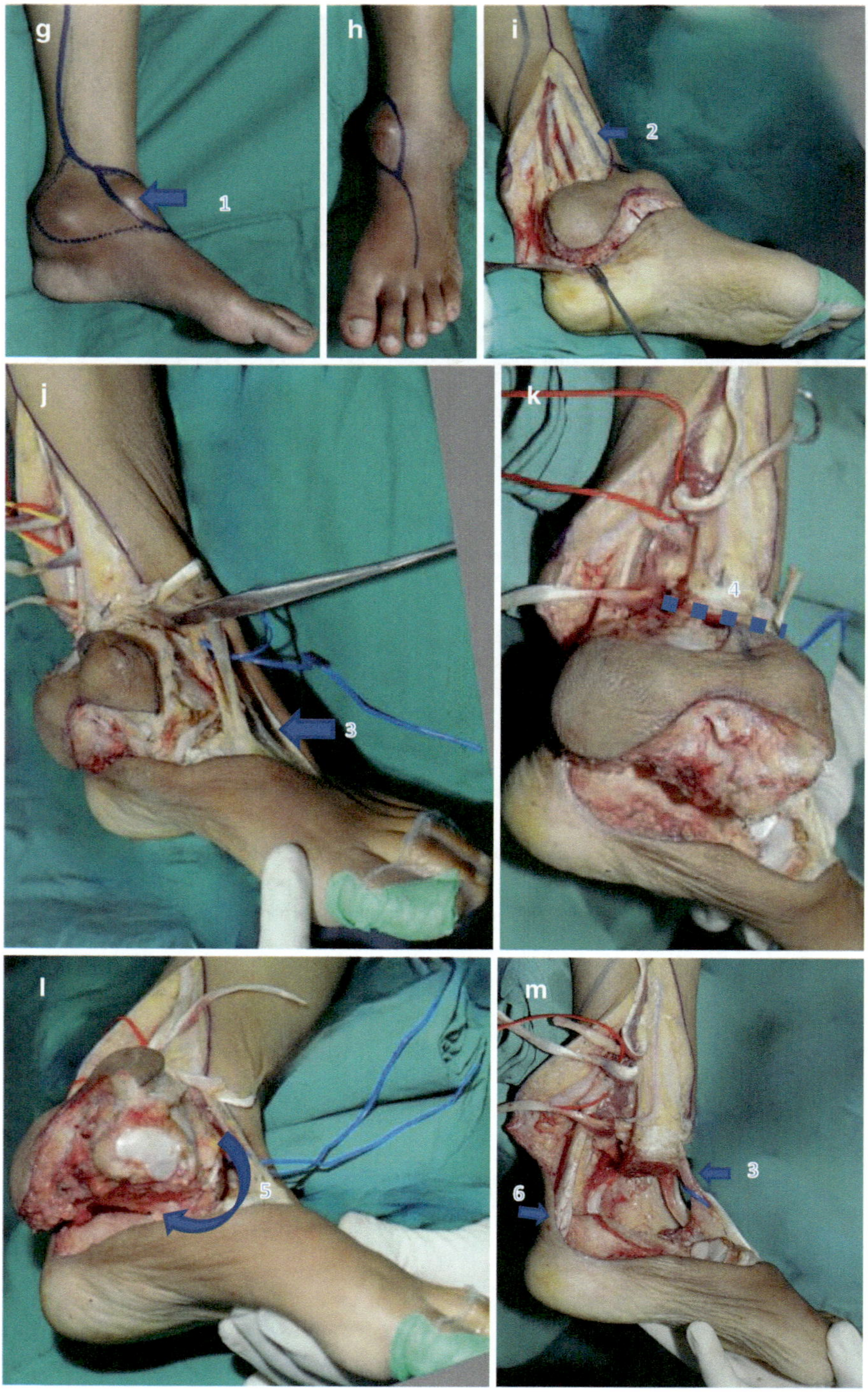
g
1
h
i
2
j
3
k
4
l
5
m
3
6

1. Biopsy scar and skin infiltration remove in total with talus
2. Saphenous vein
3. Tibialis anterior vessels
4. Tibia osteotomy
5. Talus was mobilised from lateral structure after osteotomy tibia, navicular and subtalar joint
6. Achilles tendon

Wide resection of the talus was achieved by resecting beyond the tibiotalar, subtalar, and talonavicular joints, which incorporated the adjacent bones. The extensile anterior skin flap method was utilised, with mobilisation of the anterior and posteromedial neurovascular bundles and tendons prior resection. The Achilles and flexor hallucis tendons, in close vicinity to the talus's posterior facets, were mobilised and protected before the distal tibia and fibula osteotomy at the level of the distal syndesmosis. The osteotomy of the distal tibia-fibula, navicular, and calcaneal bones created a space for free mobilisation of the entire talus. Valgus stress and eversion of the foot at the proximal ankle created a wide window for final detachment of the talus from the surrounding structures laterally (Fig. 5g–m).

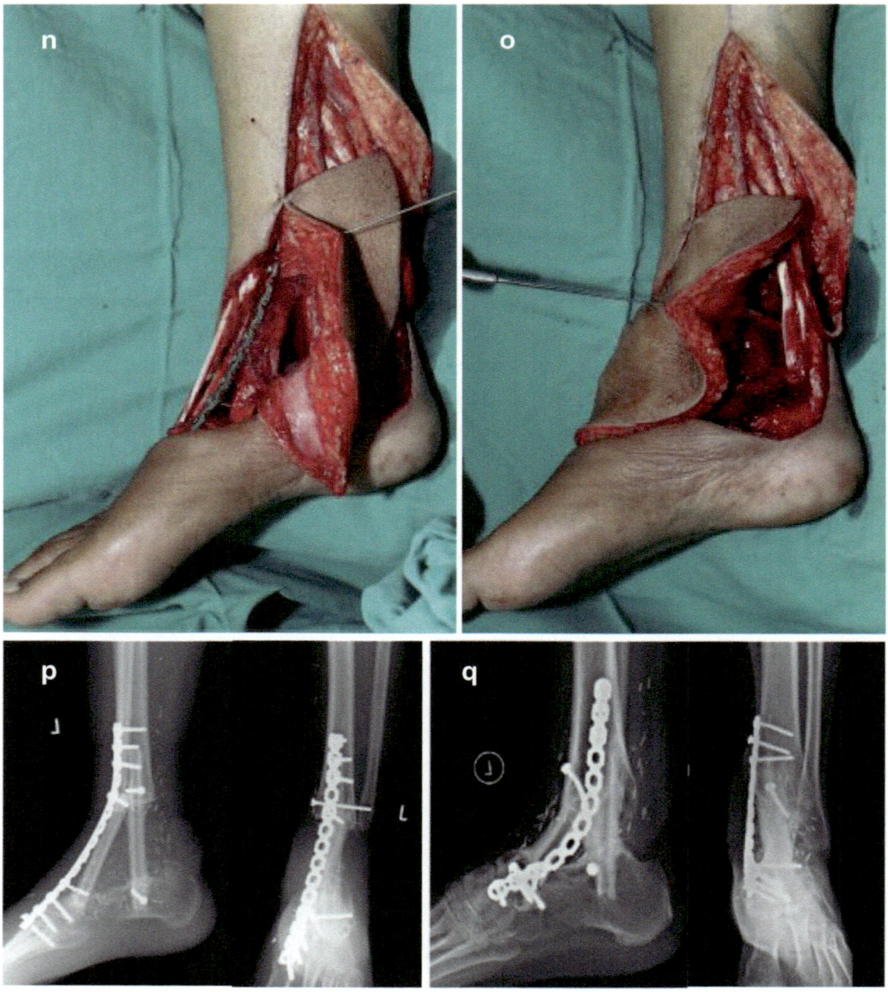

- Fibula hypertrophy is anticipated after 2 years, and solid ankle fusion is anticipated

Reconstruction method utilised two bony struts from the osteotomised fibular bone, or so-called double-barrel fibula, configured in a wide-based triangular framework resembling a stable pyramid. The first strut forming the tibia-calcaneum bridge provides stability, weight loading, and length, while the second strut at the tibia-navicular bridge maintains the hindfoot and midfoot stability and supports the medial arch. The stability of this triangular shape reconstruction also resists angular and rotational stress (Fig. 5n–r).

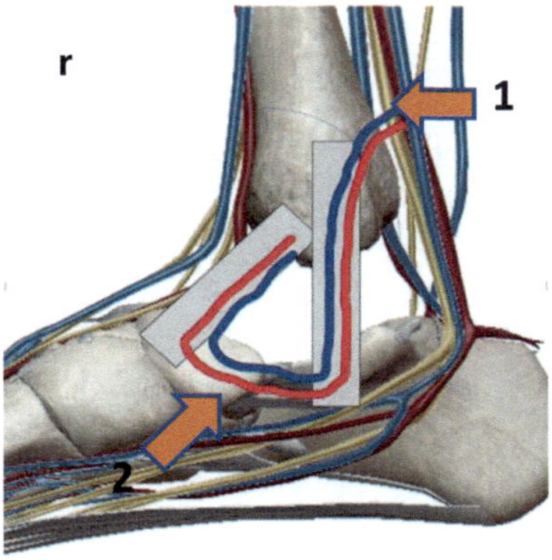

1. End to site anastomosis peroneal to posterior tibial vessels
2. Fibula osteotomy and mobilisation of peroneal artery to prevent kinking of vessels

Calcaneal Resection with DCIA Reconstruction

The calcaneum is an extremely rare location for primary malignancy. Wide oncological margin is difficult, as there are no true anatomical boundaries, and the hind foot compartment is narrow and tight. Below-knee amputation is an option in majority of cases, especially when the heel pad is involved. Surgery is limited to symptomatic aggressive benign bone tumour or low-grade malignancy when the tumour is confined to the intraosseous part or there is minimal extraosseous involvement.

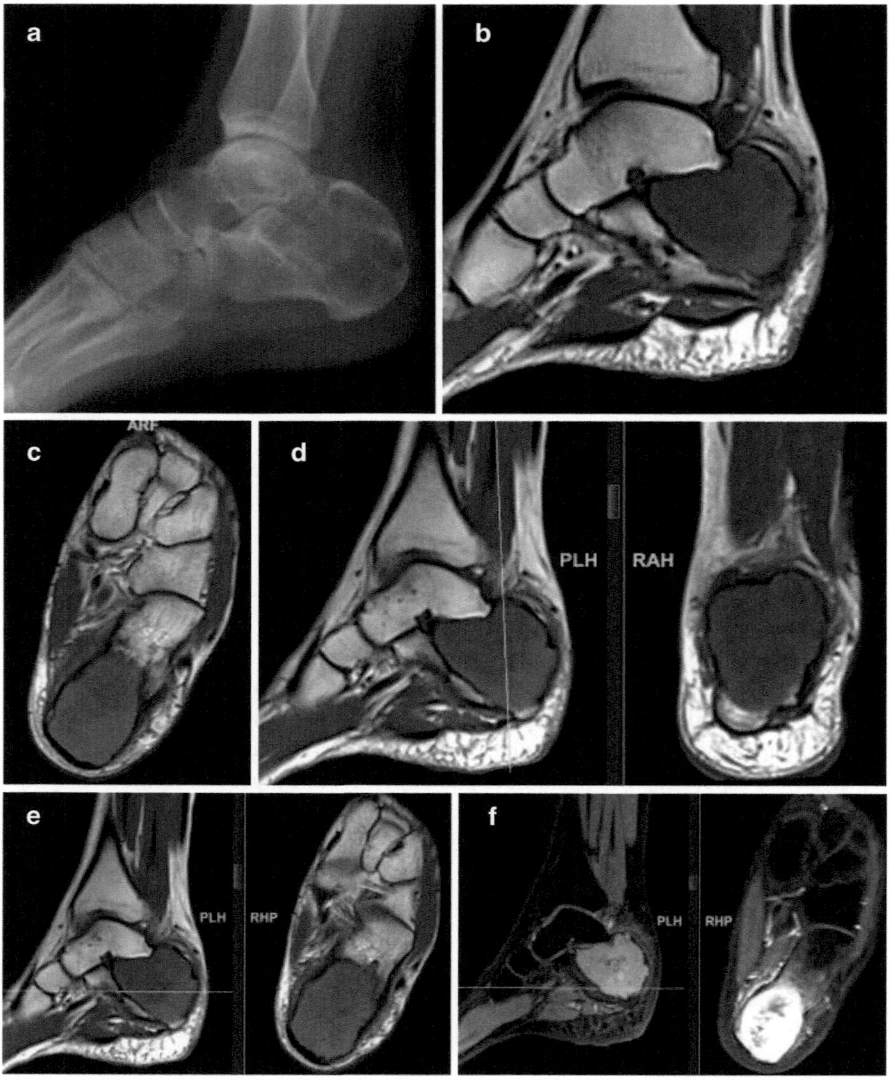

Evaluation of the heel pad, subtalar joint, calcaneal-cuboid joint, abductor hallucis, and plantar fascia attachment for tumour involvement is crucial to minimise contamination during surgery. Medial neurovascular structures are closely attached to the calcaneum (Fig. 6a–f).

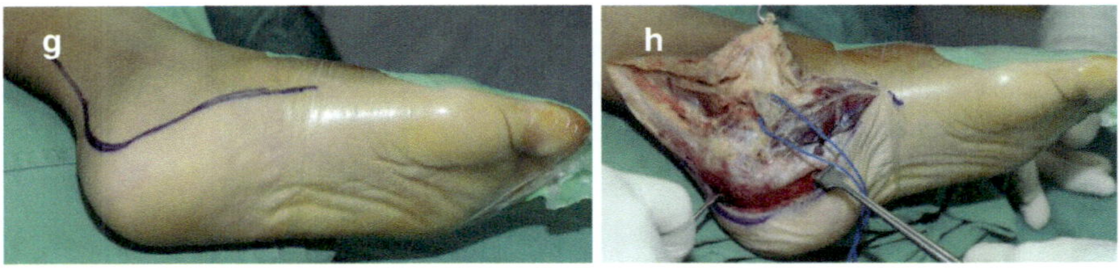

The posterior tibia neurovascular structures are approached through an extensile medial approach up to the junction of the medial and lateral plantar nerve. The calcaneal cuboid joint is identified distally by detachment of the abductor hallucis muscle and plantar fascia from the calcaneal attachment. The entire calcaneum is exposed by reflecting the heel pad proximally and distally. Care must be taken to not violate the periosteum for margin and posterolateral blood supply of the heel pad (Fig. 6g–j).

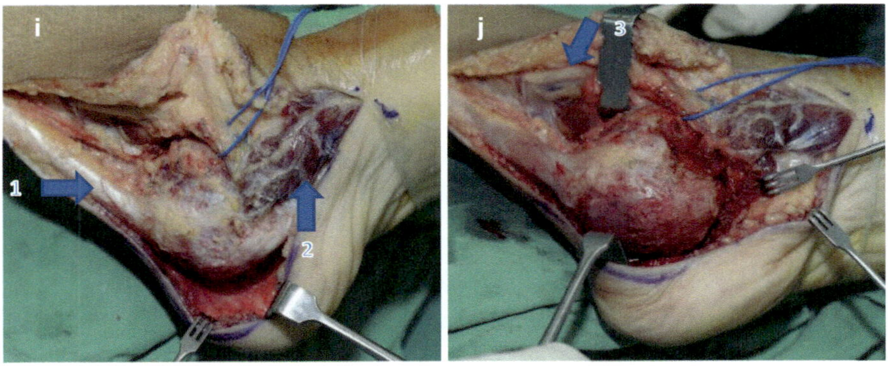

Subtalar joint is identified by reflecting all the flexor tendons from its fibro-osseous tunnel, and subsequently, the Achilles tendon is resected at the calcaneal attachment. Intraarticular resection at the talocalcaneal and calcaneal-cuboid joint helps to deliver the tumour (Fig. 6k–n).

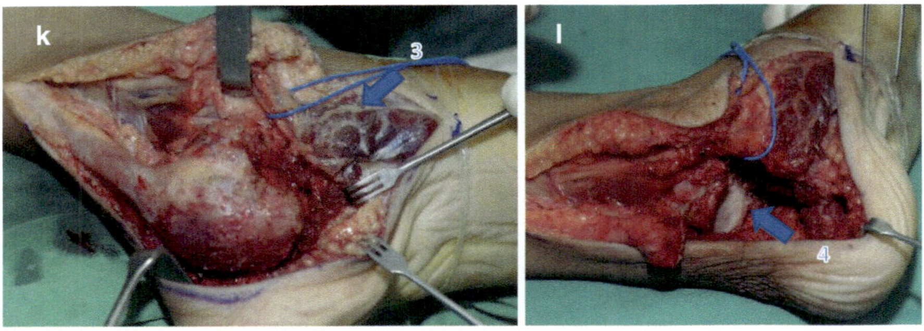

1. Achilles tendon
2. Abductor hallucis attachment
3. Posterior tibial neurovascular structures
4. Subtalar joint

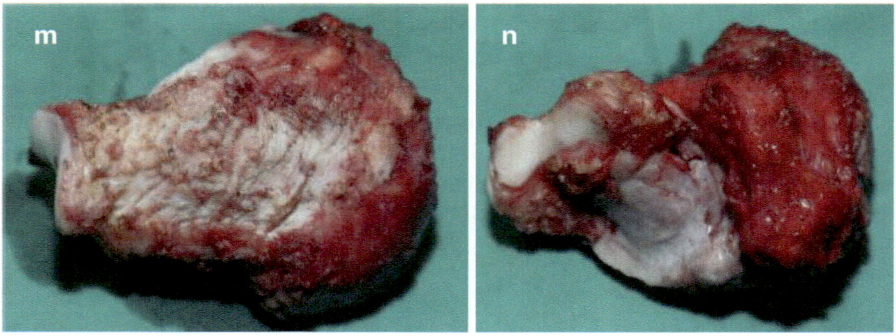

The osteocutaneous vascularised iliac graft is a good donor for heel reconstruction, as it can be shaped as the heel and fused to the talus and cuboid. Hypertrophy of the graft will subsequently improve the function and stability of the foot. Perforators to the iliac crest and skin are identified and confirmed with a Doppler. The entire flap is based on the circumflex iliac artery supply (Fig. 6o–t).

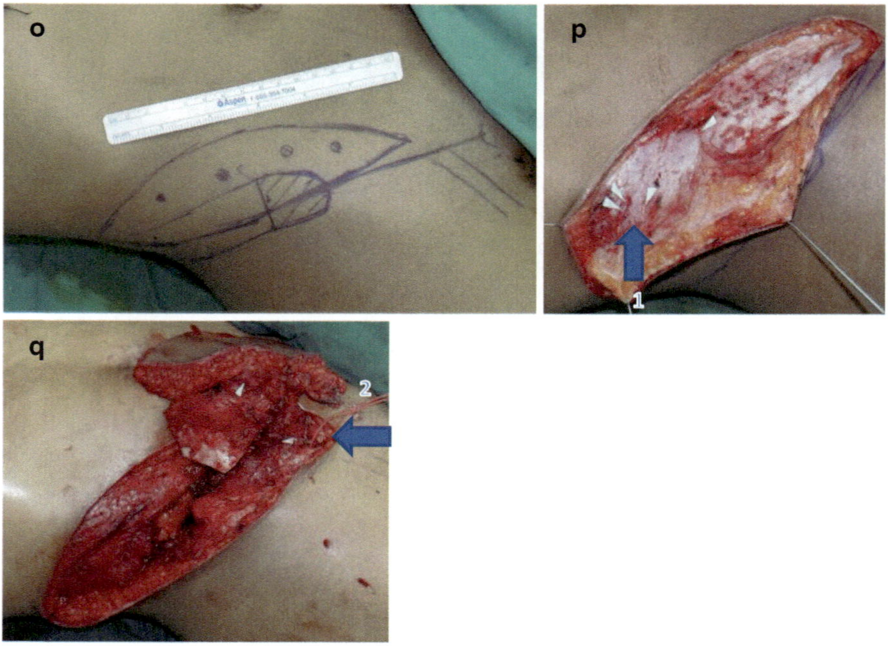

1. Perforator vessels of DCIA
2. Dorsal circumflex iliac artery

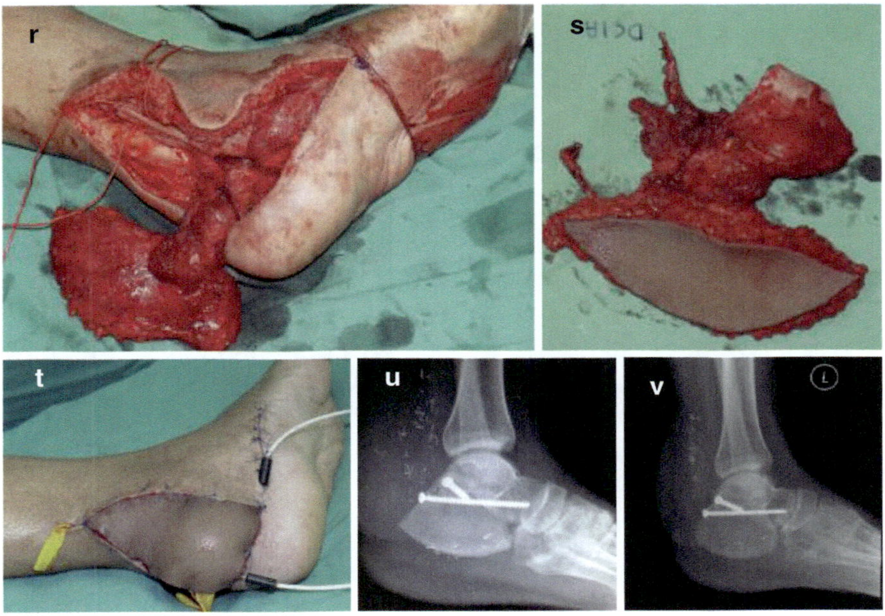

Calcaneal 'Vascularised iliac crest' hypertrophy 2 years after surgery (Fig. 6u, v).

Patients underwent debulking procedures at 2 years postoperatively to address the bulky flap and returned to regular nonimpact sporting activities (Fig. 6w–y).

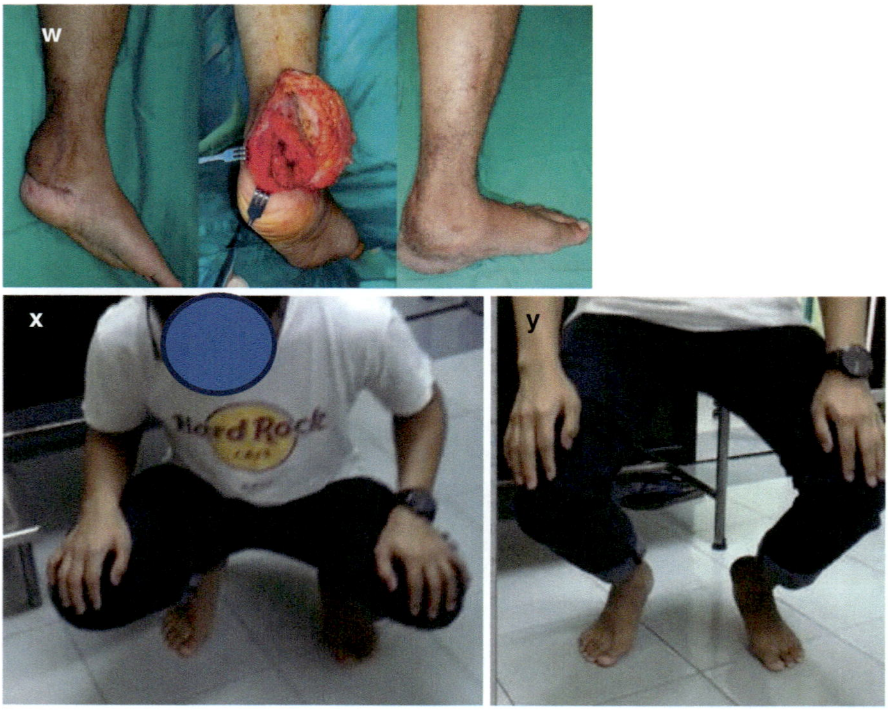

Acknowledgements The author thanks Professor Wan Azman Wan Sulaiman, Professor Arman Zaharil Mat Saad, and Professor Ahmad Sukari Halim from the Plastic Reconstructive Unit at Universiti Sains Malaysia and MSU Medical Centre, Management and Science University, for their contributions and team members for managing the patients. All plastic, reconstructive, and microsurgical procedures were performed by the team members.

Suggested Reading

1. Bahamonde Munoz L, Escudero HM. Massive chondroblastoma of the talus: treatment with en bloc talectomy and tibiocalcaneal arthrodesis: long-term follow-up of a case. Foot Ankle Spec. 2017;10(3):274–7.
2. Özer E, Aycan OE, Er ST, Tanrıtanır R, Arıkan Y, Kabukçuoğlu YS. Primary tumor and tumor-like lesions of bones of the foot: single-center experience of 166 cases. J Foot Ankle Surg. 2017;56(6)
3. Özger H, Alpan B, Topalan M. Biological reconstruction of the foot: free vascular iliac flap. In: Orthopaedic surgical oncology for bone tumors. Springer Nature Switzerland AG; 2022. p. 357–67.
4. Kadam AB, Dhamangaonkar AC. Giant cell tumor of talus: T-construct method of bone grafting. Foot Ankle Spec. 2017;10(4):364–7.
5. Rosli MA, Ismail WFW, Sulaiman WAW, Zin NAM, Halim SA, Johar FM, Saad AZM, Halim AS. Calcaneal reconstruction with free deep circumflex iliac artery osteocutaneous flap following aggressive benign bone tumor resection. Foot Ankle Int:1–9.

6. Roslia MA, Sulaimana WAW, Ismail WFW, Yahaya S, Saad AZM, Wan Z, Halim AS. Functional outcomes in total talus reconstruction with triangular double-barrel free fibula flap following oncological resection: a retrospective case series review. J Plast Reconstruct Aesthet Surg. 2022;13:22.
7. Özger H, Eralp L, Türker M, et al. Surgical treatment of malignant tumors of the foot and ankle. Int J Clin Oncol. 2005;10:127–32.
8. Win TT, Balqis N, Faisham WI. Osteosarcoma of the Talus. A rare location of the tumor with literature review. Ann Pathol Lab Med. 2016;3

Intercalary Resection and Reconstruction

Wan Faisham Nu'man Bin Wan Ismail,
Ferdiansyah Mahyudin, Mohammad Hardian Basuki,
Istan Irmansyah Irsan, Achmad Fauzi Kamal,
Vivek Ajit Singh, Azura Mansor, Nor Faissal Yasin,
and Ajay Puri

Introduction

Limb salvage surgery with intercalary resection is performed when safe oncological margins are achievable, if tumour extent allows for preservation of adjacent joints. It can be performed for primary as well as metastatic bone tumours; however, reconstructions of the diaphysis after the resection of bone tumours are surgically demanding.

W. F. N. B. W. Ismail (✉)
Prince Court Medical Center, Kuala Lumpur, Malaysia

Orthopaedic Oncology Reconstructive Unit, Universiti Sains Malaysia,
Kubang Kerian, Kelantan, Malaysia

F. Mahyudin · M. H. Basuki
Orthopaedic and Traumatology Department, Faculty of Medicine of Universitas Airlangga/
Dr. Soetomo General Academic Hospital, Surabaya, Indonesia

I. I. Irsan
Department of Orthopaedic Surgery, Saiful Anwar Hospital, Brawijaya University,
Malang, Indonesia

A. F. Kamal
Department of Orthopaedic and Traumatology, Faculty of Medicine Universitas Indonesia/
Dr. Cipto Mangunkusumo General Hospital, Jakarta, Indonesia

V. A. Singh · A. Mansor
Department of Orthopaedic Surgery, Faculty of Medicine, University Malaya,
Kuala Lumpur, Malaysia

N. F. Yasin
Department of Orthopaedic Surgery, Faculty of Medicine, University Malaya,
Kuala Lumpur, Malaysia

A. Puri
Department of Surgical Oncology, Tata Memorial Centre, Mumbai, India

A. Puri, W. F. N. B. W. Ismail (eds.), *Atlas of Orthopedic Oncology Volume 2*,
https://doi.org/10.1007/978-981-95-8962-3_10

The options for reconstruction include the following:

- Intercalary endoprosthetic reconstructions
- Three-dimensional printed custom prostheses
- Massive bone allograft
- Reimplanting sterilised tumour bone using extracorporeal radiation or cryotherapy with liquid nitrogen
- Vascularised free fibula

Surgical Anatomy

Understanding muscle coverage attachment for the middle femur is important for resection planning and assessing the possibility of tumour extension.

- The vastus intermedius is an important muscle that covers the entire anterior femur from the articularis genu suprapatellar region. This muscle can be removed completely with the femur, especially for distal femur sarcoma.
- Medially, it is attached to the pectineus, adductor brevis, and adductor longus and magnus.
- Posteriorly, the entire femur is covered by loose areolar tissue, and the short head of the biceps is attached to the lateral border of the femur.

Anatomical barriers against tumour extension for intercalary tibial resection are as follows:

- Thick periosteum prevents subcutaneous and skin infiltration and attachment of soleus muscle medially must be evaluated for infiltration.
- The tibialis posterior and flexor digitorum longus muscles originate from the proximal tibia and must be included in the surgical margin with posterior tumour extension.
- The tibialis anterior muscle and other leg extensors in the anterior compartment.

The entire humerus is covered by muscle that provides an anatomical barrier for tumour extension

- Brachialis muscle covers the anterior part of the distal humerus and protects the neurovascular bundle and biceps muscle.
- Medial and lateral triceps originate at the posterior humerus and provide a good cuff of the muscle for wide margin surgery.
- All tendinous attachments and the common flexor and extensor origins of the forearm must be carefully evaluated for tumour extension.
- Deltoid is attached at the deltoid tuberosity at the anterolateral surface of the humerus.

Assessments

Careful preoperative evaluation for intramedullary extension and soft tissue infiltration in the diaphyseal region is important for the final decision of resection margin. The surgical plan and approach are based on the direct extension of the tumour into soft tissue and proximity to major neurovascular bundles.

Intercalary Allograft Fibula Composite Reconstruction of Femur Diaphysis

Intracalary osteosarcoma of the midshaft femur in an 8-years-old girl responding well to chemotherapy was presented. The resection margin was predetermined by MRI, and allograft fibula composite reconstruction was used for long-term biological outcome (Fig. 1a–e). Long distal femur locking plate was used and contralateral distal femur epiphysiodesis was planned.

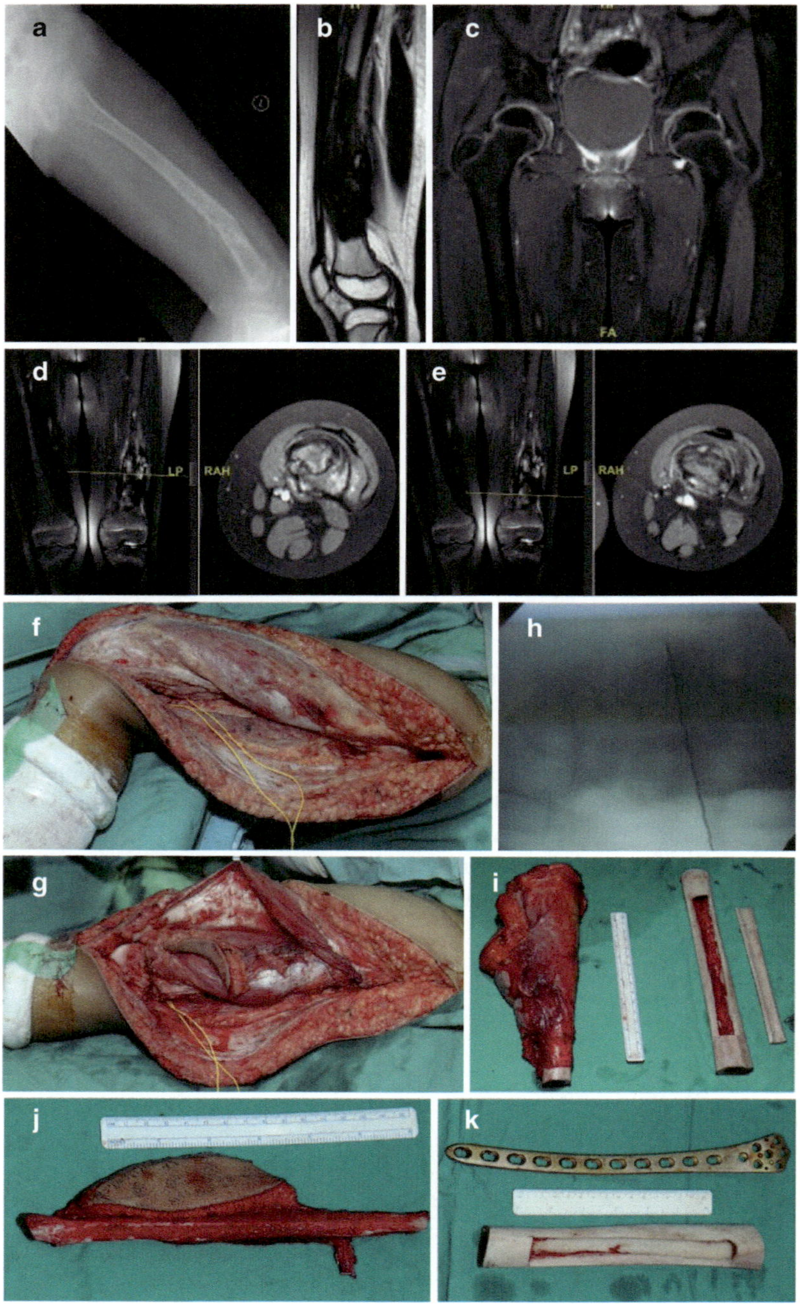
a
b
c
d
LP
RAH
e
LP
RAH
FA
f
h
g
i
j
k

Resection through lateral approach was carried out, whereby the entire vastus intermedius and partial vastus medialis was included in the margin. Intraoperative imaging confirmed resection level prior to bone resection (Fig. 1f–h). The intraoperative planning involved the use of allograft, vascularised fibula graft, and plate using the 'Capanna method'. The peroneal vesels were anastomosed to remnant branch of vastus intermedius (Fig. 1i–m).

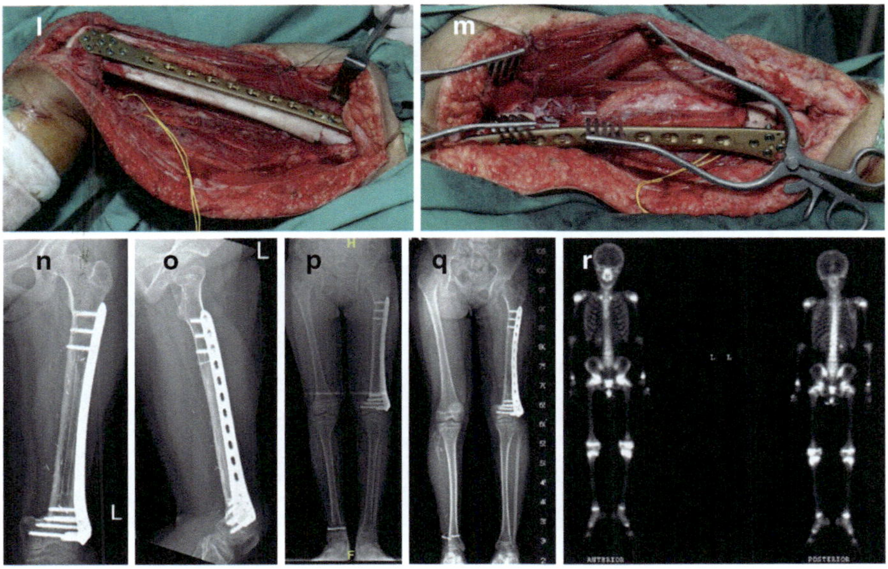

Radiograph showed full incorporation of graft. Scanogram at the age of 10 and 13 revealed 3 cm shortening; however, the patient is comfortable with a shoe raise. Total incorporation and revascularisation of graft was demonstrated on staging bone scan 3 years later (Fig. 1n–r).

Intercalary Resection with Physeal Preservation and Distal Femur Allograft Reconstruction

Osteosarcoma mid-shaft femur with spared distal femur growth plate was reconstructed with intercalary allograft. The proximal junction was complicated by non-union and collapse with implant failure. The vascularised fibula graft was used to splint the posterior medial segment to prevent further collapse and induce union, and the allograft was maintained. There is total incorporation of vascularised graft to allograft, and long-term biological incorporation was anticipated.

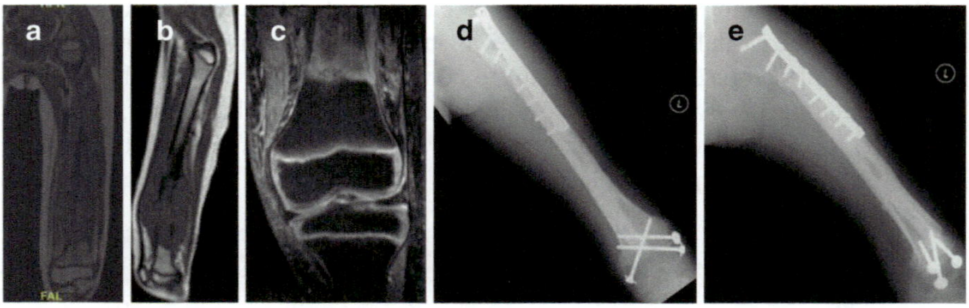

Osteosarcoma in a 10-year-old girl was managed by intercalary resection with preservation of epiphyseal part, reconstructed with cemented allograft and fixed with multiple screws distally and DCP plate for proximal stability (Fig. 2a–e).

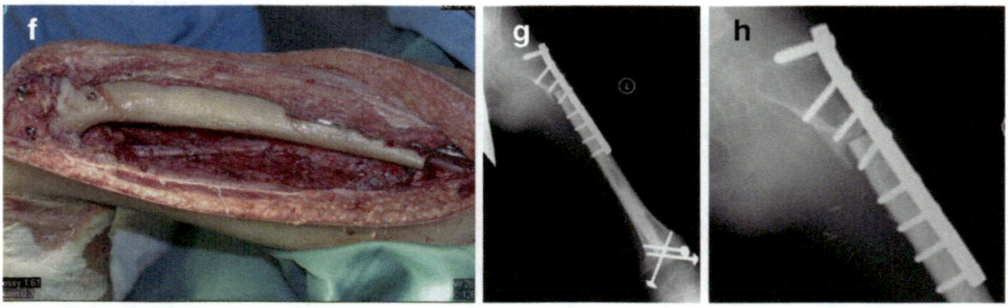

Junctional non-union and late collapse of metaphyseal area of allograft are known complications and potential causes of failure for this method of reconstruction (Fig. 2f–h). Salvage procedures with vascularised fibula graft can prevent further collapse and improve union. Long plate for stabilisation protection of entire allograft is also an option to prevent late failure and collapse.

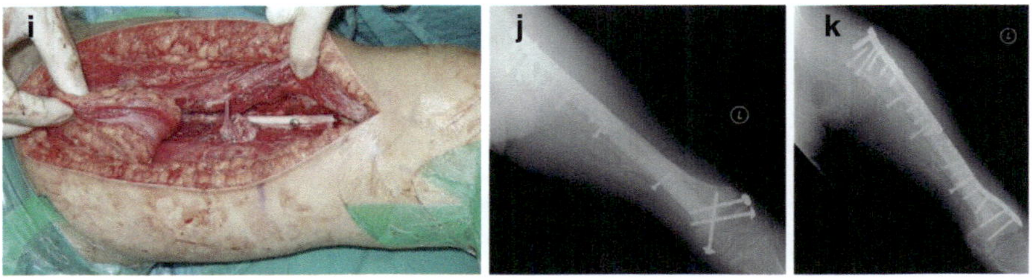

Non-union and collapse of the medial allograft lead to varus deformity of proximal fragment. An onlay vascularised fibula graft over the posterior medial femur was done. Full incorporation and retention of reconstruction were achieved 10 years after primary reconstructive surgery (Fig. 2i–k).

Intercalary Osteosarcoma with Recycled Bone Reconstruction Using Liquid Nitrogen

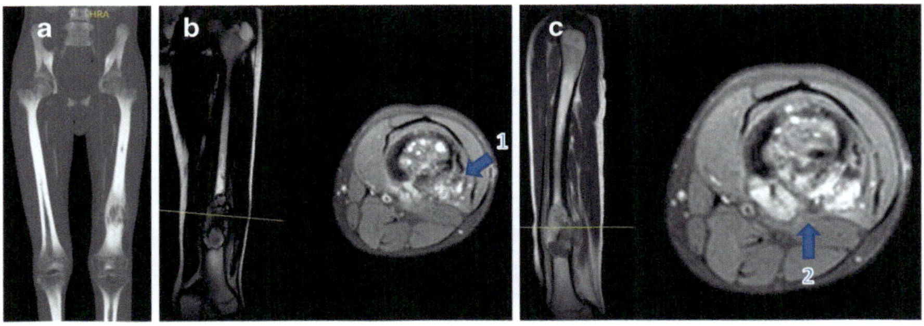

Intercalary osteosarcoma of the distal third of the femur responded well to chemotherapy. The soft tissue involvement was confined to vastus intermedius, and origin of short head biceps was removed as oncological margin (Fig. 3a–d).

- Vastus intermedius
- Short head of biceps

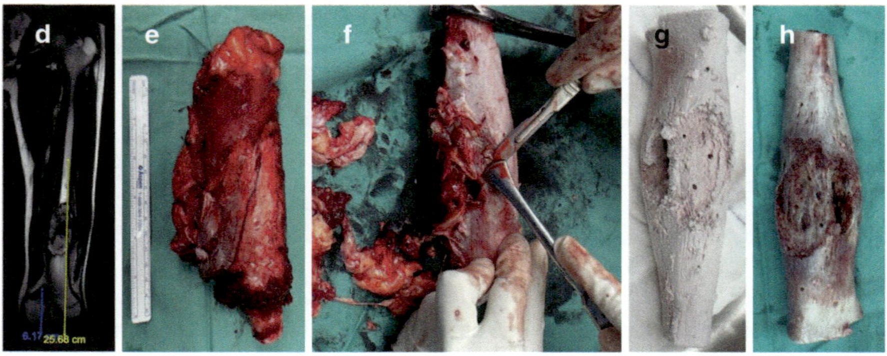

Recycling process using liquid nitrogen cryotherapy

- Resection with cuff of normal tissue (Fig. 3e)
- Remove soft tissue and ream intramedullary content (Fig. 3f)
- Cryotherapy (Fig. 3g, h)
- Final processed bone

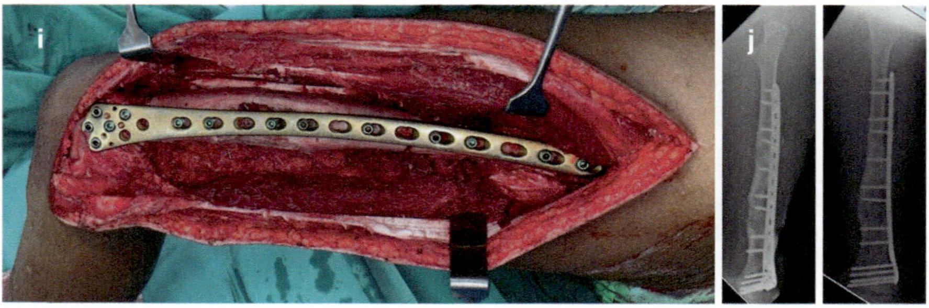

Final stabilisation with long distal femur locking plate, X-ray showed union at 6 months (Fig. 3i, j).

Intercalary Endoprosthesis Reconstruction

A 15-year-old boy presented with Ewing's sarcoma of the left midshaft femur. He underwent neoadjuvant chemotherapy, followed by wide resection and replacement with a diaphyseal prosthesis (Fig. 4a–e).

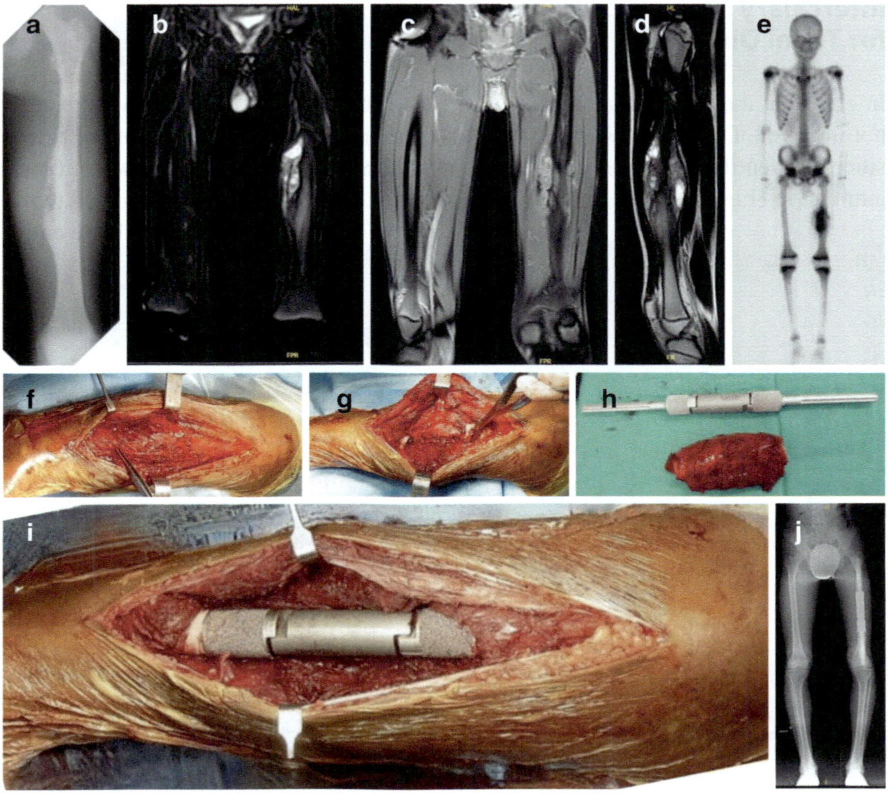

A wide resection was carried out. The defect is reconstructed with a diaphyseal prosthesis. First, a trial prosthesis is carried out to determine the correct limb length. Once the length is determined, the final prosthesis is cemented in (Fig. 4f–j).

There are two challenges associated with this form of reconstruction.

1. Preserving adequate proximal and distal segments to accommodate the proximal and distal stems. Short stems with supporting side plates can be used as an alternative.
2. Reducing the prosthesis post-cementation due to the tight soft tissue if the actual length is to be maintained. The prosthesis must be reduced before the hardening of the cement to allow for the adjustment in its rotatory alignment. Designs of implants with Interlocking segments with side screws enable easier reduction.

Intercalary Physeal-Sparing Allograft Reconstruction for Tibial Diaphysis

In children, the epiphyseal segment can be preserved whereby the growth plate is not involved. Detailed MRI evaluation and intraoperative radiographs/image intensifier for identification of anatomical landmarks is important to prevent tumour contamination (Fig. 5a–e).

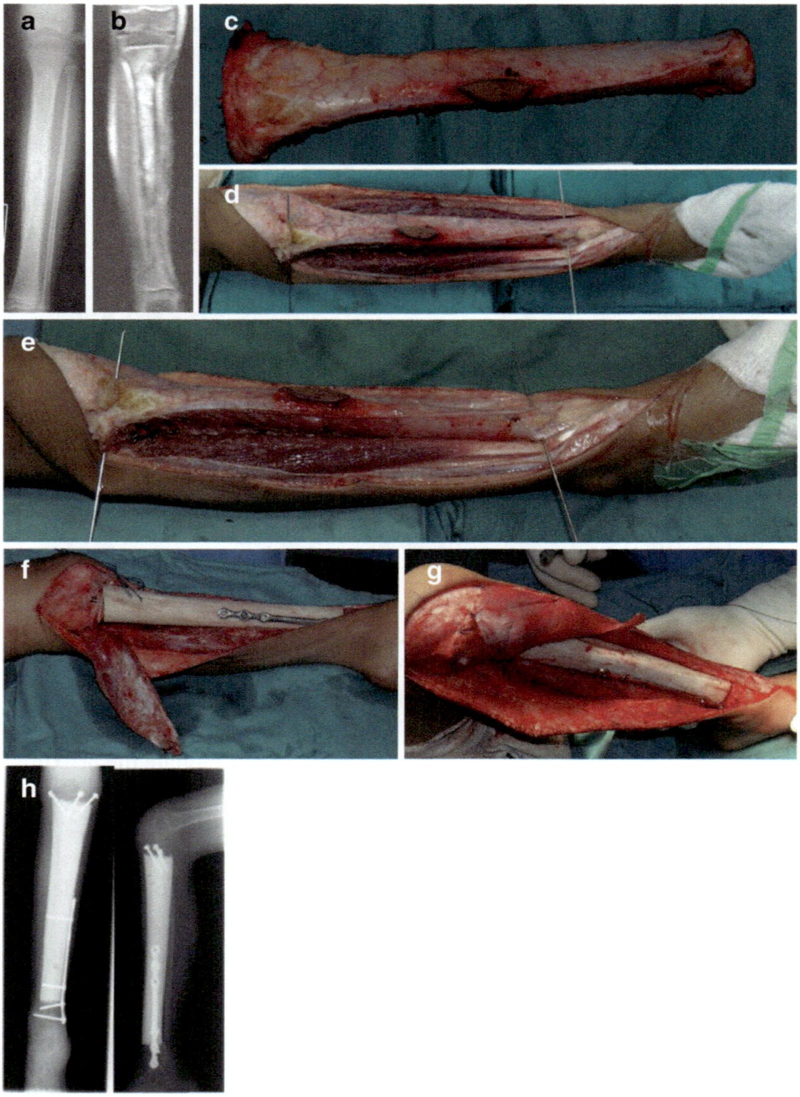

Stabilization of epiphyseal segment to allograft was achieved with multiple screws and plate to the remnant diaphysis. The contralateral epiphysiodesis was done at 6 months to minimise limb length discrepancy. Final allograft incorporation was achieved (Fig. 5f–j).

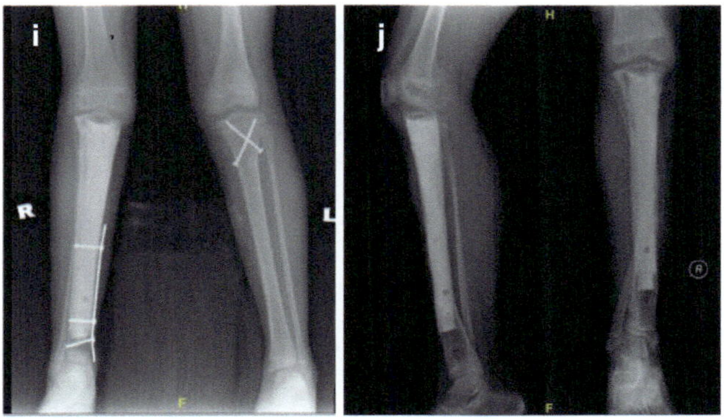

Diaphyseal Adamantinoma with Extraosseous Extension Reconstructed with Intercalary Allograft and Vascularised Fibula Composites

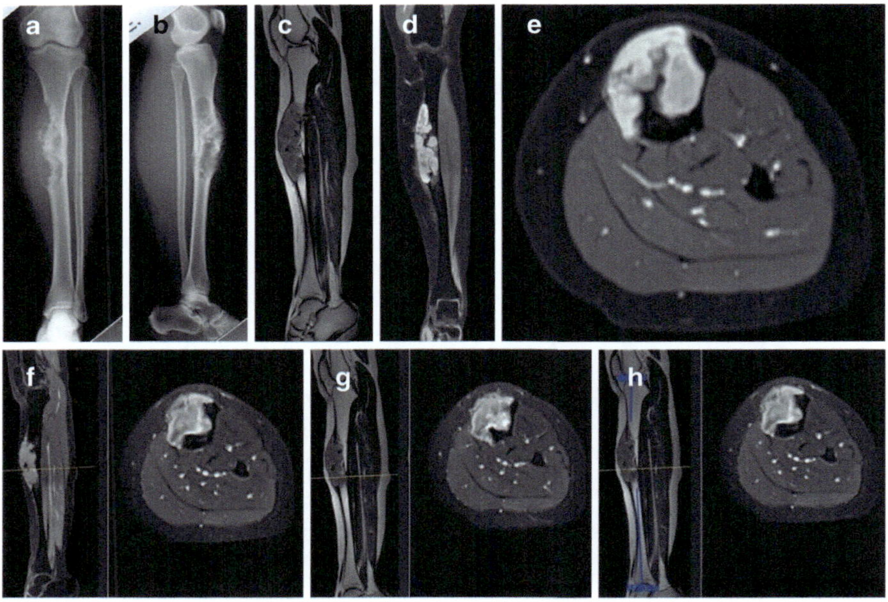

Diaphyseal adamantinoma was identified with extraosseous extension to the subcutaneous tissue, soleus, and tibialis posterior attachment. Measurement of the intramedullary extension from the joint line is an intraoperative reference for accurate level of resection (Fig. 6a–h).

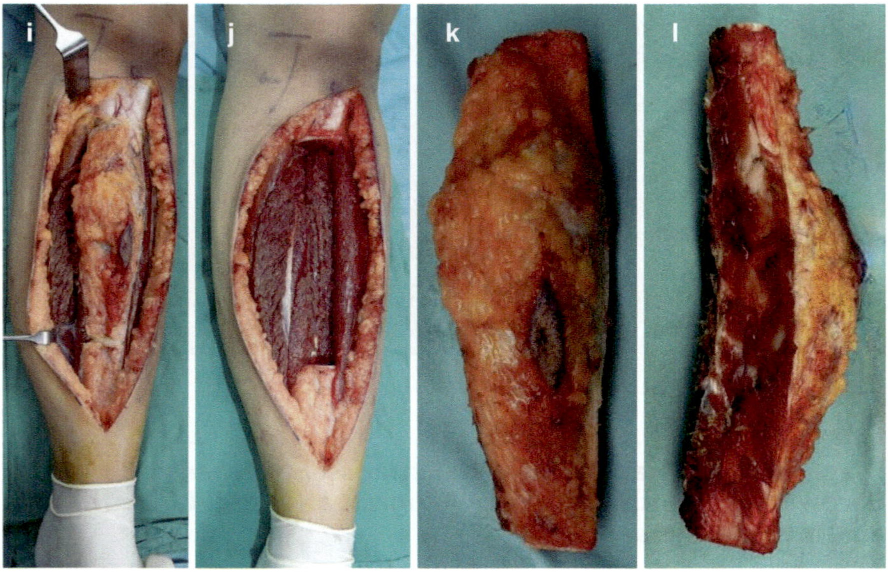

Biopsy scar, subcutaneous tissue, cuff of soleus, and tibialis posterior muscle were included as tumour margin (Fig. 6i-l).

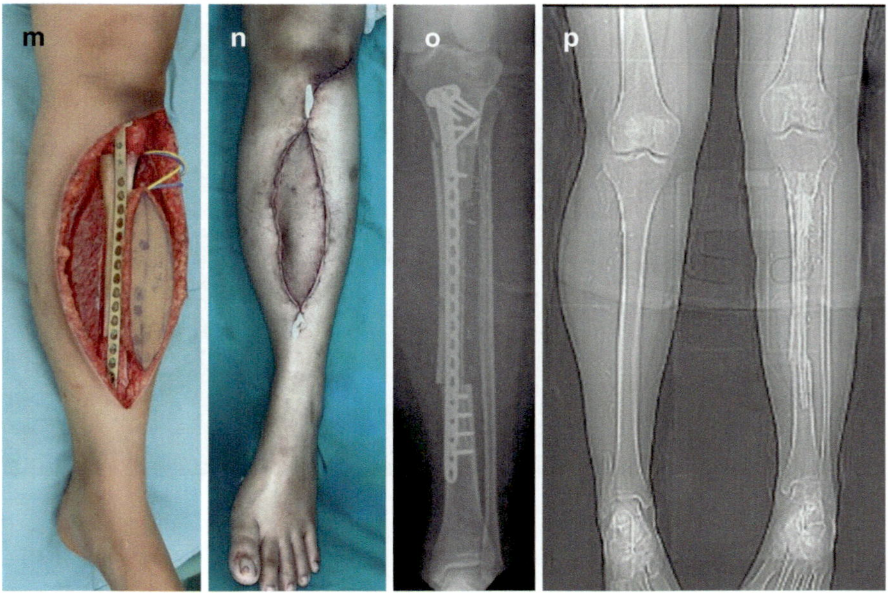

Reconstruction of post resection tibia defect with long segment allograft and vascularised fibula graft composite 'Campanna technique'. The peroneal vessels were anastomosed to anterior tibial vessels, and the entire construct was stabilised with a proximal tibia locking plate (Fig. 6m–p).

Intercalary Tibia Resection with Epiphyseal Preservation and Reconstruction Using Recycled Cryotherapy Technique

A 13-year-old boy presented with osteosarcoma of right proximal tibia with epiphyseal preservation resection intercalary resection (Fig. 7a–c).

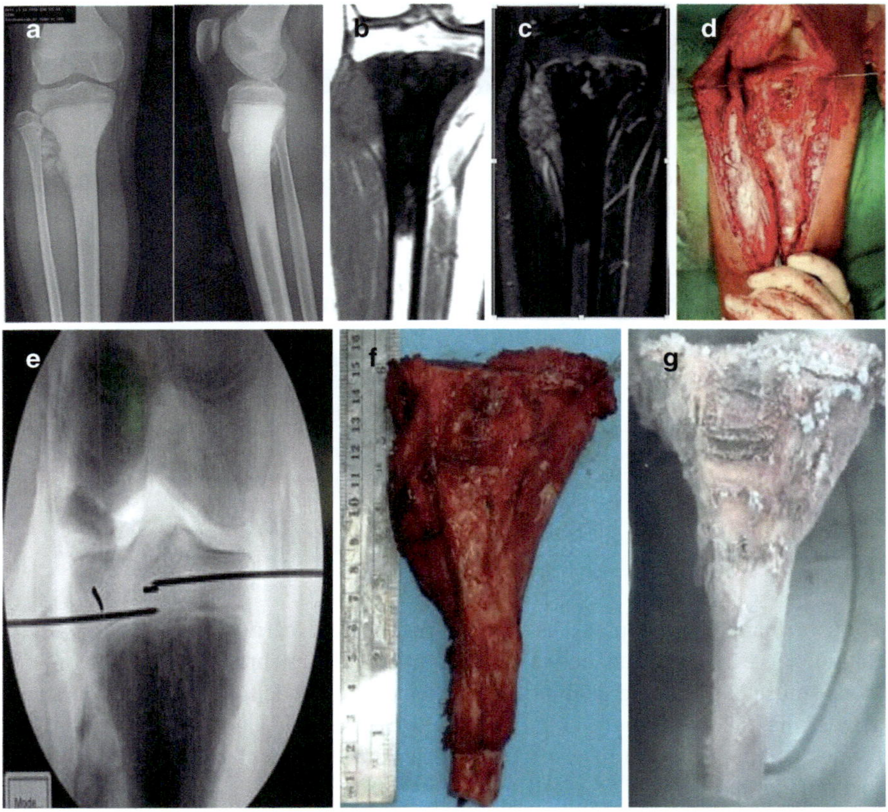

Bone resection was done above epiphyseal plate after elevation the patella tendon, the soft tissue and extracortical extension of the tumour was cleared prior cryotherapy with liquid nitrogen (Fig. 7d–g).

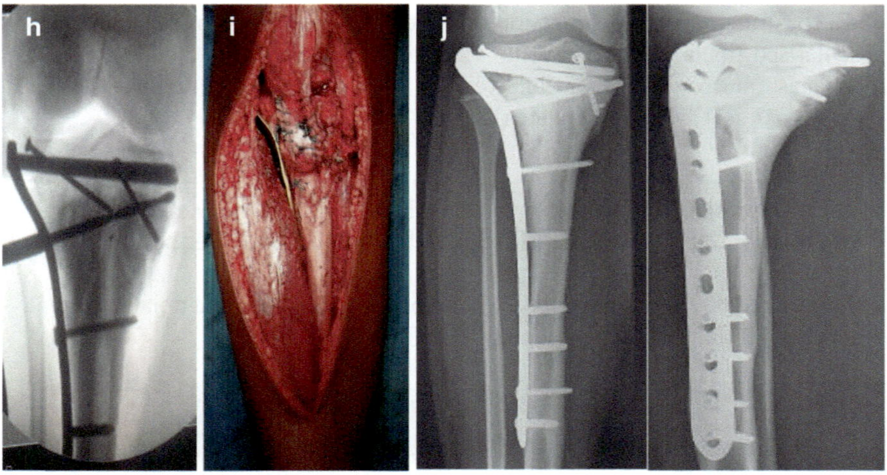

The recycled bone was stabilised with anterolateral locking compression plate; X-ray at 2 years showed full union at the junction and revascularisation of reimplanted tibia segment (Fig. 7h–j).

Humerus with Intercalary Allograft Reconstruction

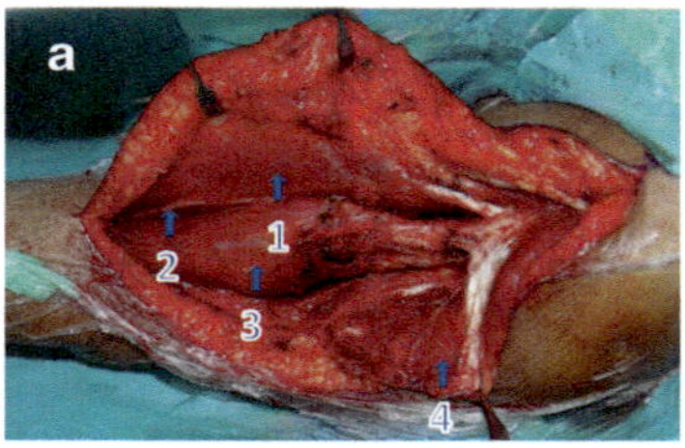

The brachialis muscle provides a good oncological barrier for tumour margin. Radial nerve is explored between brachioradialis and brachialis muscle plane, biceps muscle is elevated from brachialis plane, and the deltoid attachment is transacted from tuberosity with cuff of tissue. Proximal and distal osteotomy is performed for mobilisation of shaft from posterior attachment of medial and lateral triceps (Fig. 8a).

1. Biceps
2. Musculocutaneous nerve
3. Brachialis
4. Deltoid
5. Radial nerve

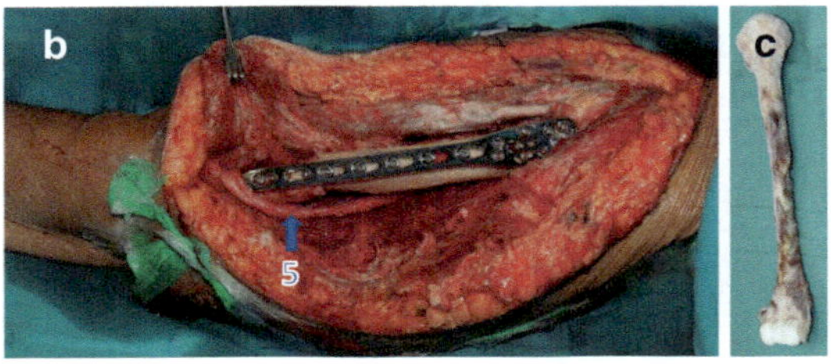

Intercalary allograft reconstruction was stabilised with proximal humerus plate (Fig. 8b, c).

Intercalary Resection of Distal Humerus and Reconstruction Using Recycle Cryotherapy Technique

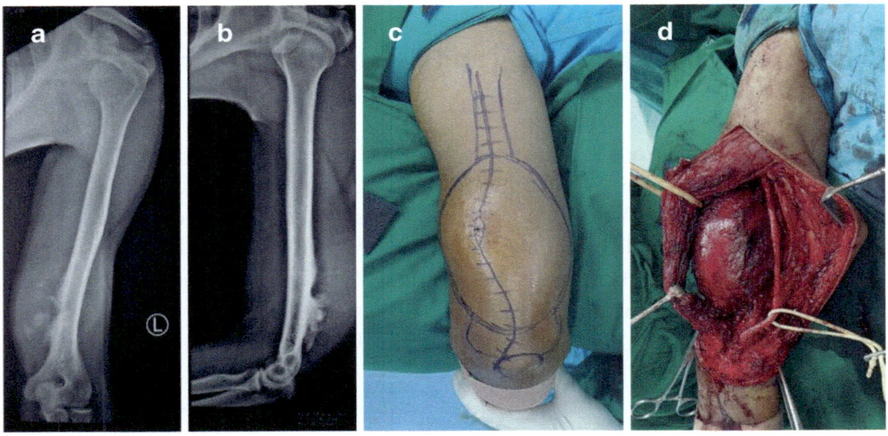

A case of parosteal osteosarcoma on posteromedial aspect of distal humerus with extensive posteromedial soft tissue extension was presented; however, distal humeral condyle was not involved (Fig. 9a, b).

Intercalary resection of distal humerus was done with cuff of medial and lateral triceps muscle after mobilisation of ulnar nerve and long head of triceps with tendon. Distal osteotomy was done above the olecranon fossa with 1 cm margin from distal tumour extension (Fig. 9c–f).

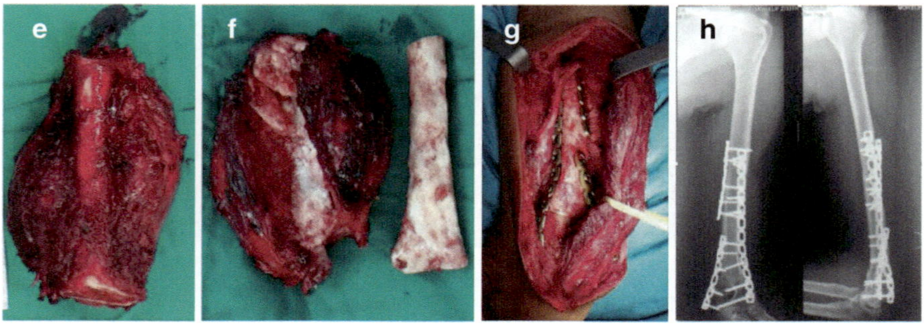

The segment of humerus was treated with liquid nitrogen for tumour sterilisation and stabilised with long lateral plate and two medial plates across osteotomy sites. Two years after surgery, osteotomy sites united with good function and elbow movements (Fig. 9g, h).

Extracorporeal Radiotherapy and Reimplanting Sterilised Tumour Bone

Under aseptic precautions, all the soft tissue, including the periosteum, is stripped from the specimen, which is resected respecting oncologic principles. The bone specimen is wrapped in Vancomycin soaked mops and sterile polyethylene surgical drapes, placed in a sterile container, and irradiated to a dose 50 Gy/1 fraction. On returning to the operative room, the marrow contents are reamed and the bone specimen lavaged with a high-speed pulsatile lavage system to remove residual marrow tissue. The specimen is realigned with the host bone and stabilised with suitable internal fixation.

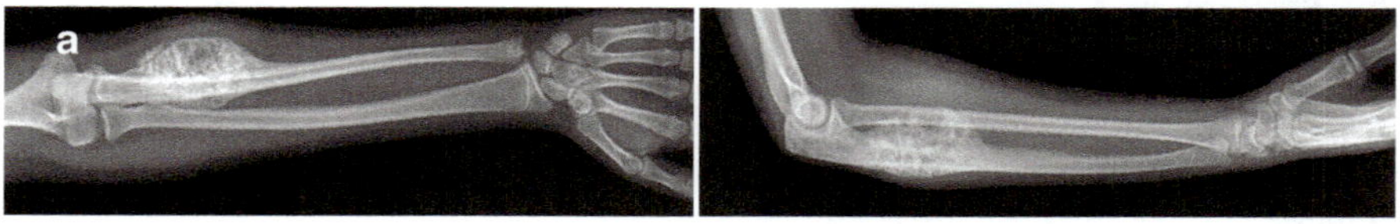

Preoperative X-ray of osteosarcoma ulna which extended just short to the articular surface proximally (Fig. 10a).

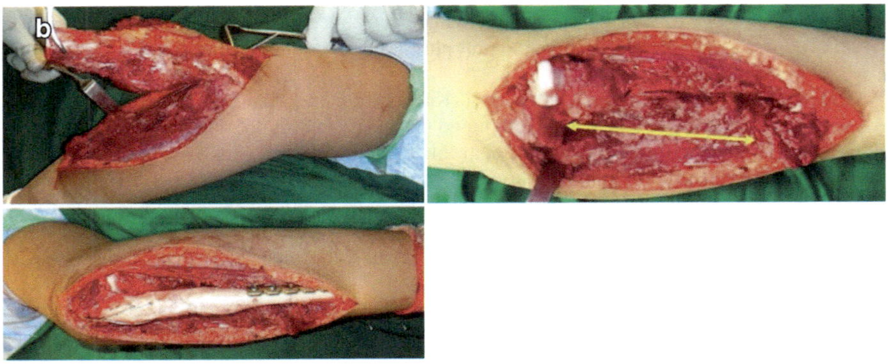

Intraoperative images showing resection of the intercalary ulna, extent of defect, and stabilisation of the irradiated bone after reimplantation (Fig. 10b).

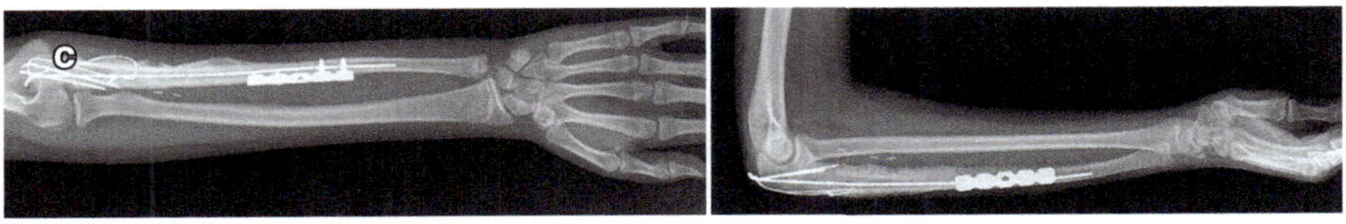

Four years postoperative X-ray (an intramedullary K wire was used at index surgery as an internal splint for the irradiated bone) (Fig. 10c).

Acknowledgement The author thanks Professor Ismail Munajat, Dr. Emil Fazliq Mohd and Professor Abdul Razak Sulaiman for managing limb length discrepancy in pediatric sarcoma patient using contralateral epiphysiodesis methods. Special contribution for microsurgical procedures by Professor Wan Azman Wan Sulaiman, Professor Arman Zaharil Mat Saad and Professor Ahmad Sukari Halim from the Plastic Reconstructive Unit at Universiti Sains Malaysia and MSU Medical Centre, Management and Science University.

Suggested Reading

1. Errani C, Ceruso M, Donati DM, Manfrini M. Microsurgical reconstruction with vascularized fibula and massive bone allograft for bone tumors. Eur J Orthop Surg Traumatol. 2019;29(2):307e311.
2. Fuchs B, Ossendorf C, Leerapun T, Sim FH. Intercalary segmental reconstruction after bone tumor resection. Eur J Surg Oncol. 2008;34(12):1271e1276.
3. Aponte-Tinao L, Farfalli GL, Ritacco LE, Ayerza MA, Muscolo DL. Intercalary femur allografts are an acceptable alternative after tumor resection. Clin Orthop Relat Res. 2012;470(3):728e734.
4. Agarwal M, Puri A, Gulia A, Reddy K. Joint-sparing or physeal sparing diaphyseal resections: the challenge of holding small fragments. Clin Orthop Relat Res. 2010;468(11):2924e2932.
5. Campanacci DA, Puccini S, Caff G, et al. Vascularised fibular grafts as a salvage procedure in failed intercalary reconstructions after bone tumour resection of the femur. Injury. 2014;45(2):399e404.

6. Campanacci DA, Totti F, Puccini S, et al. Intercalary reconstruction of femur after tumour resection: is a vascularized fibular autograft plus allograft a long- lasting solution? Bone Joint J. 2018;100-B(3):378e386.
7. Higuchi T, Yamamoto N, Nishida H, et al. Knee joint preservation surgery in osteosarcoma using tumour-bearing bone treated with liquid nitrogen. Int Orthop. 2017;41(10):2189e2197.
8. Zekry KM, Yamamoto N, Hayashi K, et al. Intercalary frozen autograft for reconstruction of malignant bone and soft tissue tumours. Int Orthop. 2017;41(7):1481e1487.
9. Capanna R, Campanacci DA, Belot N, et al. A ne`w reconstructive technique for intercalary defects of long bones: the association of massive allograft with vascularized fibular autograft. Long-term results and comparison with alternative techniques. Orthop Clin North Am. 2007;38(1):51e60.

Bone Tumour Resection and Reconstruction: Upper Limb

Scapulectomy

Wan Faisham Nu'man Bin Wan Ismail

Introduction

Malignant tumour of the scapula is rare. Diseases include chondrosarcoma, Ewing's sarcoma, osteosarcoma, and metastatic disease, particularly thyroid, where surgery is undertaken to improve overall outcome. Wide resection of the scapula for malignant tumour is aimed at achieving local control and preservation of upper limb function. Reconstructions following a scapulectomy are to provide a stable shoulder for good elbow and hand function.

Surgical Anatomy

The scapula is a thin, flat triangular-shaped bone placed on the posterolateral aspect of the thoracic cage. It articulates with the humerus at the glenohumeral joint, and with the clavicle at the acromioclavicular joint.

The coracoid process is a hook-shaped bone structure that projects anterolaterally from the superior aspect of the scapular neck and acts as a critical anchor for many tendons, including the tendons of the pectoralis minor, coracobrachialis, and short head of the biceps brachii muscles. Ligamentous attachments to the surrounding bones—coracoclavicular, coracohumeral, coracoacromial ligaments—need to be released during a scapulectomy.

The acromion process extends from the spine of the scapula and origin of the acromial head of the deltoid muscle. It articulates with the clavicle and is stabilised

W. F. N. B. W. Ismail (✉)
Prince Court Medical Center, Kuala Lumpur, Malaysia

Orthopaedic Oncology Reconstructive Unit, Universiti Sains Malaysia, Kubang Kerian, Kelantan, Malaysia

A. Puri, W. F. N. B. W. Ismail (eds.), *Atlas of Orthopedic Oncology Volume 2*,
https://doi.org/10.1007/978-981-95-8962-3_11

with strong ligaments. The deltoid muscle origin must be detached from the acromion, and ligament to the clavicle must be free for total scapulectomy.

The scapula is covered by compartment of muscles originating on its anterior and posterior surface, which act as oncological anatomical barriers:

- Anterior: subscapularis
- Posterior: infraspinatus, supraspinatus, and teres major and minor

The parascapular muscle, which is attached to the scapula, has the potential to be infiltrated by the tumour, particularly large tumour with soft tissue extension, and must be evaluated prior to resection for surgical margin.

- Medial: trapezius, rhomboid major, and minor serratus posterior
- Lateral: teres major and minor and lateral border of the latissimus dorsi
- Scapular spine: posterior group of the deltoid muscle and trapezius

The tendon part of the rotator cuff covers the entire glenoid and neck of the scapula and is attached to the tuberosity of the humerus and integrated with the joint capsule. The head *of* the proximal humerus is contained within the compartment surrounding the scapula by the rotator cuff muscles. Evaluation of joint involvement or contamination for intraarticular or extraarticular resection is important due to its close proximity of periarticular structures to the joint.

Vessels and Nerve

- The subclavian and axillary artery is situated anterior to the scapula above the subscapularis muscle and is accompanied by the brachial plexus below the clavicle. The subclavian vessels branch into the suprascapular, dorsal scapular, and circumflex scapular arteries and create an extensive network over the superior and posterior border of the scapula. These vessels must be properly secured, ligated, and clipped for scapulectomy.
- The axillary nerve arises from the posterior cord situated anterior to the subscapularis muscle. It travels towards the lower border of the subscapularis and exits the axilla through the quadrangular space, together with the posterior humeral circumflex artery and vein. The axillary nerve is outside the compartment should be spared for some abduction function of the deltoid.
- The thoracodorsal artery, terminal branch of the subscapular artery, runs inferomedial along the lateral border of the scapula and passes posteriorly deep to the latissimus dorsi muscle. It is accompanied by the thoracodorsal nerve from the posterior cord of the brachial plexus. The vessels are important to be preserved in large tumours with soft tissue extension for local rotational flap cover.

Assessment

Scapula tumours commonly originate from the metaphyseal part of the scapula around the scapula neck and glenoid. The subscapularis and rotator cuff provide good anatomical boundaries for tumour margin. Assessment of direct infiltration to its surrounding structures is important to minimise contamination and achieve wide margin.

Structures to be carefully evaluated on an MRI:

- Entire scapula blade, acromion, and coracoid process
- Shoulder joint and rotator cuff tendon and its tuberosity attachment
- Acromion clavicular joint
- Muscle attachment to the scapula as outlined above
- Axillary artery and brachial plexus in cases with anterior extension and breech in the subscapularis
- Lymph node within the infraclavicular region

Solitary Scapular Thyroid Metastases

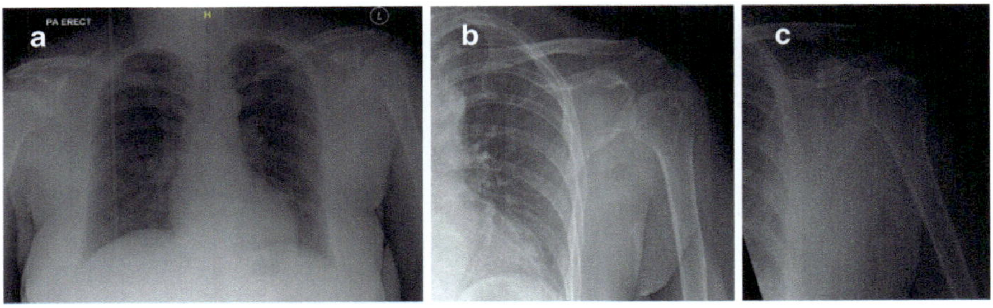

A 34-year-old female with a 3-year history of follicular thyroid carcinoma underwent total thyroidectomy and tyrosine replacement. She complained of chronic shoulder pain and X-ray showed expansile lytic lesion of the scapulae (Fig. 1a–c). Thyroid scan showed no other bony metastases (Fig. 1d).

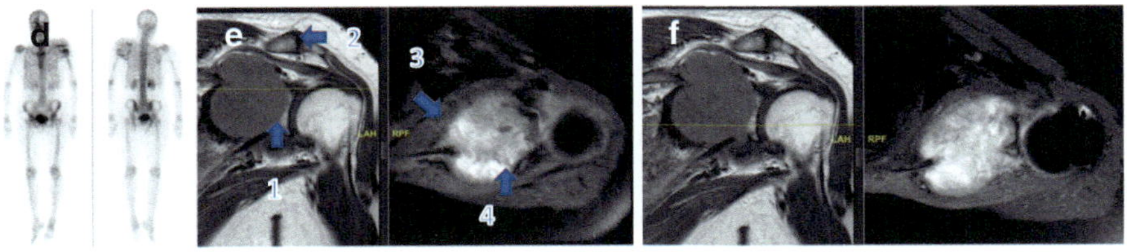

MRI revealed expansile lesion confined to the metaphyseal, neck, and glenoid. The coracoid process was also involved. There was no joint contamination, and it was confined within the subscapularis and rotator cuff margin (Fig. 1e, f).

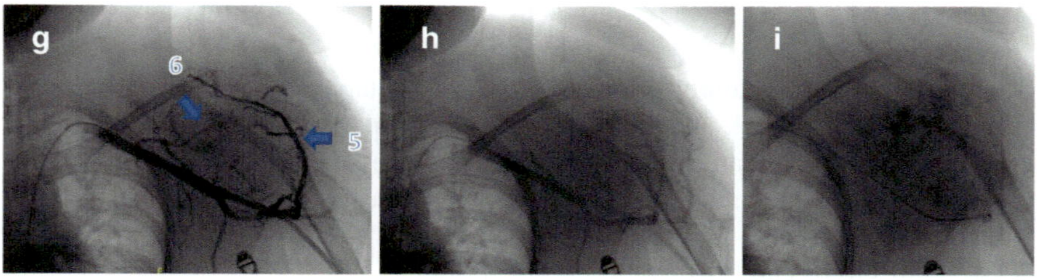

Angio-embolisation was performed to minimise tumour vascularity prior to surgery (Fig. 1g–i). A total scapulectomy with Tikhoff-Linberg reconstruction was done to control local disease (Fig. 1j, k).

1. Glenoid tumour abutting to subchondral bone
2. Acromion-clavicular joint free
3. Subscapularis
4. Infraspinatus
5. Posterior circumflex humeral artery
6. Suprascapular anastomosis

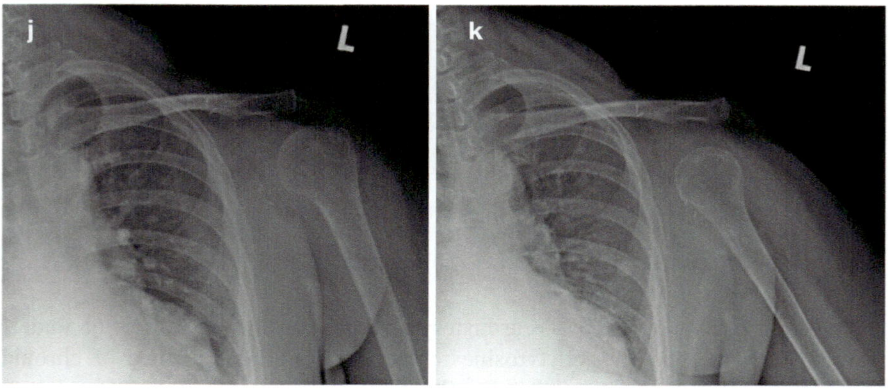

Scapula Chondrosarcoma—Wide Resection and 'Tickhoff-Lindberg' Procedure

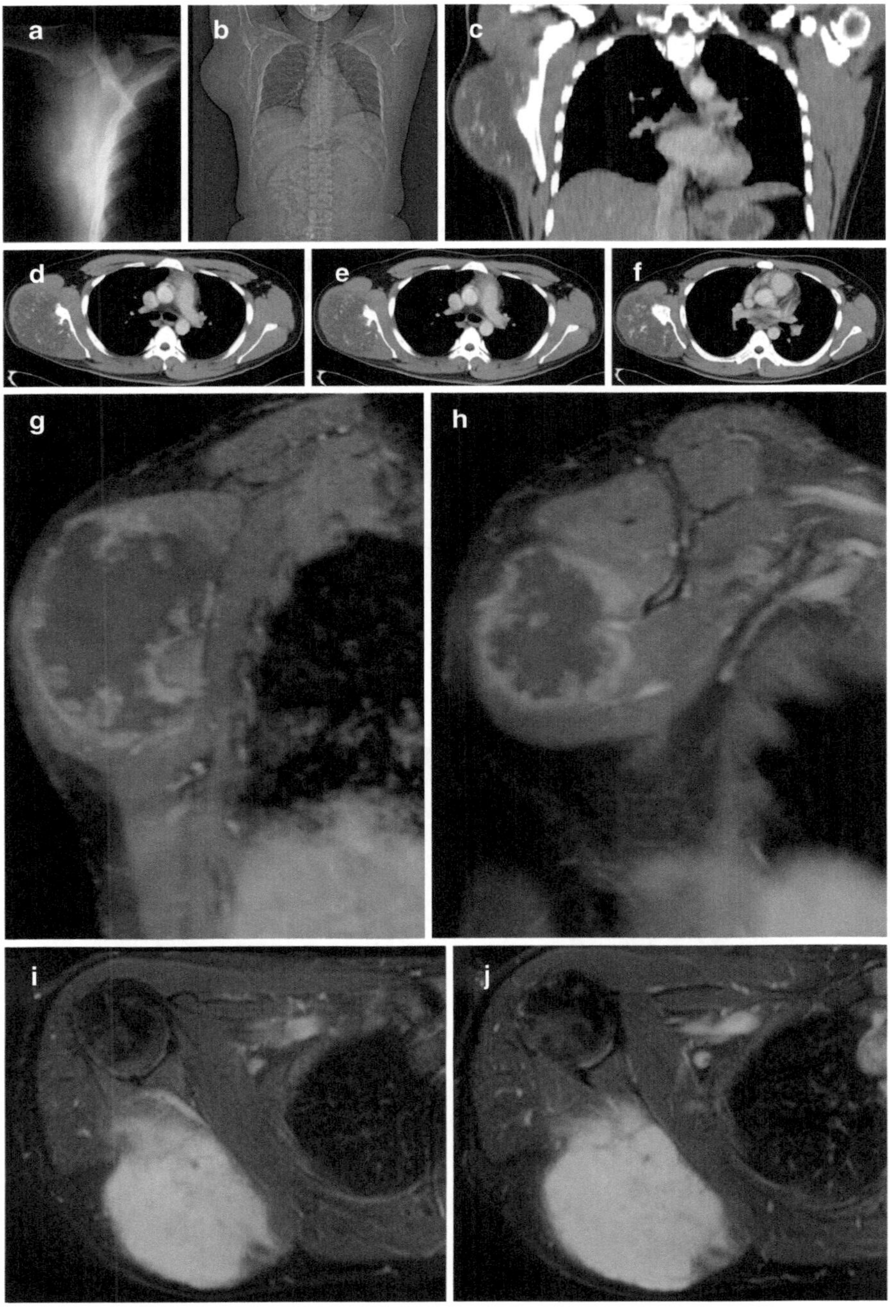

Chondrosarcoma arising from an exostosis on outer surface of the scapula. It involved the entire scapular blade to the neck of glenoid; however, the coracoid and acromion were spared. The supraspinatus muscle and infraspinatus muscle were involved. In addition, the inner table was spared, and the surrounding soft tissue was not involved (Fig. 2a–j).

Surgical Steps: Intraarticular Scapulectomy

The patient was in a lateral position with good padding over the contralateral shoulder and bony prominences. An extensile approach was used from the tip of the scapula curve anteriorly to the coracoid process for anterior exposure. A skin flap is created to expose the entire periscapular muscle. The superficial muscle deltoid, trapezius, latissimus dorsi, and platysma are detached from the scapula attachment to expose the deep layer of muscle (Fig. 2k–m).

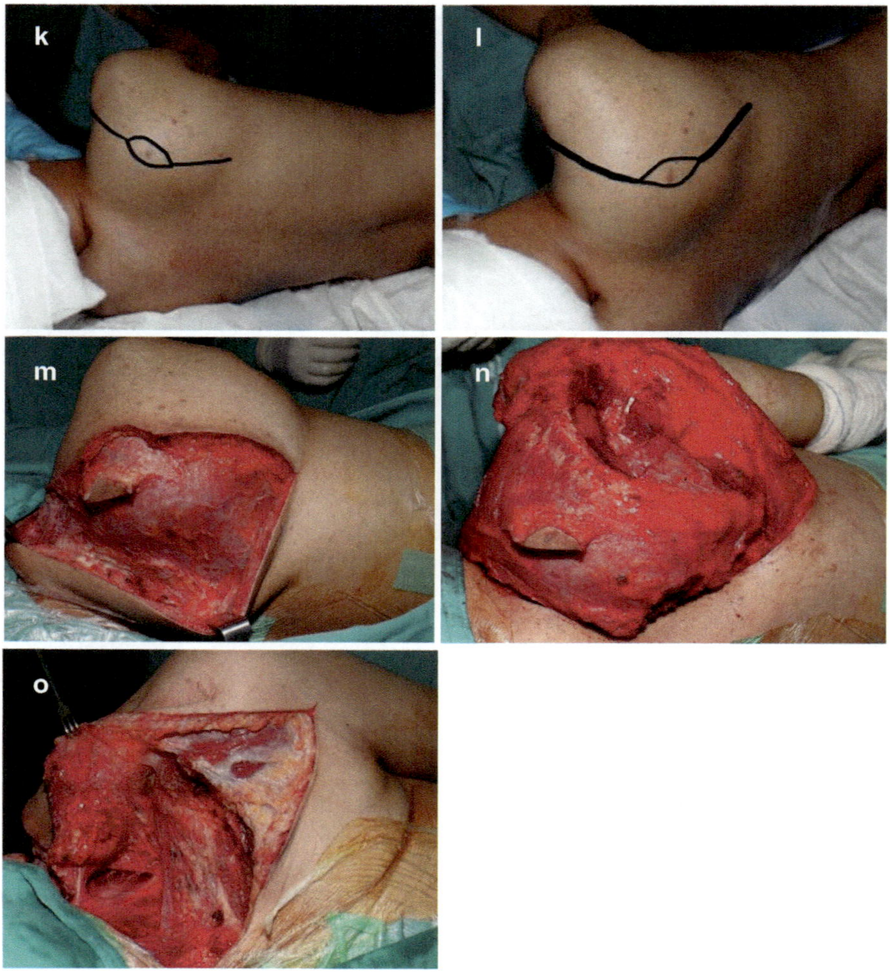

Anteriorly, the pectoralis major and anterior deltoid were detached from the clavicle to expose the coracoid process. The entire deltoid was subsequently mobilised laterally from the acromion to expose the humeral head and rotator cuff tendon. Both the rhomboid and levator scapulae muscles were detached from the medial scapula border. The plane between the subscapularis and thoracic cage is created to lift the entire scapulae laterally (Fig. 2n–q).

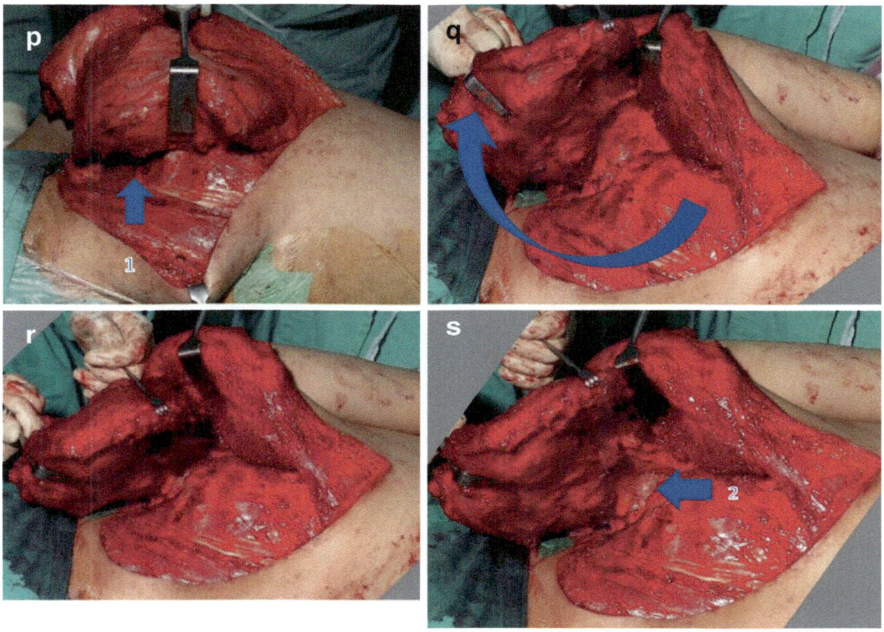

1. Rhomboid major and minor and levator scapulae attachment
2. Subclavian-axillary vessels and brachial plexus

The entire scapula is freed from the anterior aspect by detaching the conjoint tendon from the coracoid process. Subsequently, the tendon of the supraspinatus, infraspinatus, and subscapularis and joint capsule from the head of the humerus were transacted for intraarticular resection. The acromion is freed from the acromioclavicular joint for final scapulectomy (Fig. 2r–t).

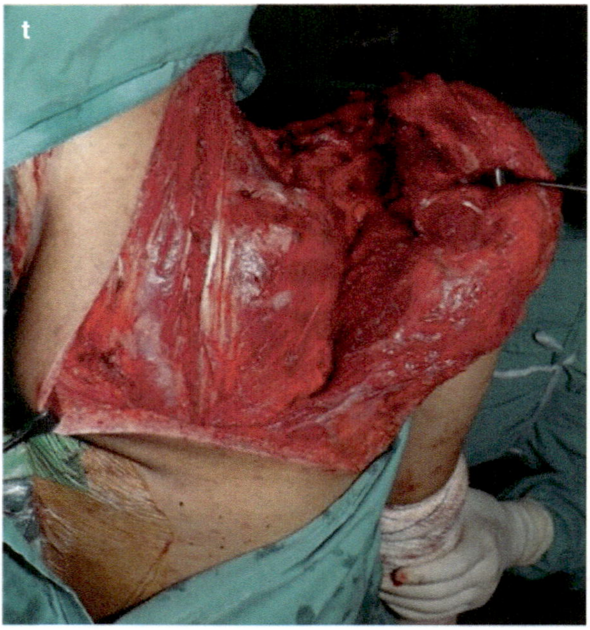

Options of Reconstruction

- Endoprosthesis reconstruction
- Suspension arthroplasty

Tickhoff-Lindberg 'suspension arthroplasty' reconstruction whereby the humeral head is attached to the lateral clavicle with tape. The head is medialised to facilitate muscle closure and the remaining deltoid is attached to the clavicle and remnant of the periscapular muscle (Fig. 3a–e). It provides a stable shoulder with minimal abduction and flexion for good elbow and hand function. Overall, functional outcome is low to average.

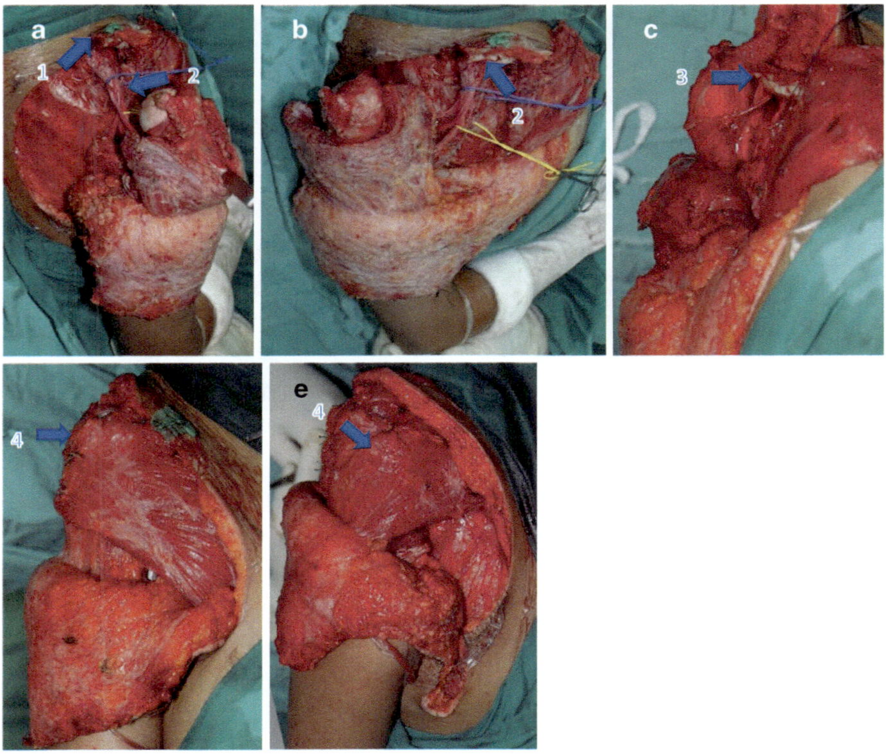

1. Remnant of the lateral clavicle
2. Axillary vessels and brachial plexus
3. The humeral head is stabilised to the lateral clavicle using Mersilene tape
4. Pectoralis major was sutured to the deltoid muscle

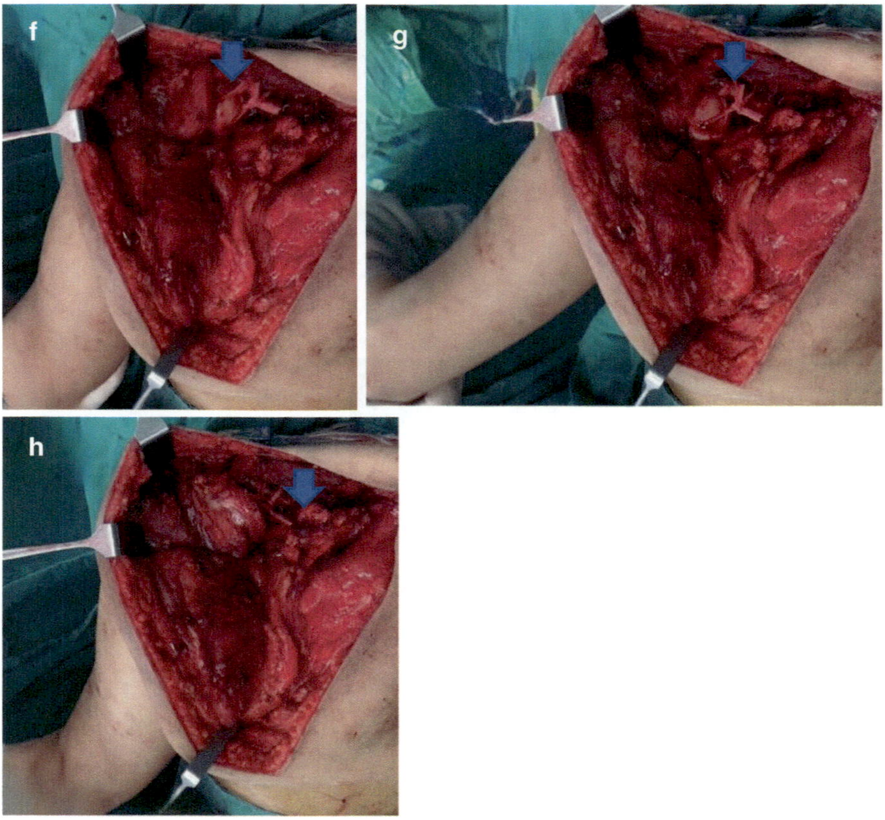

Stability of the reconstruction was tested through a range of motion of abduction and rotation with telescoping forces (Fig. 3f–h).

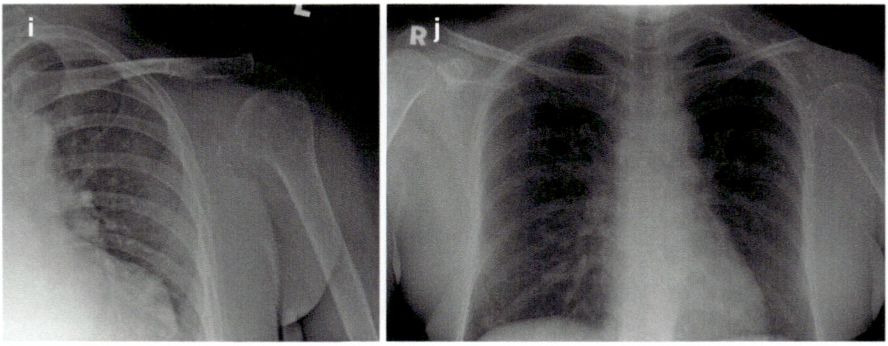

Late reconstruction failure due to lateral clavicle fracture (Fig. 3I, j).

Suspension arthroplasty resulted in low functional score due to loss of fulcrum for abduction and forward flexion. Medialisation of the deltoid and primary apposition with the pectoralis created a stable scar for protection suspension; however, it left the shoulder stiff.

Resection of Scapula Exostoses

Exostosis of the inner table of the scapula caused pain due to chronic irritation of scapulothoracic articulation; additionally, pressure effect on the thoracic cage also led to rib deformity (Fig. 4a–e).

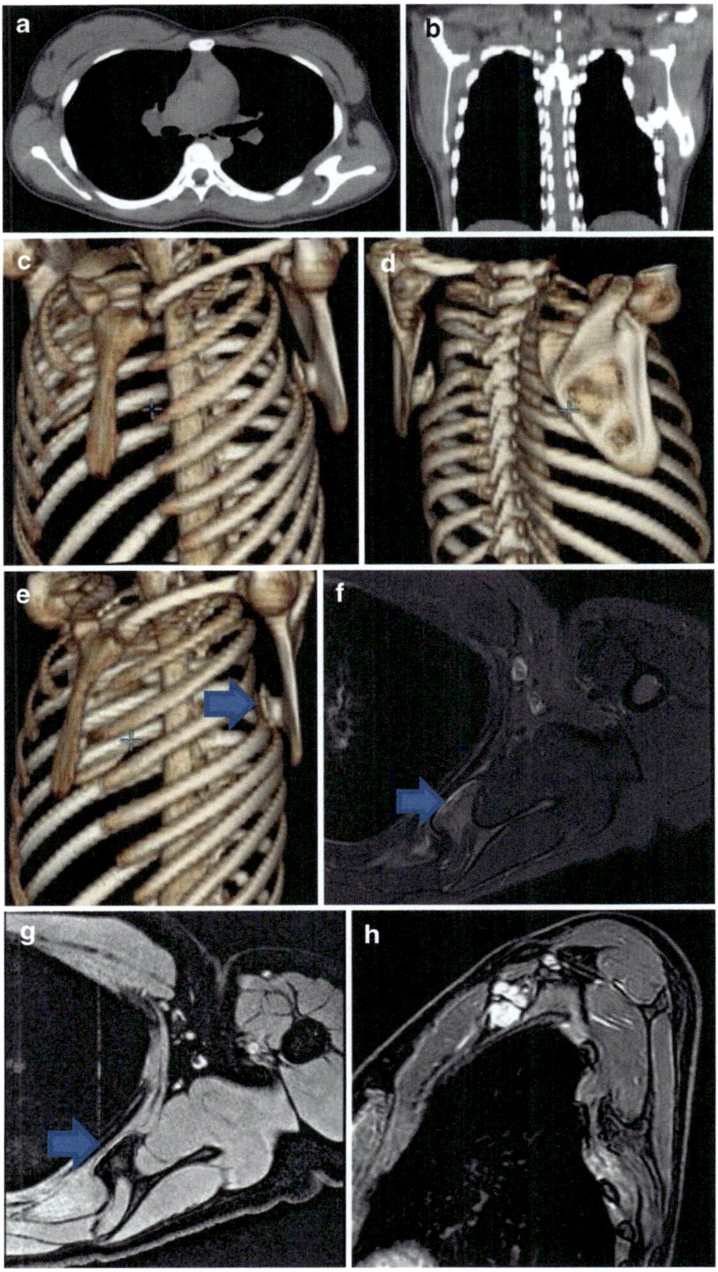

MRI was done to evaluate the cartilage cap thickness and rule out malignancy (Fig. 4f–h).

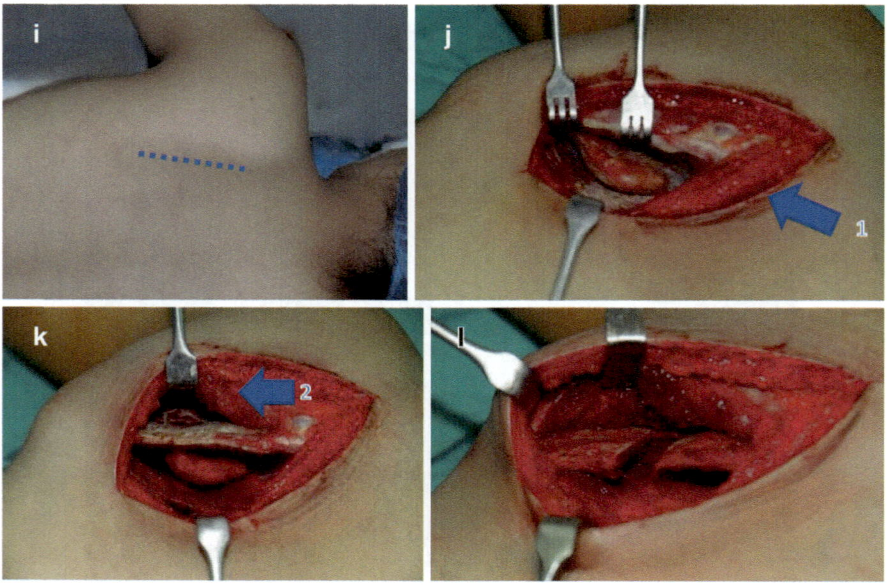

- Trapezius muscle
- Infraspinatus muscle

The sessile stalk was identified at the inner wall of the scapula after mobilisation of subscapularis muscle. A guided saw osteotomy was then performed over the entire base of exostosis for final mobilisation and complete removal of exostosis (Fig. 4i–l).

Partial Scapulectomy and Glenoid Using Computer-Guided Bony Resection

A case of benign myoblastic tumour involving inferior border of scapula up to the scapula spine and extending to 1/3 of the inferior glenoid (Fig. 5a–i). In view of benign and aggressive behaviour, a narrow bony margin was planned with glenoid resection to minimise surgical morbidity.

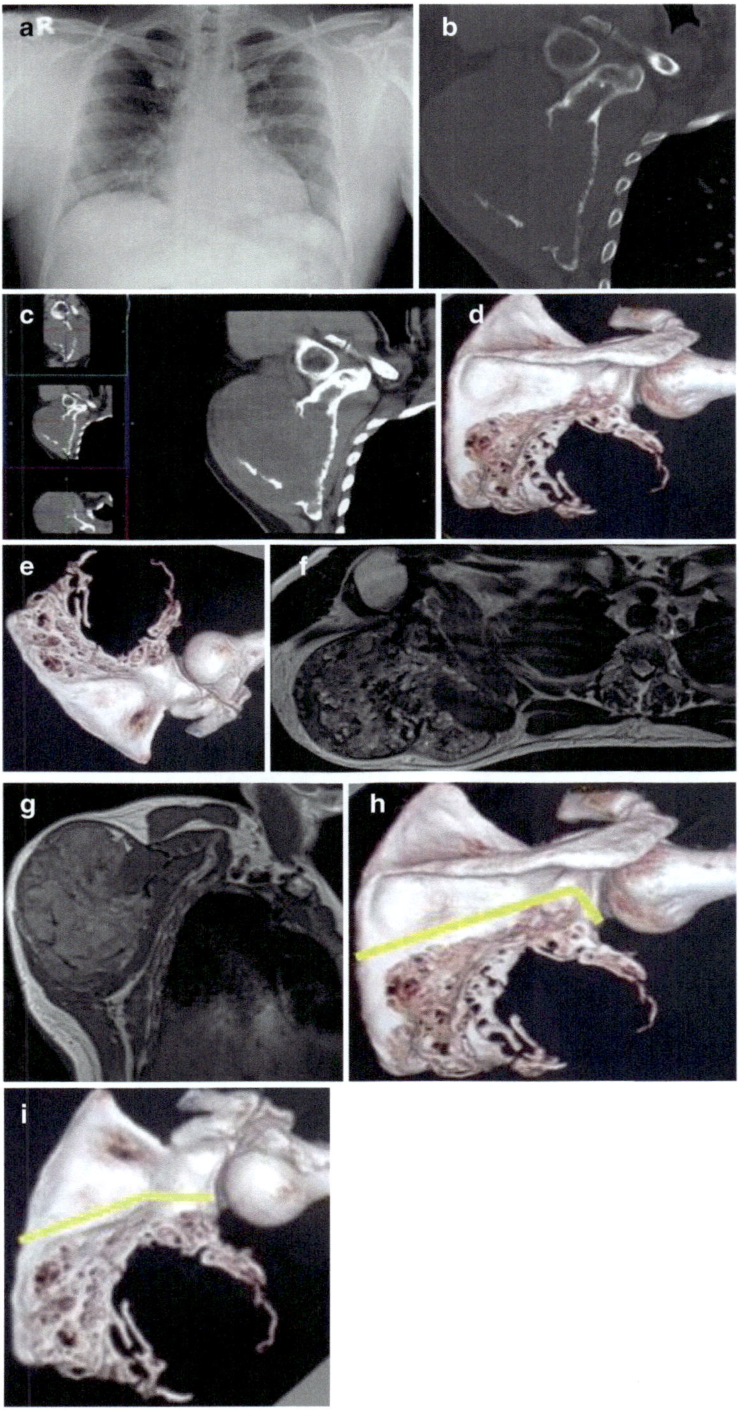
a R
b
c
d
e
f
g
h
i

The navigation-guided resection was aimed for complete resection of scapula below scapula spine with 1 cm margin and inferior half of the scapula with 5 mm margin. Two plane resection lines were planned to achieve complete resection margin (Fig. 5j–m).

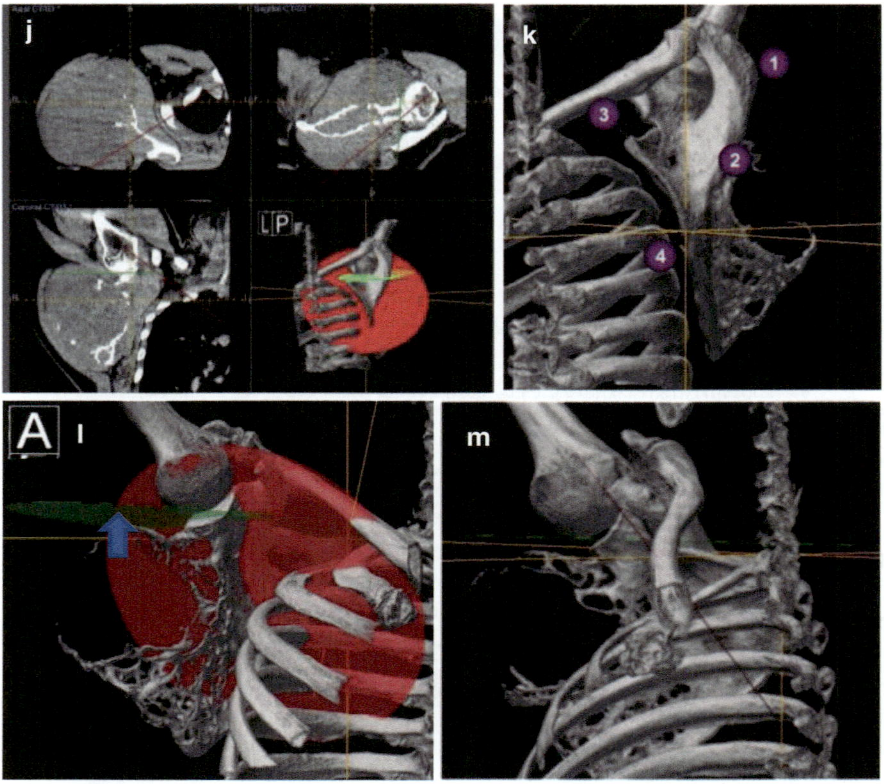

Intersection line of horizontal cut below the scapula spine to the partial glenoid cut

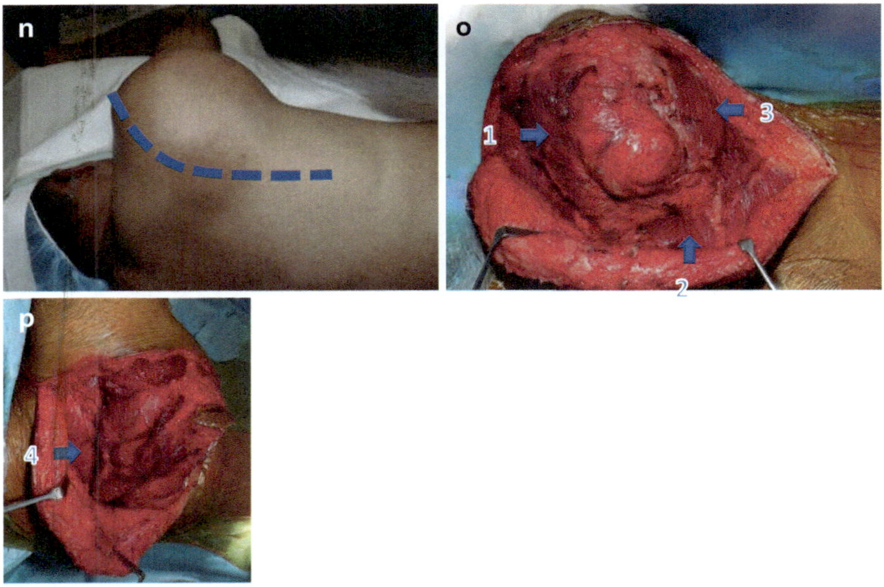
n
o
1
2
3
p
4

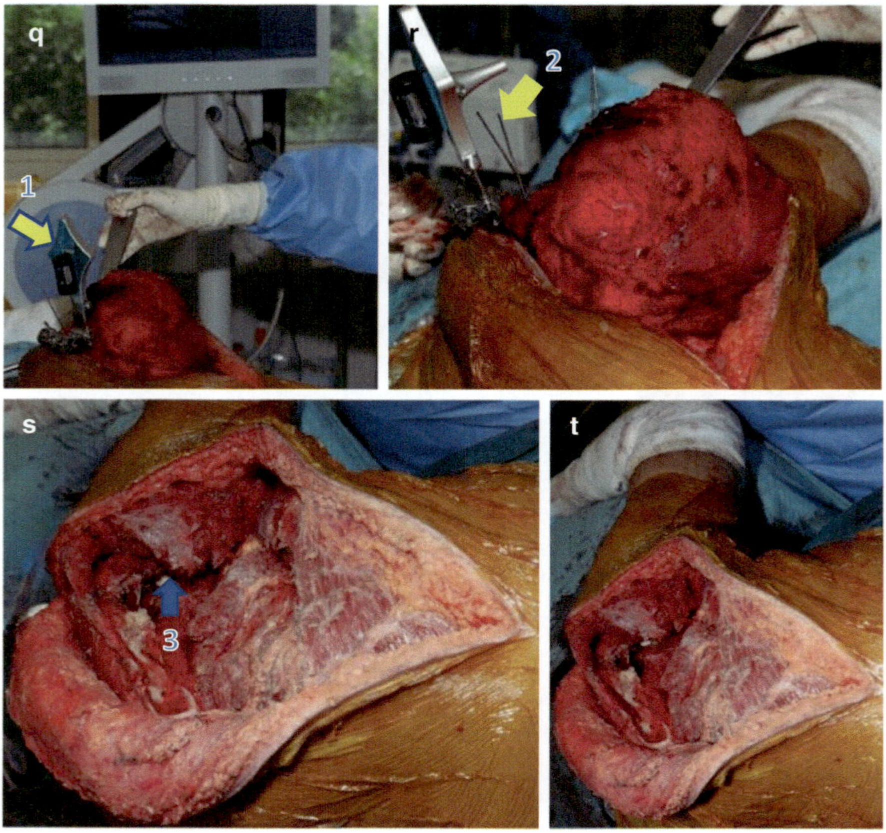

Incision involves creating medial and lateral flap of scapula for exposure to the coracoid process. The fist layer muscle trapezius and deltoid were elevated from medial border and scapula spine. All muscles attached to the lower border of scapula were detached—rhomboid, latissimus dorsi, and teres origin and attachment. The lower border of scapula was elevated from chest wall together with subscapularis muscle as anterior margin (Fig. 5n–p).

1. Deltoid origin at scapula spine
2. Trapezius muscle
3. Teres major
4. Supraspinatus muscle

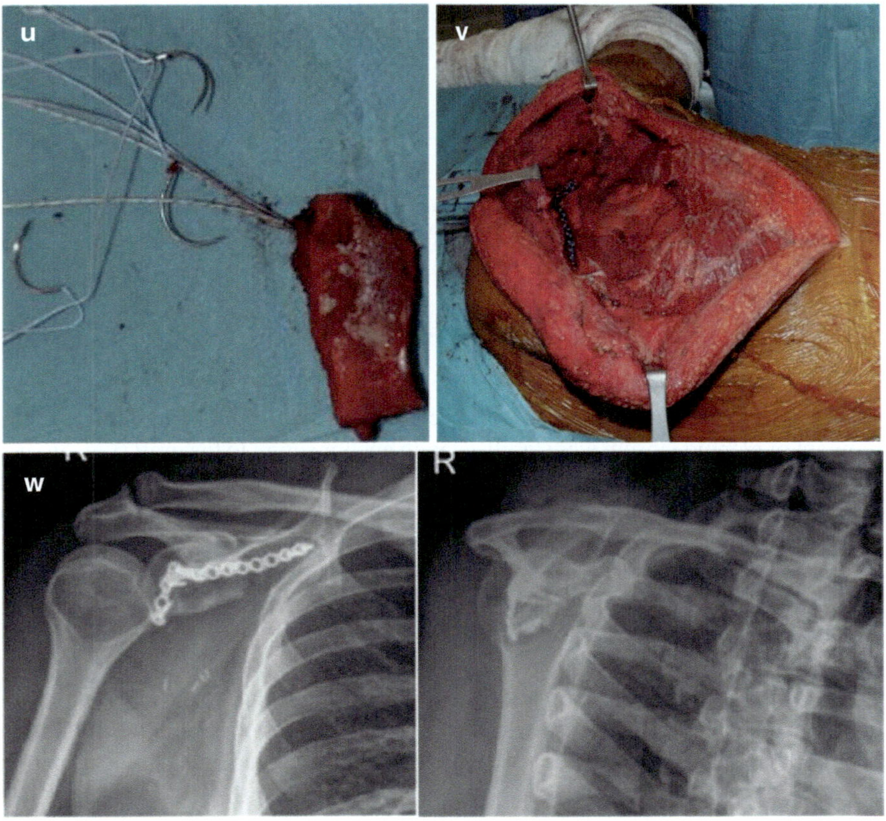

The tracker stabilised at the scapula spine, and 4-point bony references were identified for anatomical confirmation. Subsequently, multiple K-wires were inserted to outline the site and direction of osteotomy (Fig. 5q–t).

1. Tracker stabilised at the scapula spine
2. Multiple K wire as guidance for osteotomy
3. Humeral head and remnant of glenoid labrum

x

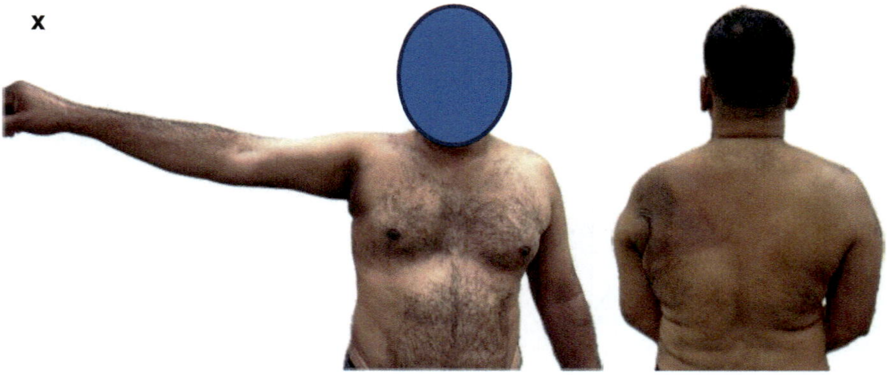

The inferior border of scapula was reconstructed with iliac bone graft and the remnant of glenoid labrum was stabilised with anchor suture to the graft (Fig. 5u–w). Two years after surgery and local radiotherapy, the patient was able to have good functional shoulder (Fig. 5x). Text supposed to be below the reconstruction procedure.

Resection of Acromion and Lateral Clavicle

This is a case of chondroid lesion of acromion with soft tissue extension to posterior deltoid, supraspinatus, and infraspinatus muscle. There is medial extension to the lateral clavicle and posterior deltoid which should be included as surgical margin (Fig. 6a–e).

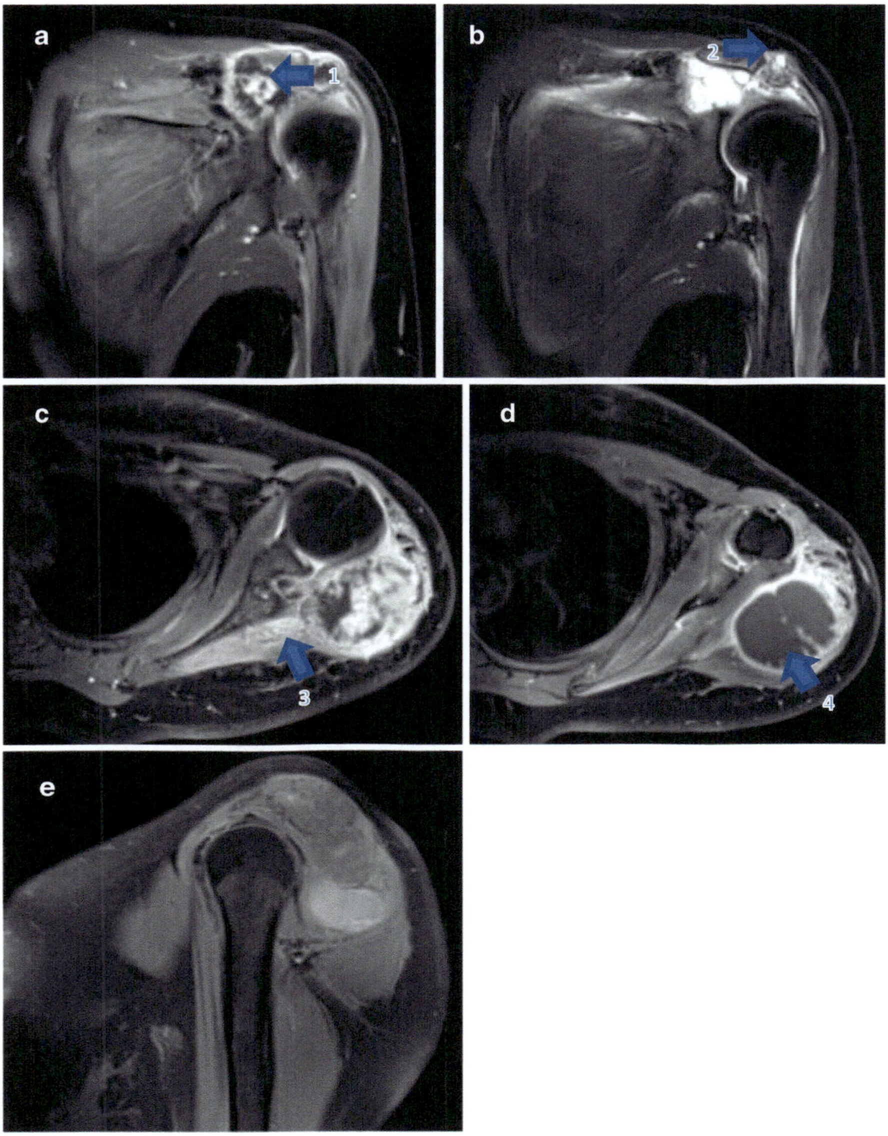

1. Acromion
2. Acromion-clavicular joint
3. Supraspinatus
4. Posterior deltoid

Fasciocutaneous flaps were created to expose the entire shoulder, posteriorly below the scapula origin of deltoid and below clavicle anteriorly. The posterior deltoid was detached from deltoid origin at the scapula spine and its insertion at the humeral tuberosity for good margin. The entire supraspinatus and infraspinatus were removed subperiosteally, and finally the scapula spine was detached from scapula for mobilisation of entire acromion with remaining soft tissue attached. The lateral clavicle was removed as part of margin due to acromion-clavicular joint involvement (Fig. 6f–i).

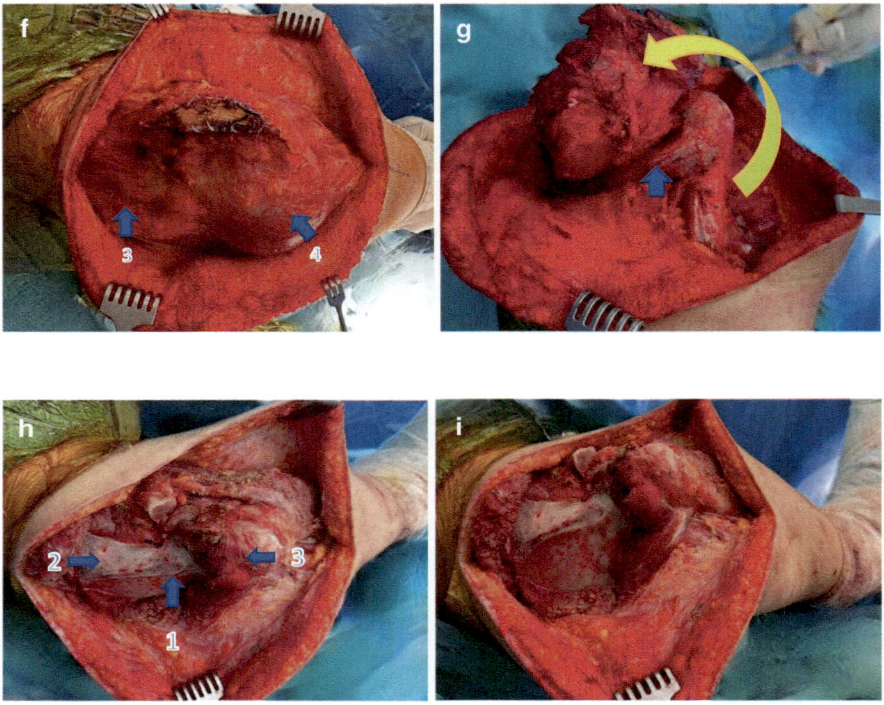

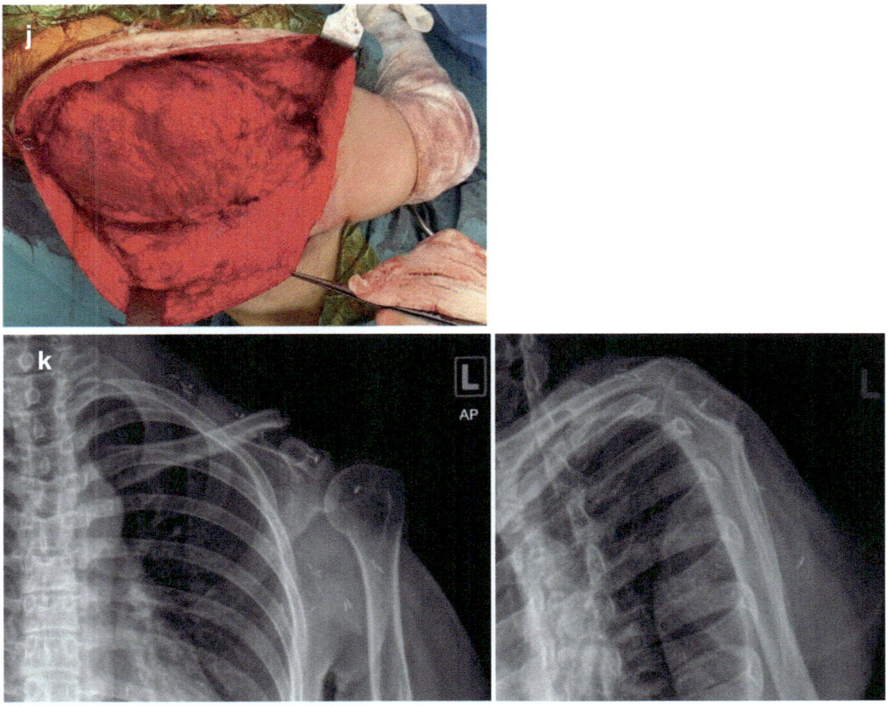

- Remnant scapula spine
- Suprascapular fossae
- Humeral head

Rotational latissimus dorsi flap was performed to cover the exposed scapula and clavicle, shoulder padding and contour and motorised to the remnant rotator cuff tendon and deltoid to strengthen shoulder abduction (Fig. 6j, k)

Scapular Prosthesis

Scapula prosthesis created a stable articulation fulcrum for the shoulder joint and results in lateralisation for deltoid function. Key structures to be protected are the axillary nerve and posterior circumflex vessels to the deltoid.

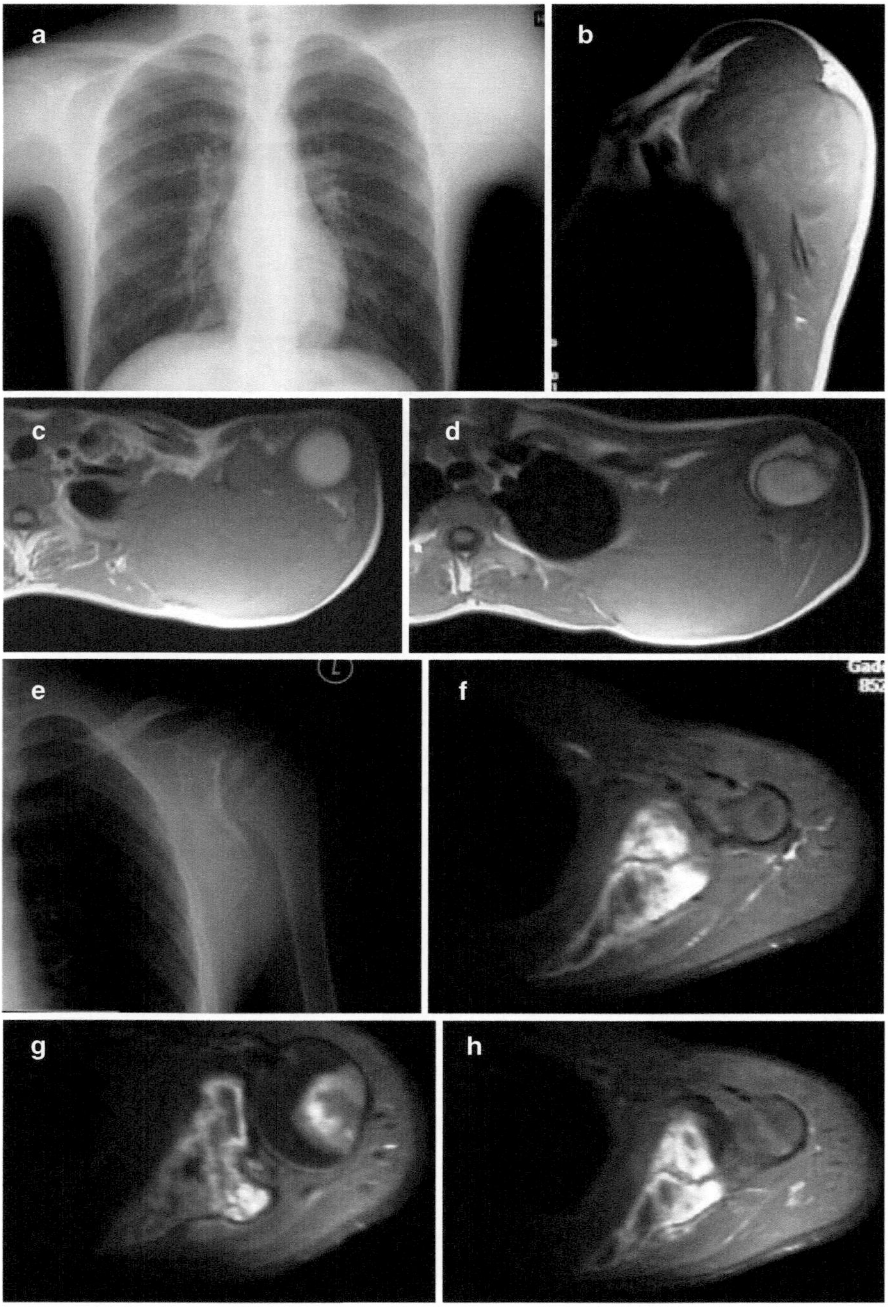

A 17-year-old boy with Ewing's scapula that responded well to chemotherapy with almost 100% necrosis on restaging. The initial MRI revealed the entire scapula involved with massive soft tissue oedema entire scapulae. Post-chemotherapy MRI showed complete resolution of the soft tissue component (Fig. 7a–h).

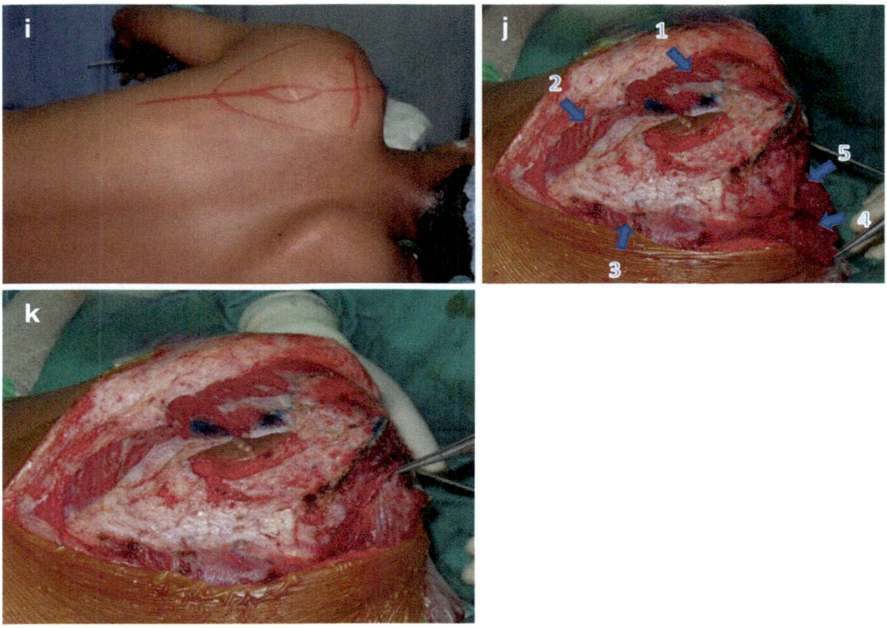

The entire muscle mass enveloping and attached to the scapula was planned for excision as part of the oncological margin (Fig. 7i–k).

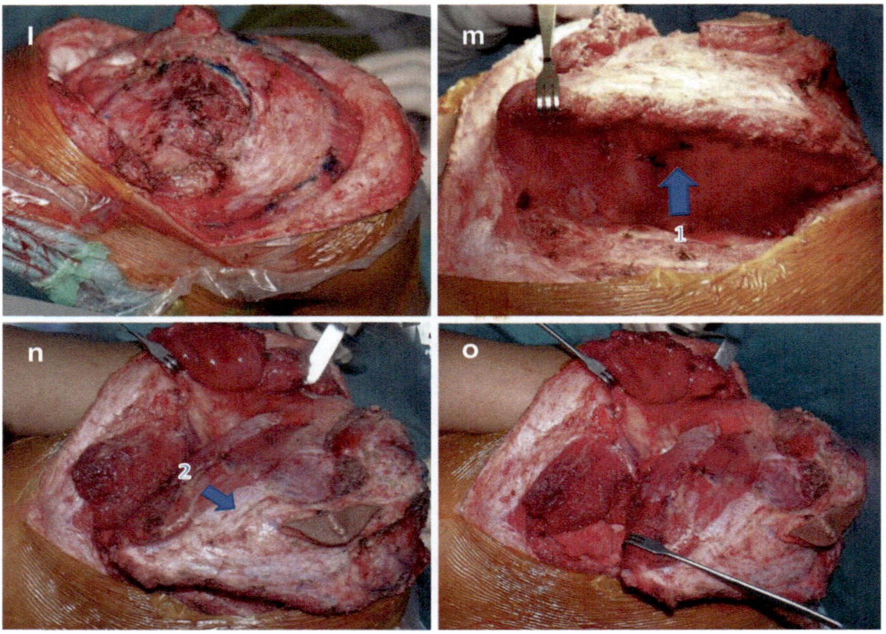

1. Deltoid-scapula origin
2. Teres major and minor
3. Rhomboid major and minor
4. Trapezius
5. Levator scapula

The trapezius muscle is detached from the medial and superior border of scapula to expose the second layer of muscles. The scapula was mobilise superior and lateral maintaining the subscapularis as an oncological border. The teres major and minor and deltoid are detached from the lateral border until the tendon of the rotator cuff and head are identified (Fig. 7l–q).

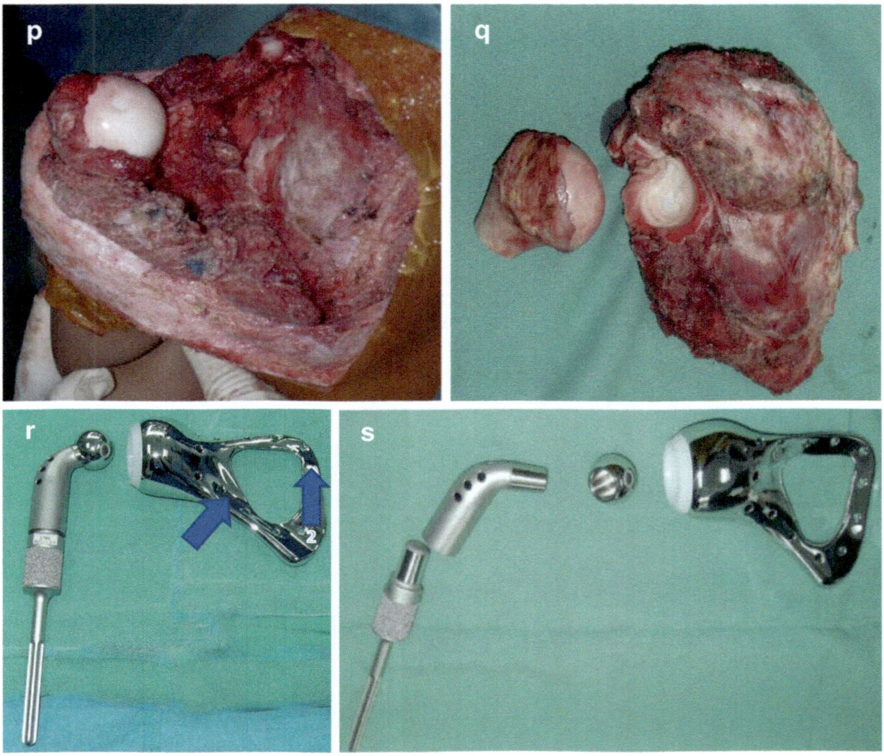

Para scapula muscle anatomical margin

1. Subscapularis muscle
2. infraspinatus

The entire scapula was mobilised anteriorly, all the tendons attached to the coracoid process and ligaments were detached to release the scapula from the clavicle and surrounding structures.

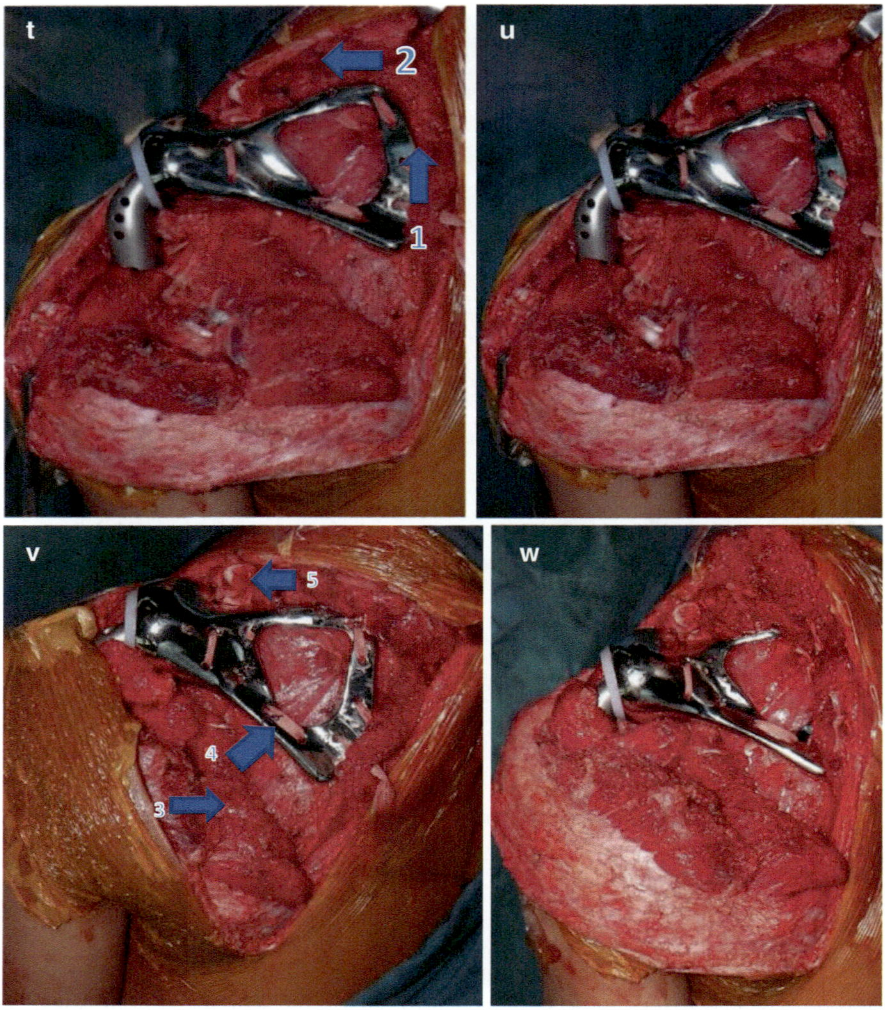

A custom-made constrained scapula requires resection of the proximal humerus below the tuberosity as all the rotator cuffs muscles were removed as oncological margin. It was designed with multiple small holes over the border for soft tissue reconstruction to stabilise the scapula (Fig. 7r, s).

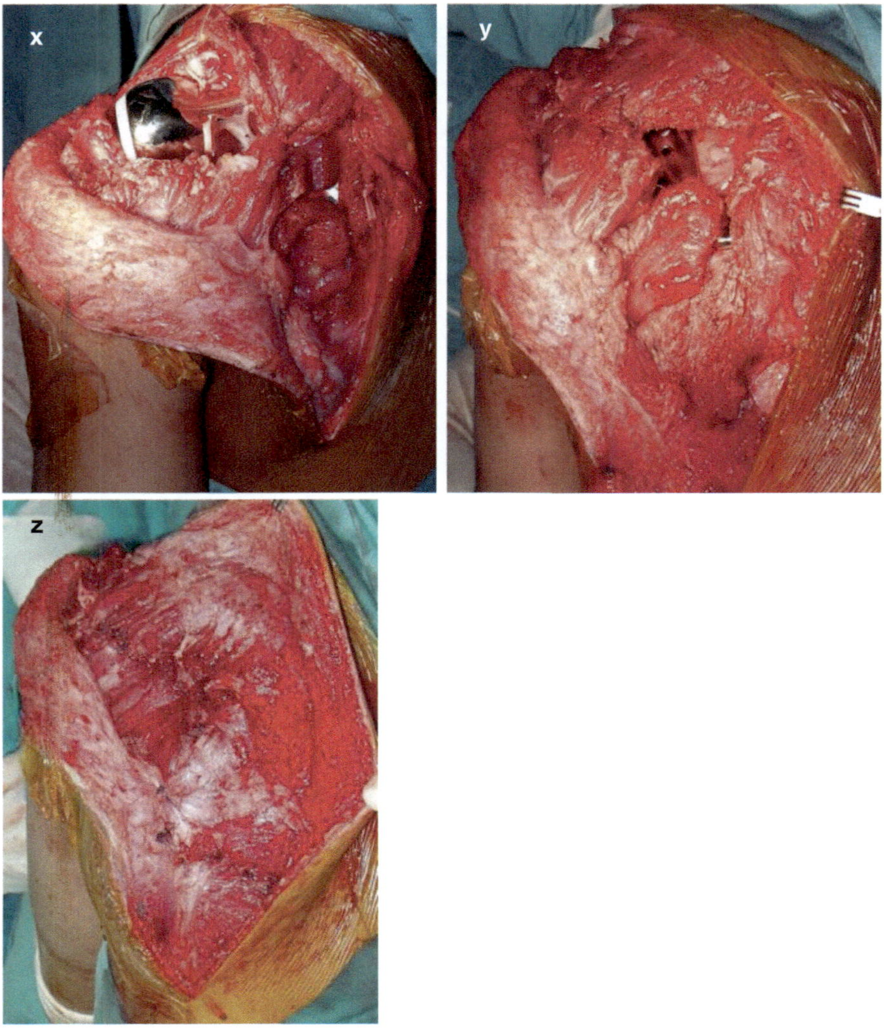

The scapula prosthesis was stabilised and sutured to remaining scapula stabiliser muscles (Fig. 7t–w):

1. Rhomboid major and minor
2. Levator scapulae
3. Teres minor and major
4. Intercostal muscle
5. Clavicle

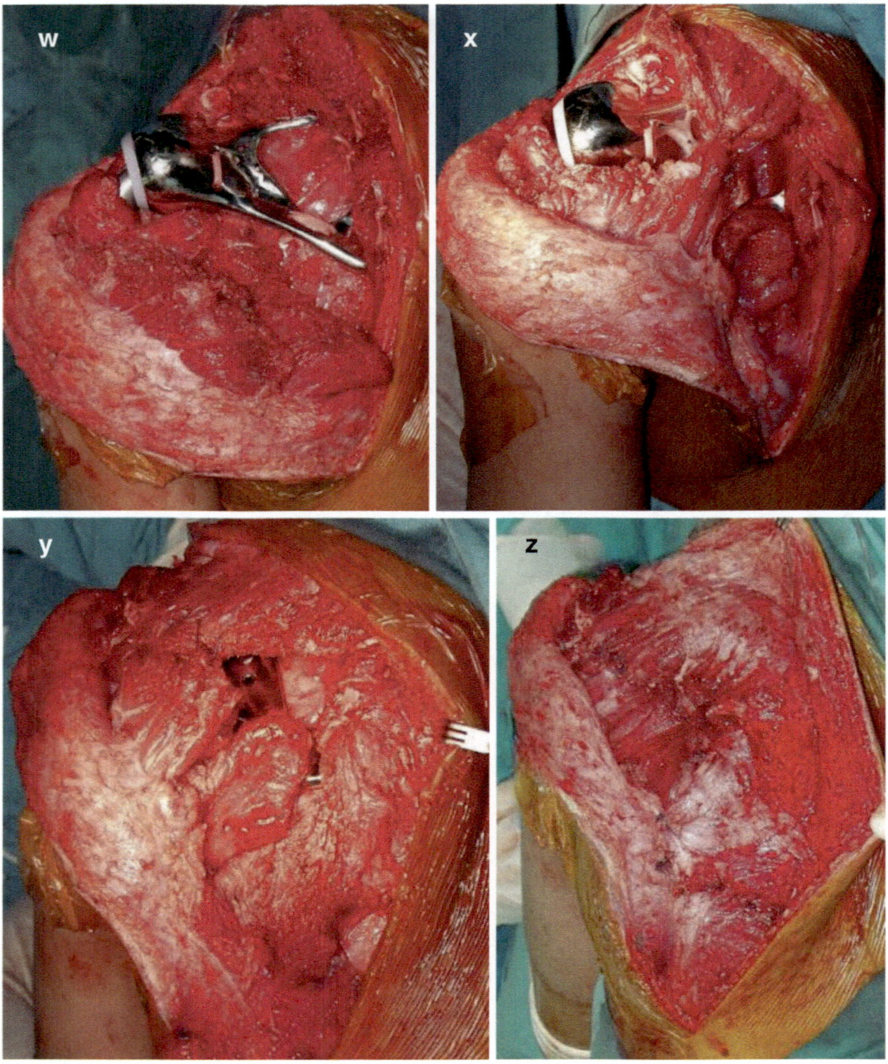

Reconstruction of the posterior deltoid to the remnant trapezius is possible as the scapula prosthesis is smaller and in a medial position compared to original scapula (Fig. 7t–z). Deltoid and shoulder contour were maintained (Fig. 7aa–ac).

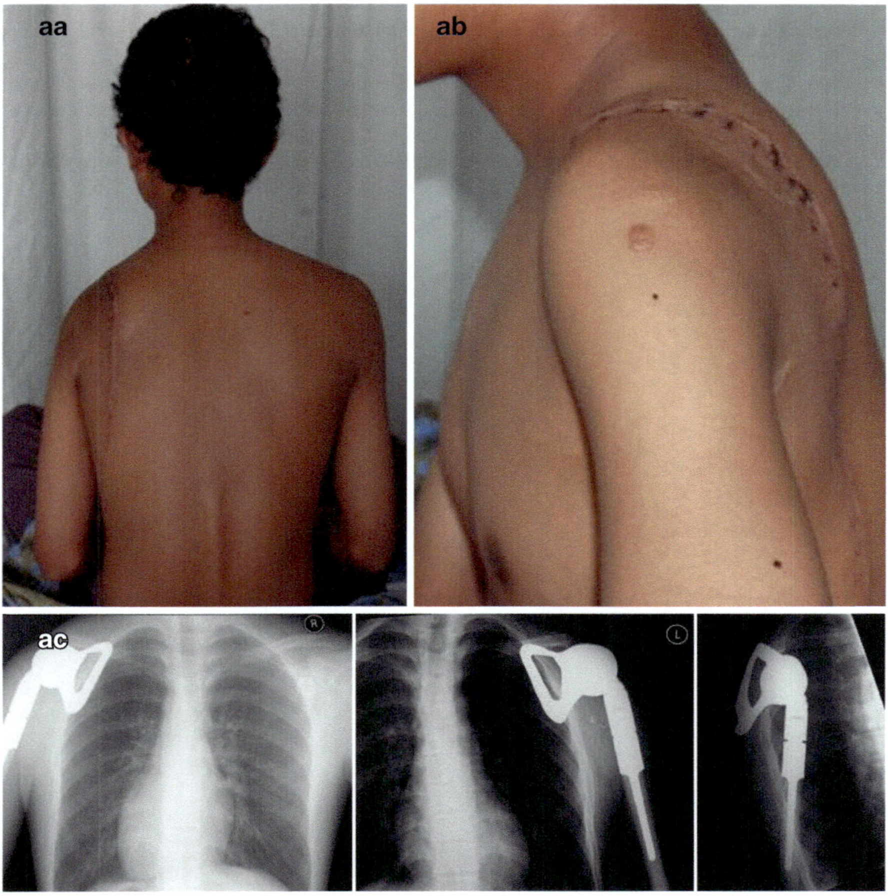

Suggested Reading

1. Hayashi K, Karita M, Yamamoto N, Shirai T, Nishida H, Takeuchi A, Kimura H, Miwa S, Tsuchiya H. Functional outcomes after total scapulectomy for malignant bone or soft tissue tumors in the shoulder girdle. Int J Clin Oncol. 2011;16(5):568–73.
2. Ippolito JA, Thomson JE, Lesson MC, Monson DK, Aboulafia A, Benevenia J. Endoprosthetic total scapula replacement versus suspension arthroplasty following tumor resection. J Surg Oncol. 2018;
3. Benevenia J, Cavanaugh Z, Ippolito J, Thomson J, Guinand L. Implant reconstruction of the shoulder girdle: scapular prosthesis. In: Orthopaedic surgical oncology for bone tumors. Springer Nature Switzerland; 2022. p. 391–9.
4. Mavrogenis AF, Mastorakos DP, Triantafyllopoulos G, Sakellariou VI, Galanis EC, Papagelopoulos PJ. Total scapulectomy and constrained reverse total shoulder reconstruction for a Ewing's sarcoma. J Surg Oncol. 2009;100(7):611–5.

5. Mayil Vahanan N, Mohanlal P, Bose JC, Gangadharan R, Karthisundar V. The functional and oncological results after scapulectomy for scapular tumours: 2-16-year results. Int Orthop. 2007;31(6):831–6.
6. Papagelopoulos PJ, Mavrogenis AF. Total scapulectomy and reconstruction using a scapular prosthesis. In: Master techniques in orthopaedic surgery orthopaedic oncology and complex reconstruction. Lippincott Williams & Wilkins, A Wolters Kluwer; 2011. p. 293–305.
7. Puchner SE, Panotopoulos J, Puchner R, Schuh R, Windhager R, Funovics PT. Primary malignant tumours of the scapula – a review of 29 cases. Int Orthop. 2014;38(10):2155–62.

Resection Proximal Humerus and Shoulder Girdle

Wan Faisham Nu'man Bin Wan Ismail

Proximal humerus is a common site for primary malignant sarcoma and metastases. The anatomical relations are complicated; however, limb salvage surgery is possible in majority of the cases and amputation is rarely performed for sarcoma. Advancement of resection and reconstruction is based on the Tikhoff-Linberg procedure, wide margin resection, and shoulder suspension reconstruction for elbow and hand function. Malawer classified the type of resection from I to VI based on tumour involvement and resection margins around the shoulder joint and scapulae girdle.

Surgical Anatomy

The anatomical barrier for tumour extension around the shoulder girdle is complex due to multiple tendon and muscle attachments. The deltoid is a good anatomical barrier for the entire proximal metaphyseal humerus. The long head of the biceps tendon that runs in the bicipital groove is usually infiltrated in high-grade sarcoma with anterior extension. The attachment of the infra- and supraspinatus and subscapularis must be carefully evaluated for direct tumour infiltration. The tumour over the meta-diaphyseal region must be evaluated for direct infiltration to the pectoralis major, latissimus dorsi, and teres major insertions.

- The axillary artery passes the inferior border of the axilla to form the brachial artery that runs together with the median, ulnar, and radial nerves medially.

W. F. N. B. W. Ismail (✉)
Prince Court Medical Center, Kuala Lumpur, Malaysia

Orthopaedic Oncology Reconstructive Unit, Universiti Sains Malaysia, Kubang Kerian, Kelantan, Malaysia

A. Puri, W. F. N. B. W. Ismail (eds.), *Atlas of Orthopedic Oncology Volume 2*,
https://doi.org/10.1007/978-981-95-8962-3_12

- The brachial artery supplies the biceps muscle with multiple muscular perforator branches. Care must be taken to maintain this perforator during exploration to minimise devascularisation of the biceps.
- Musculocutaneous nerve arises from the lateral cord just distal to the coracoid process, passes through the coracobrachialis, and runs between the brachialis and biceps.
- The axillary nerve travels through the quadrangular space together with the posterior circumflex artery and vein at the posterior border of the surgical neck of the humerus and runs beneath the deltoid muscle and supplies the deltoid.
- The radial nerve comes off the posterior cord of the plexus and continues anterior to the latissimus dorsi and teres major. Just distal to the teres major, the nerve courses into the posterior aspect of the arm to run between the medial and long head of the triceps.

Shoulder joint involvement determines whether the resection is intraarticular or extraarticular.

Assessment

Surgical classification of proximal humerus resection for sarcoma is based on the surgical margin and relation of the tumour to the anatomical compartment and status of the glenohumeral joint. The deltoid muscle that envelopes the proximal humerus is an important structure for oncological clearance in extra-compartment malignant tumour. MRI assessment, particularly tissue plane to the deltoid muscle and glenohumeral involvement, is an important step prior surgical resection.

MRI assessment for extraosseous tumour extension includes the following:

- Insertion of the tendon to the proximal humerus: subscapularis, supraspinatus, infraspinatus, pectoralis major, latissimus dorsi, and teres major
- Sarcoma with anterior extension: coracobrachialis and straight head and long head biceps tendon
- Sarcoma with posterior extension: long head triceps
- Shoulder capsule and glenoid joint
- Extension beyond the shoulder joint through the subscapularis, supraspinatus, and infraspinatus muscle and tendon

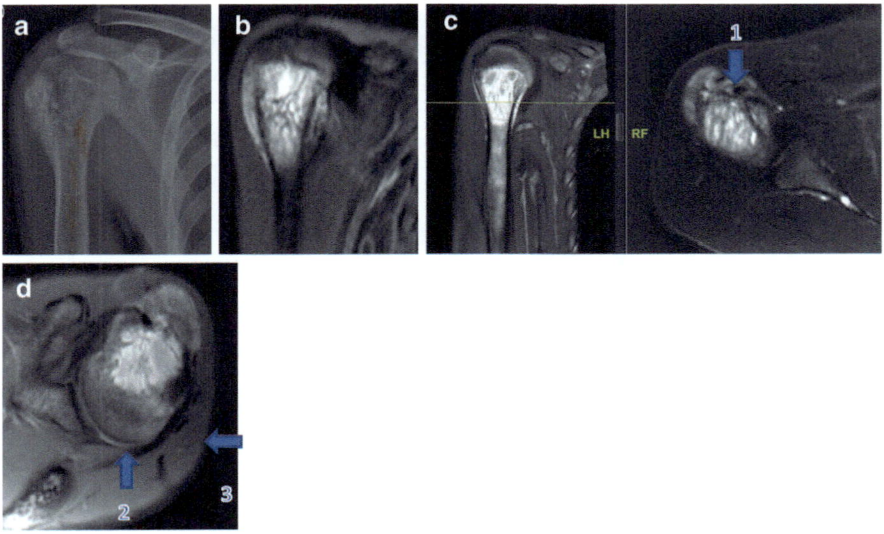

1. Long head biceps within bicipital groove
2. Free shoulder joint
3. Posterior deltoid

The osteosarcoma of the proximal humerus responded well to neoadjuvant chemotherapy with extension of the anterolateral compartment of the deltoid. The posterior plane to the deltoid was still intact. The long head of the biceps was involved; however, the glenohumeral joint was free (Fig. 1a–d).

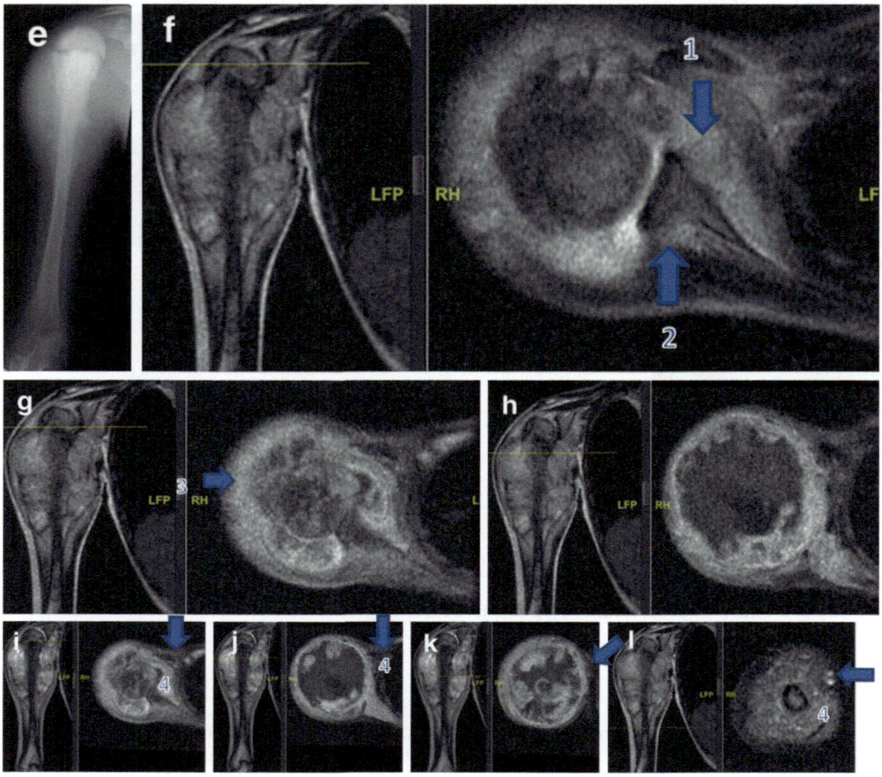

1. Subscapularis muscle involvement
2. Supraspinatus muscle involvement
3. Entire deltoid infiltrated by sarcoma
4. Brachial artery with major nerve from axillary fossae to mid arm

Proximal humerus osteosarcoma with poor response to chemotherapy showed extensive tumour extension to the entire deltoid. The subscapularis muscle and glenohumeral joint were involved with tumour extension. Type V resection involved extraarticular resection and parts of scapula to achieve good oncological clearance (Fig. 1e–l).

Simple Resection of Proximal Humerus Osteosarcoma (Type I)

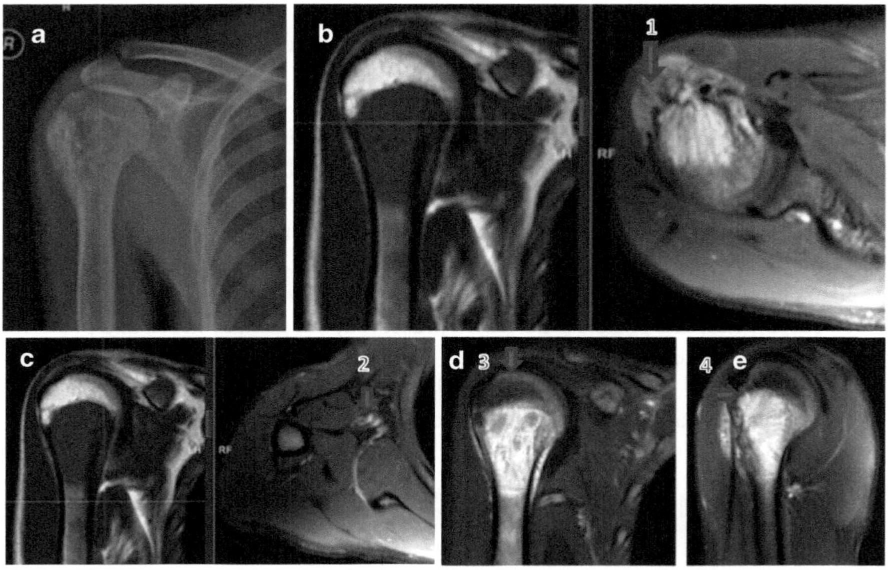

1. Osteosarcoma extension to anterior deltoid with clear plane to posterior deltoid muscle
   (Fig. 2a–e)
2. Brachial neurovascular structures
3. Supraspinatus tendon—free from tumour extension
4. Greater tuberosity

Surgical Steps (Fig. 2f–p)

Surgical steps technique for intraarticular resection of proximal humerus sarcoma that has responded to chemotherapy with minimal anterior extraosseous extension.

The anterior approach utilises the deltopectoral approach, which includes excision of the biopsy scar as part of the surgical margin.

- The pectoralis major is released from humerus insertion and reflected medially.
- The conjoined tendon is detached from the coracoid process for visualisation of the second layer structure and identification of tendon attachment.
- The pectoralis major, coracobrachialis, and biceps muscles are reflected medially with the neurovascular structure.

- Care must be given to the lateral plexus whereby the musculocutaneous nerve will pierce the coracobrachialis and biceps muscles and supply it for elbow flexion.
- Additional release of the pectoralis minor will expose the axillary space. The axillary artery and vein and infraclavicular part of the brachial plexus can be explored completely.
- The long head of the biceps is cut at the level of pectoralis major insertion as it lies closely in the bicipital groove and is usually infiltrated by an extraosseous anterior tumour.
- The attachment of the latissimus dorsi and teres major are also detached from the humerus by external rotation of the entire humerus. The medial structures are also completely released.
- In cases where the posterior deltoid is preserved, the axillary nerve and posterior circumflex humeral artery are explored and protected. Distal humerus osteotomy and release of all rotator cuff muscle through intraarticular resection helps manipulate the axillary nerve and vessels that supply the deltoid.

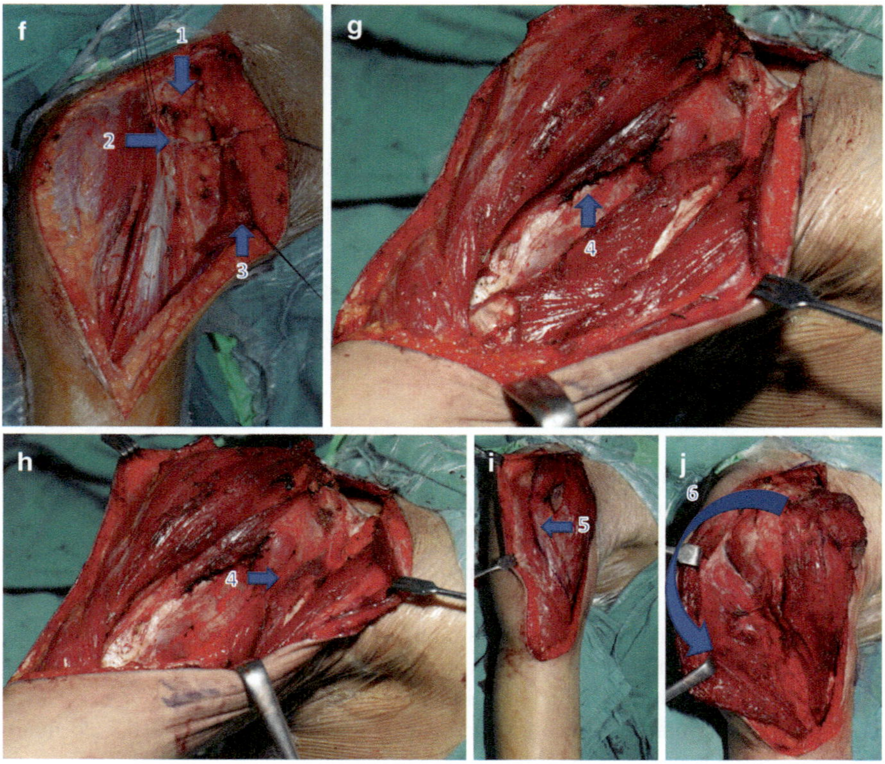

1. Coracoid process
2. Conjoin tendon—coracobrachialis, biceps, and pectoralis minor

3. Pectoralis major muscle detached from humeral insertion
4. Long head biceps in bicipital groove
5. Plan anterior deltoid resection as margin
6. Mobilisation of posterior deltoid

The anterior deltoid muscle and biopsy scars, which were confirmed infiltrated on MRI, were removed in total as the oncological margin. Posterior deltoid with posterior axillary vessels and nerve were mobilised from the proximal humerus (Fig. 2h–j). The oncological barrier by thick periosteum was adequate to maintain quality margin.

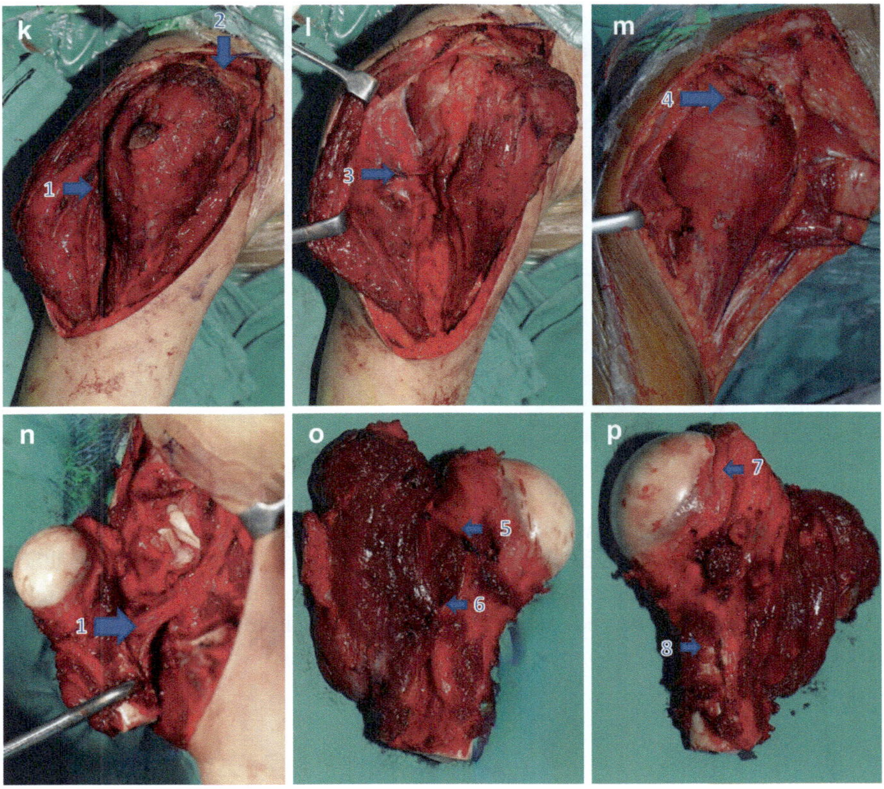

1. Posterior circumflex humeral artery
2. Acromion
3. Rotator cuff tendon—supraspinatus and infraspinatus
4. Arcuate artery from posterior circumflex humeral artery
5. Lesser tuberosity and remnant subscapularis
6. Bicipital groove and long head biceps

7. Greater tuberosity and rotator cuff tendon insertion
8. Insertion of teres major

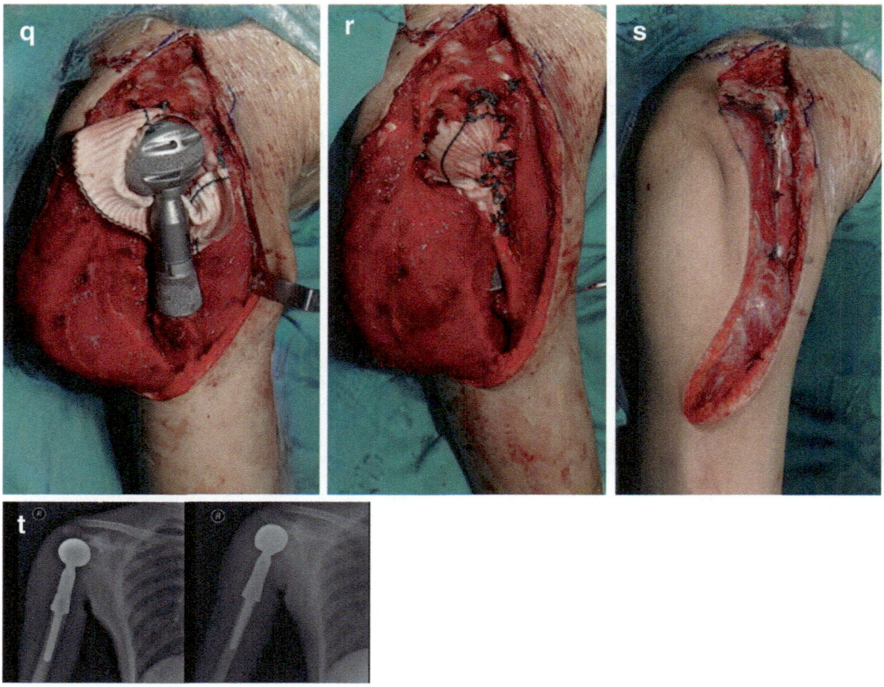

The final reconstruction with cemented proximal humerus endoprosthesis and stability of shoulder joint was provided by purse string PTFE vascular graft attached to remaining capsule and glenoid labrum. The remnant of rotator cuff was attached to the prosthesis, the conjoin tendon was reattach to coracoid process, and the remnant biceps tendon to the pectoralis major insertion. Deltoid was mobilised anteriorly and interrupted close to the pectoralis muscle insertion (Fig. 2q–t).

Options for Bone Reconstruction

Few options have been described for reconstruction of osseous defect for the proximal humerus:

- Endoprosthesis
- Reimplantation of sterilised tumour bone using extracorporeal radiation using single 60 Gy or cryotherapy with liquid nitrogen
- Osteoarticular allograft/allograft arthrodesis/combination vascularised fibula graft

The head of the humerus is suspended, and the remaining glenoid and rotator cuff muscle were reattached to the prosthesis for function. Stability of the head of the humerus prosthesis can be achieved by purse-string suture around the head to the remaining glenoid labrum using gore-tex vascular graft, prolene mesh, or Trevira tube (Fig. 2u–w).

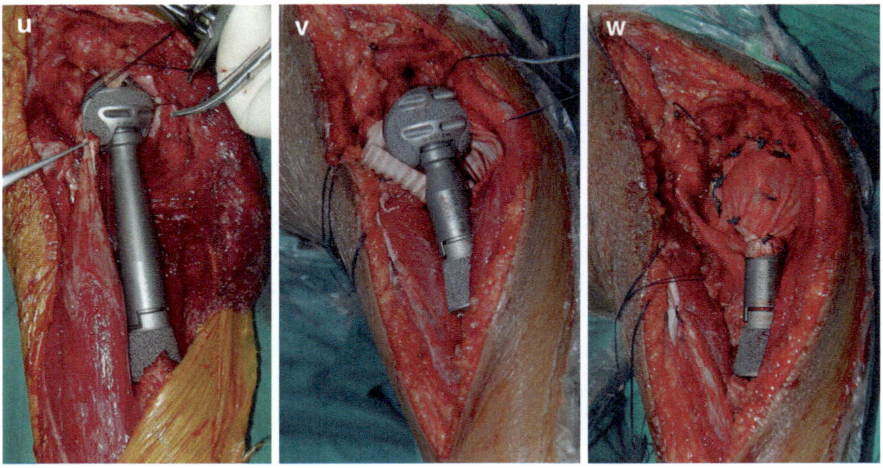

Intraosseous Chondrosarcoma with Minimal Soft Tissue Resection

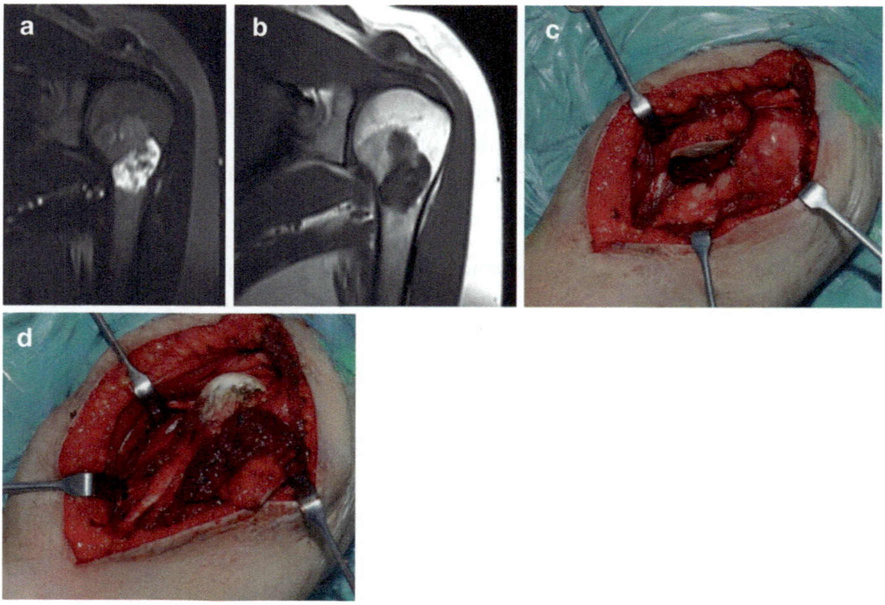

The margin for intraosseous sarcoma without soft tissue extension mainly in low-grade tumour is adequate just above the periosteum. All functional tendon and structures attached to the proximal humerus can be maintained for final reconstruction. Trevira tube is used to wrap around prosthesis for stability of shoulder and attachments of insertion rotator cuff for abduction (Fig. 3a–l).

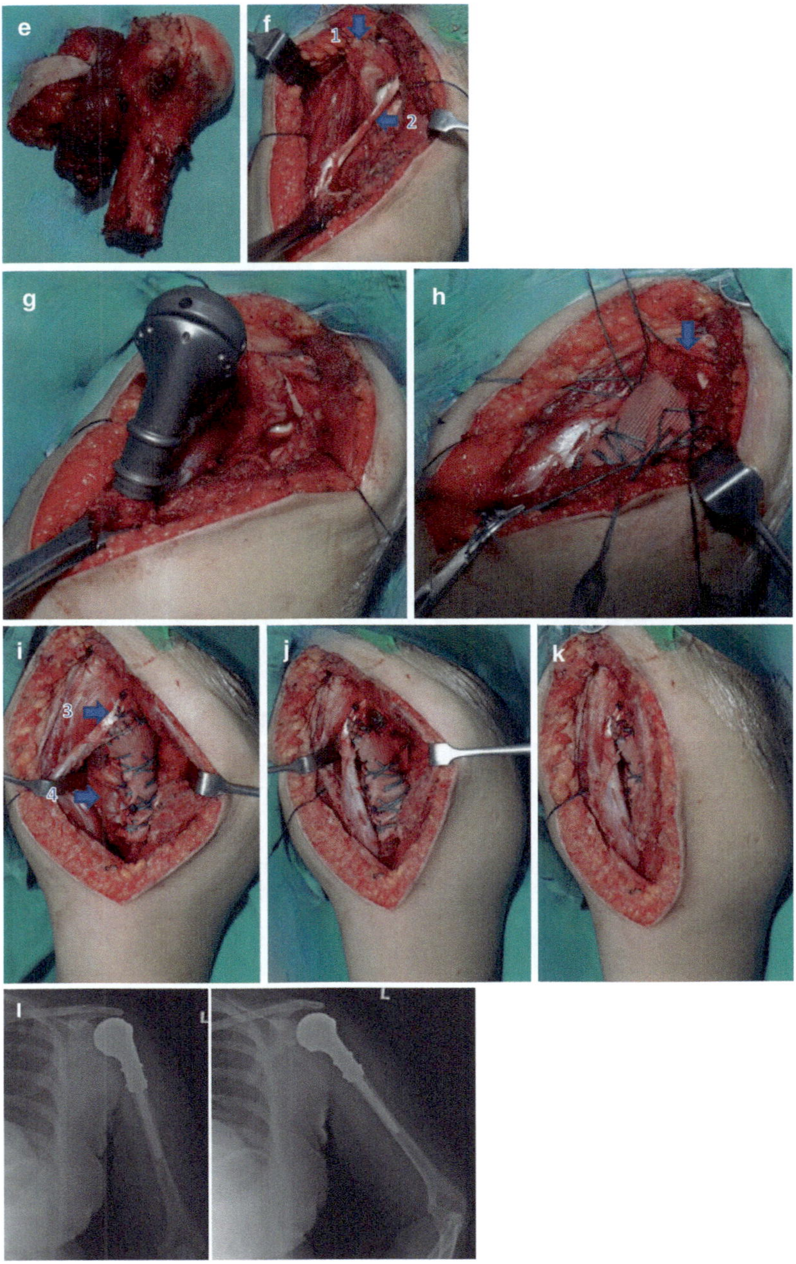

1. Infraspinatus and supraspinatus tendon
2. Long head biceps tendon
3. Reattachment of rotator cuff tendon to Trevira tube
4. Reattachment of biceps tendon

Proximal Humerus Osteosarcoma with Entire Deltoid Resection (Type II)

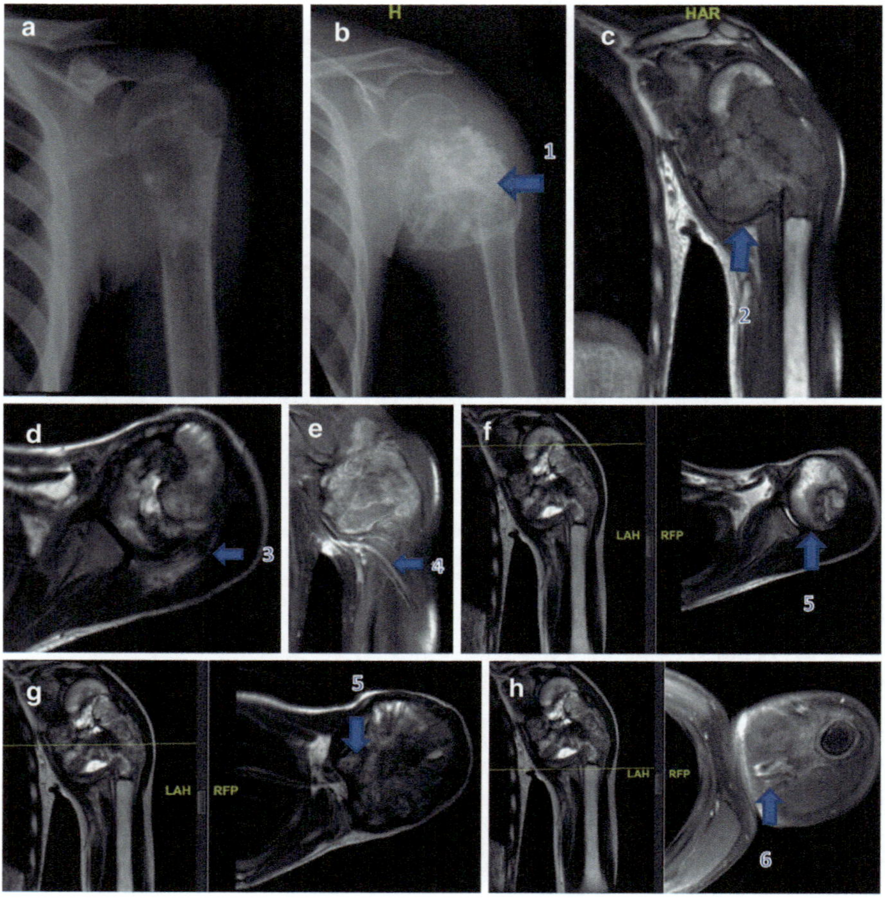

Proximal humerus with pathological fracture. The entire deltoid was involved, particularly the posterior deltoid compartment; however, the glenohumeral joint was spared. The neurovascular bundle was pushed medially, and its involvement could be traced from proximal to distal or with MRI angiography (Fig. 4a–h). In large tumours, identification of the musculocutaneous nerve is important, as primary steps before the conjoined tendon is mobilised distally for brachial vessels and nerve exploration.

1. Pathological fracture responded well to chemotherapy with union and calcification
2. Haematoma caused medial extension of tumour
3. Posterior deltoid infiltration secondary to hematoma contamination
4. Brachial artery and major nerve
5. Shoulder joint free of tumour contamination
6. Distal brachial artery abutting to the sarcoma margin

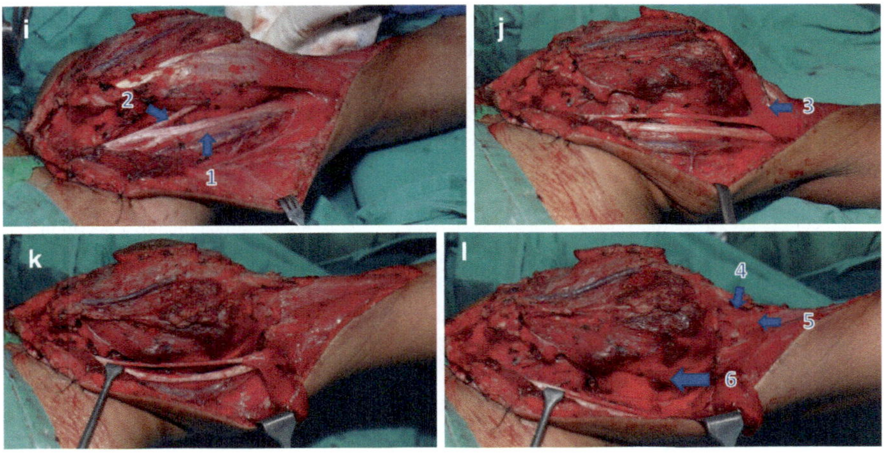

1. Median nerve and brachial artery
2. Musculocutaneous nerve
3. Biceps muscle mobilise with intact nerve
4. Deltoid insertion
5. Brachialis muscle
6. Teres major

Distal mobilization of the neurovascular structures with attached straight head biceps and coracobrachialis is important to minimise traction injury to the nerve. The biceps muscle must be mobilised medially together with the brachial artery to maintain its vascularity (Fig. 4i–l).

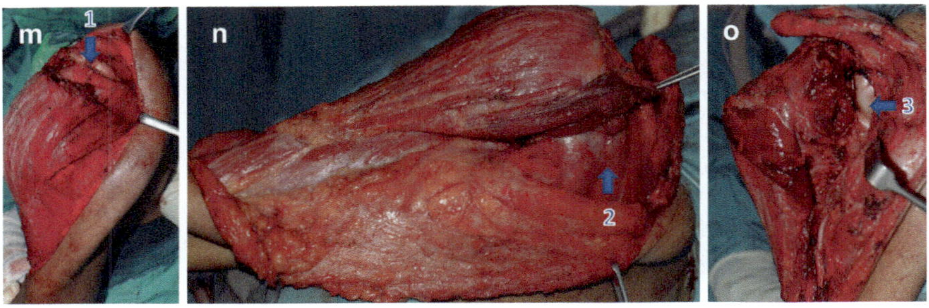

The entire deltoid was detached from the origin of the acromion, scapula spine, and clavicle. The suprascapular space was identified for intraarticular resection. The subscapularis muscle, supraspinatus, and infraspinatus were detached from the proximal humerus with margin to expose the shoulder joint (Fig. 4m–o).

1. Acromion—deltoid origin detached to expose the rotator cuff tendon
2. Infraspinatus and supraspinatus muscle and tendon
3. Circumferential detachment of rotator cuff and shoulder capsule at the labrum

The radial nerve runs through the triangular interval together with the profunda humeri vessels and crosses the proximal humerus in the posterior compartment between the long head of the triceps and humerus (Fig. 4p, q). The brachialis muscle is a good anatomical boundary and should be included as a margin in distal tumour. Securing and mobilising the radial nerve from the medial and lateral sides is important prior to distal osteotomy to prevent injury.

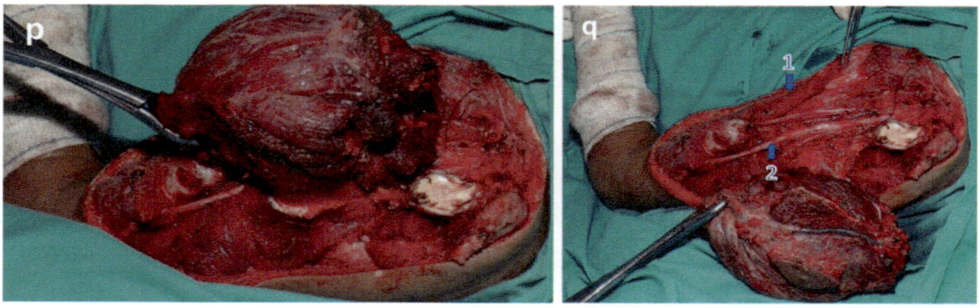

1. Biceps muscle with intact musculocutaneous nerve
2. Radial nerve

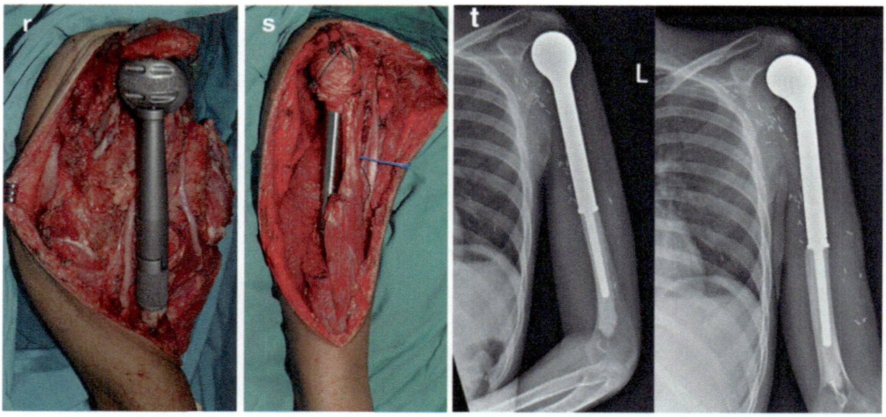

Prosthesis was stabilised by anchor suture to the acromion or prolene mesh purse-string to the remaining glenoid. The biceps tendon must be maintained in tension for good elbow flexion function. The prosthesis can be wrapped with Trevira tubes, and all tendon insertions were reconstructed anatomically for remaining function (Fig. 4r–t).

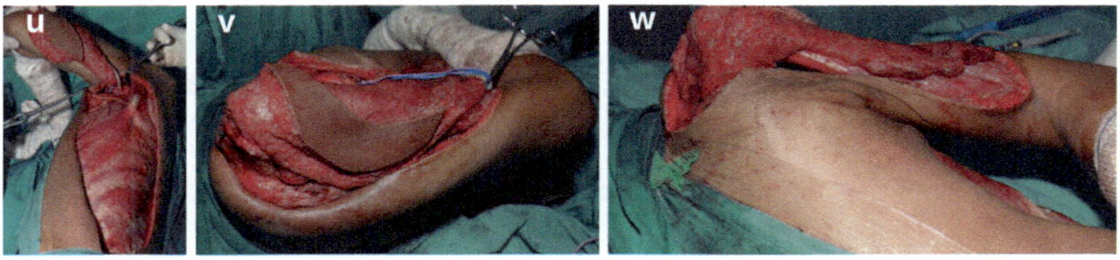

Massive resection of the entire deltoid will lead to poor soft tissue covers, flap failure, and wound dehiscence. A rotational latissimus dorsi flap is an option provided that the thoracodorsal artery was maintained, particularly in extraarticular resection of the humerus (Fig. 4u–w).

Extraarticular Resection of the Shoulder Joint

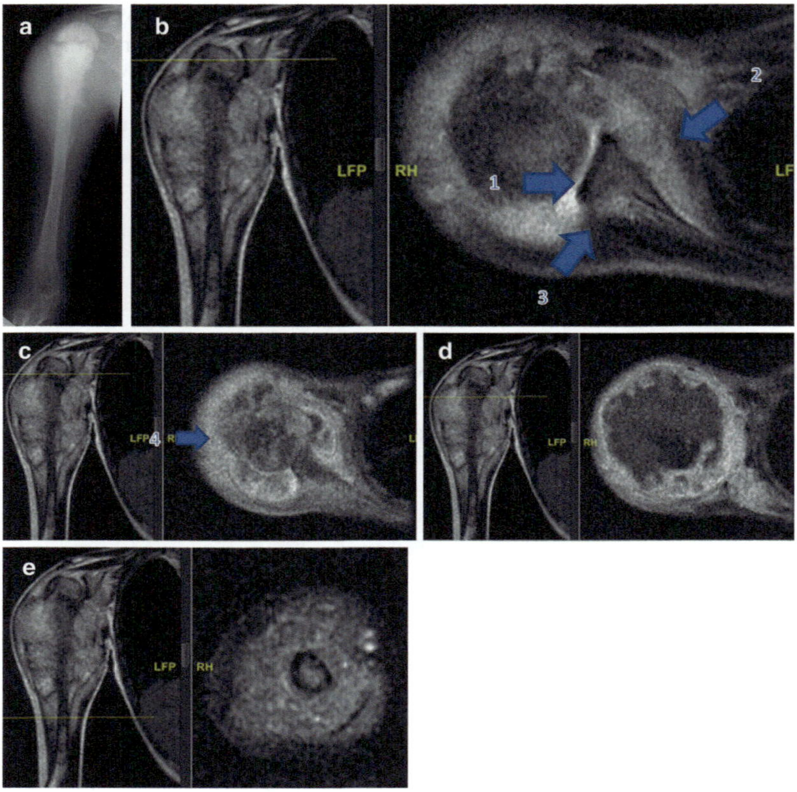

1. Shoulder joint contamination
2. Subscapularis muscle involvement
3. Supraspinatus muscle involvement
4. Entire deltoid extension

Proximal humerus osteosarcoma with poor response to chemotherapy with shoulder joint involvement (Fig. 5a–e).

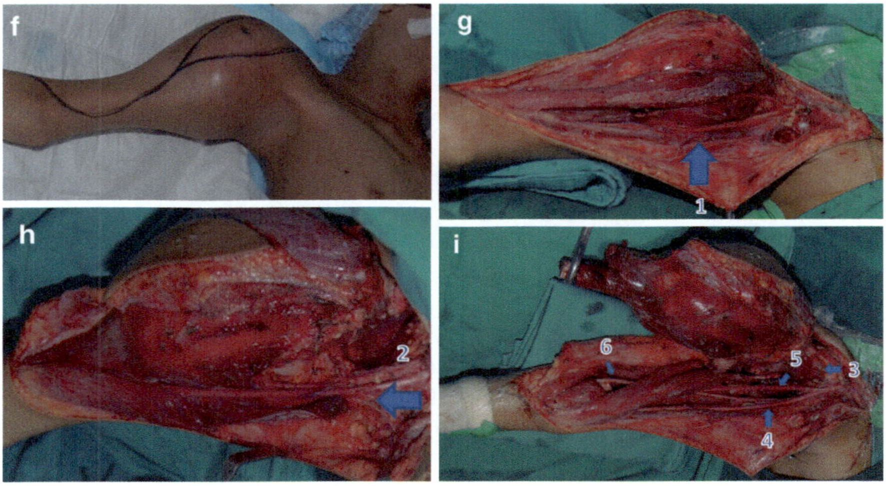

Osteotomy of the distal humerus and abduction of the shoulder should be able to identify the entire subscapularis after mobilising the subclavian vessels and brachial plexus inferiorly (Fig. 5f–i).

1. Axillary and brachial vessels and major nerve
2. Mobilisation of biceps together with intact musculocutaneous nerve
3. Subscapularis muscle
4. Median nerve
5. Musculocutaneous nerve
6. Radial nerve

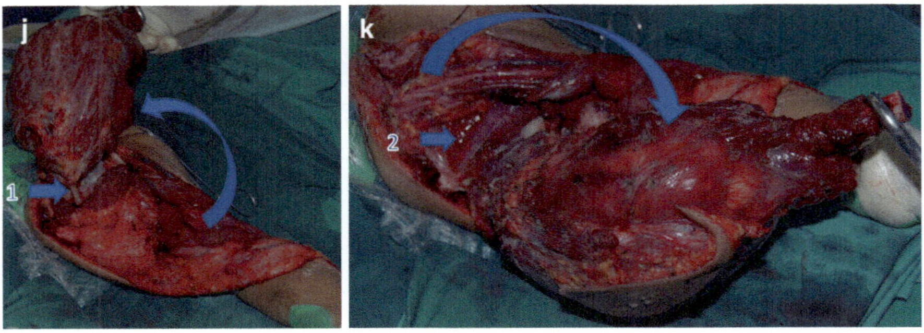

Forward flexion of the humerus will expose the entire supraspinatus and infraspinatus for muscular margin and final osteotomy. Subscapularis muscle visualisation for anterior surgical margin by abduction and extension of the humerus (Fig. 5j–n).

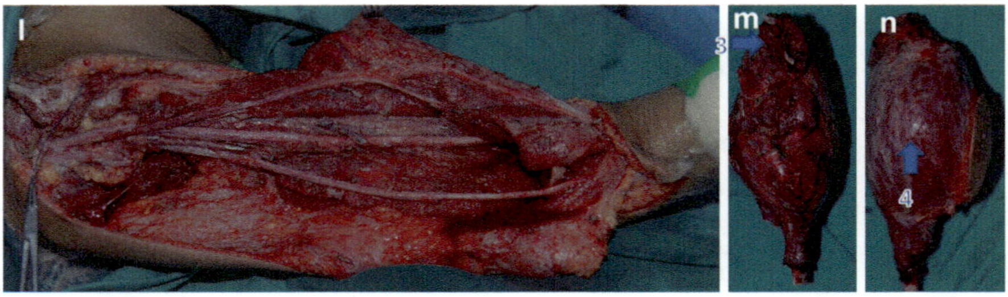

1. Scapula spine
2. Subscapularis muscle at the anterior scapula
3. Medial scapulae remove as oncological margin
4. The entire deltoid muscle includes as a margin

Reconstruction option is a combination allograft prosthesis composites due to short remnant of distal humerus for stem fixation. Allograft was stabilised with double reconstruction plate, and the humeral head prosthesis was suspended to the remaining clavicle (Fig. 5o, p).

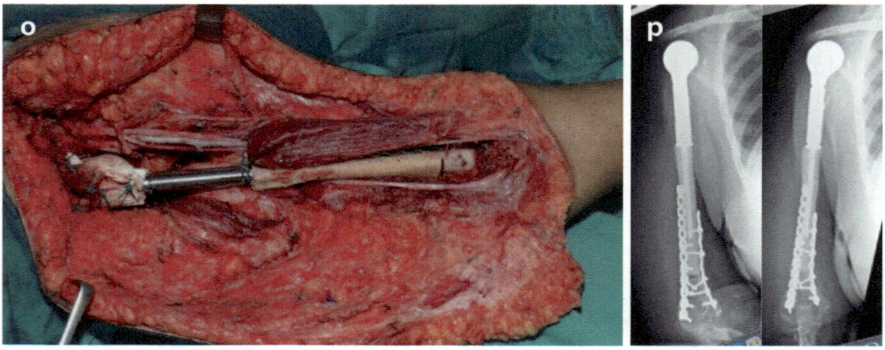

Type V Resection with Allograft Reconstruction

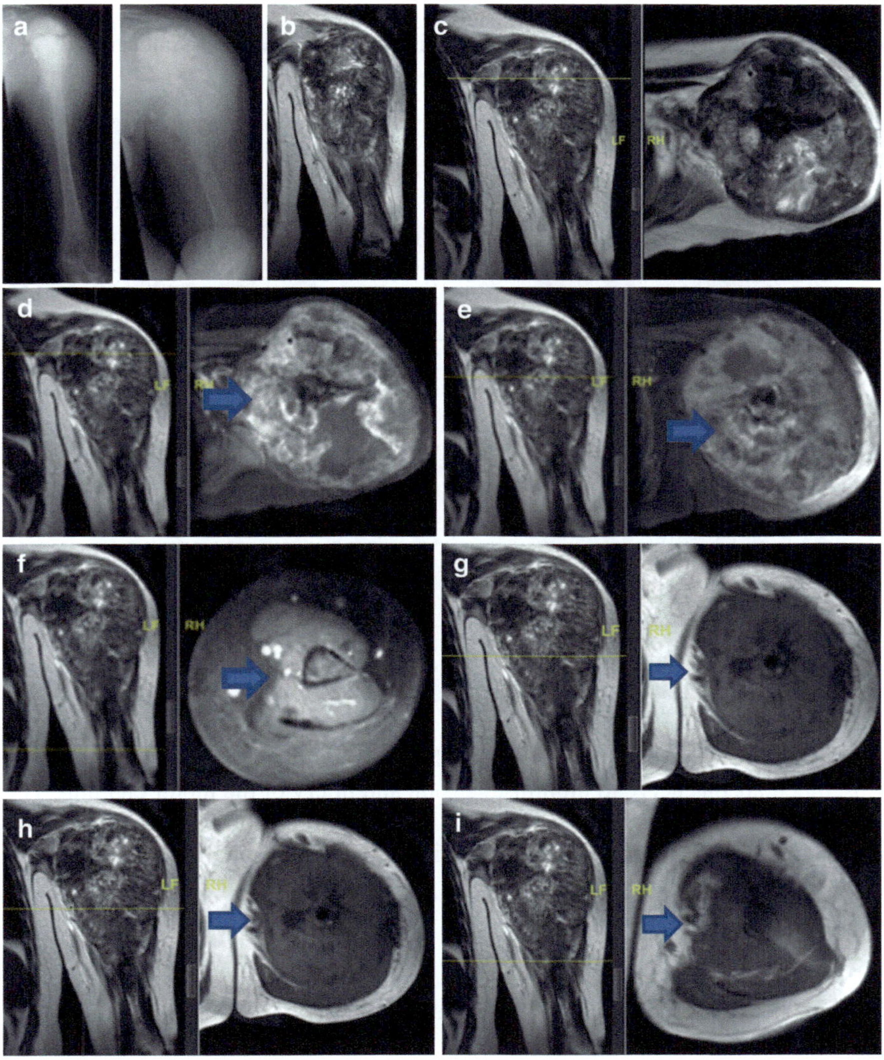

Osteosarcoma of the proximal humerus shows medullary extension to the distal humerus and soft tissue extension into the subscapularis and supraspinatus muscles (Fig. 6a–i). In proximal humerus sarcoma, the main aim of surgery is to achieve good oncological with negative microscopic margin and functional sensate upper-limb hand function. Shoulder suspension with minimal mobility required a good biceps for elbow flexion and optimum hand function. Free major distal neurovascular with intact nerve and functional biceps is important for limb salvage of proximal humerus sarcoma. The soft tissue covers for protection of reconstruction and flexibility closure, and enhanced abduction function is possible with rotational latissimus dorsi flap.

- Brachial and axillary vessels tracing for indirect evaluation of major nerve

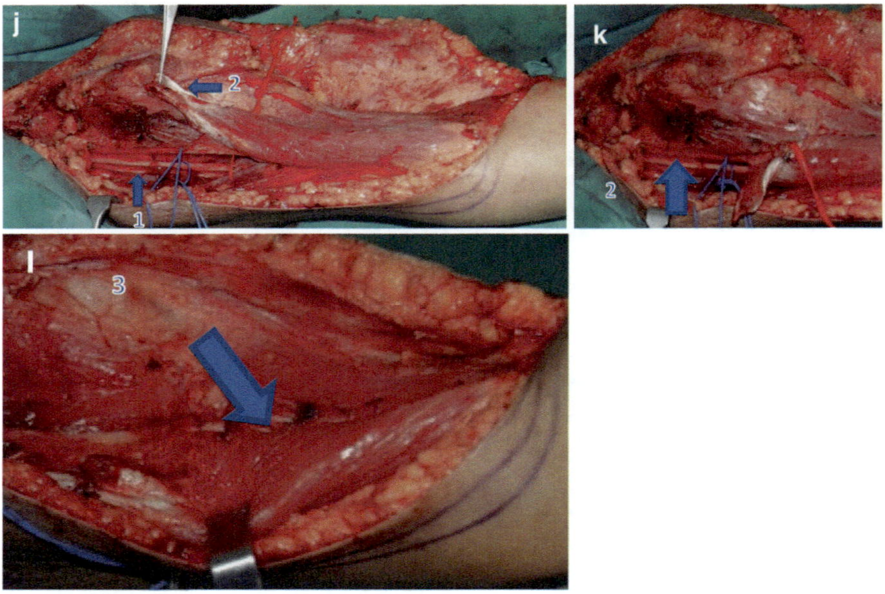

The entire biceps, long head, and straight head were mobilised medially with the musculocutaneous nerve to minimise tension and injury of the motor end unit. The brachialis muscle will provide a good cuff anteriorly for oncological border. Reconstruction with tension over prosthesis or allograft is important for strength of elbow flexor (Fig. 6j–n).

1. Brachial artery with major nerve
2. Straight head of biceps where musculocutaneus nerve pierces
3. Plane between biceps and brachialis free of adhesion and infiltration

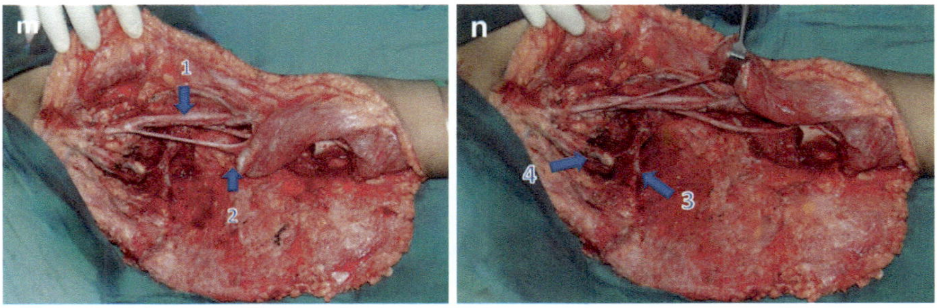

1. Brachial artery, median and ulnar nerve
2. Biceps tendon with intact musculocutaneous nerve
3. Remnant of scapula
4. Clavicle

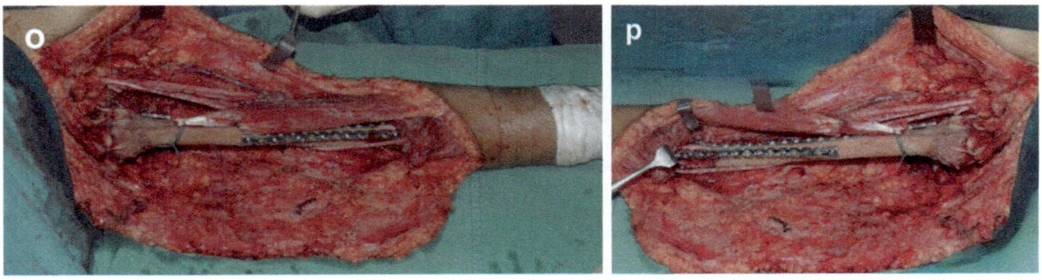

The musculocutaneous nerve with the motor unit of the biceps was intact for elbow flexion. Long segment resection was reconstructed with allograft, as short distal humerus was not suitable for prosthesis. The head of the proximal allograft was suspended to the acromion for stability suspension (Fig. 6o, p).

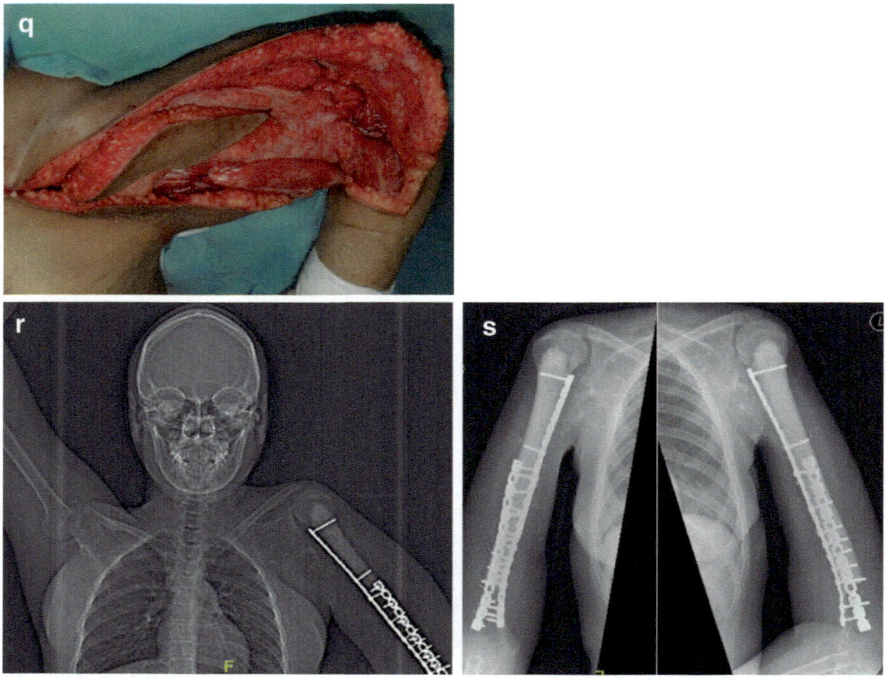

A rotational latissimus dorsi flap for soft tissue cover is used and wrapped around the allograft for vascularity to minimise infection and wound break-down (Fig. 6q–s).

Acknowledgements The author thanks Professor Wan Azman Wan Sulaiman, Professor Arman Zaharil Mat Saad, and Professor Ahmad Sukari Halim from the Plastic Reconstructive Unit at Universiti Sains Malaysia and MSU Medical Centre, Management and Science University, for their contributions and team members for managing the patients. All plastic, reconstructive, and microsurgical procedures were performed by the team members.

Suggested Reading

1. Erol B. Proximal humerus – biological reconstruction. In: Surgical oncology for bone tumors. Springer Nature Switzerland AG; 2022. p. 399–405.
2. Cladière-Nassif V, Bourdet C, Audard V, Babinet A, Anract P, Biau D. Is it safe to preserve the deltoid when resecting the proximal humerus for a primary malignant bone tumour? Bone Joint J. 2017;99-B(9):1244–9.
3. Luis Muscolo D, Ayerza MA, Aponte-Tinao LA. Proximal humeral osteoarticular allograft. In: Master techniques in orthopaedic surgery orthopaedic oncology and complex reconstruction. Lippincott Williams & Wilkins, A Wolters Kluwer; 2011. p. 317–24.
4. Gebhardt MC, Roth YF, Mankin HJ. Osteoarticular allografts for reconstruction in the proximal part of the humerus after excision of a musculoskeletal tumor. J Bone Joint Surg [Am]. 1990;72-A:334–45.

5. Gupta GR, Yasko AW, Lewis VO, et al. Risk of local recurrence after deltoid sparing resection for osteosarcoma of the proximal humerus. Cancer. 2009;115:3767–73.
6. Sanchez-Sotelo J. Proximal humeral allograft prosthetic composites. In: Master techniques in orthopaedic surgery orthopaedic oncology and complex reconstruction. Lippincott Williams & Wilkins, A Wolters Kluwer; 2011. p. 325–48.
7. van der Heijden L, Van de Sande MAJ. Implant reconstruction of the proximal humerus. In: Surgical oncology for bone tumors. Springer Nature Switzerland AG; 2022. p. 425–41.
8. Malawer MM, Sugarbaker PH, Lampert M, Baker AR, Gerber NL. The Tikhoff-Linberg procedure: report of ten patients and presentation of a modified technique for tumors of the proximal humerus. Surgery. 1985;97(5):518–28.
9. Ozaki T, Putzke M, Rödl R, Winkelmann W, Lindner N. Incidence and mechanisms of infiltration of sarcomas in the shoulder. Clin Orthop. 2001;395:209–15.
10. Rödl RW, Gosheger G, Gebert C, Lindner N, Ozaki T, Winkelmann W. Reconstruction of the proximal humerus wide resection of tumour. J Bone Joint Surg [Br]. 2002;84-B:1004–8.
11. Wittig JC, Kellar-Graney KL, Malawer MM, et al. Surgical classification system of limb-sparing resections of the shoulder girdle. Limb-sparing surgery for high-grade sarcomas of the proximal humerus. Tech Shoulder Elbow Surg. 2001;2:54–69.

Total Humerus Resection and Replacement

Wan Faisham Nu'man Bin Wan Ismail

Introduction

Total humeral resection and replacement is unusual. However, it is required when a tumour involves a large portion of the diaphysis, such as in Ewing's sarcoma, or when an extremely short segment of the distal humerus remains following adequate tumour resection. Resection of the entire humerus is required when there is an extension of the tumour from the distal or proximal humerus with extensive medullary extension or a skip lesion. The entire humerus is resected together with an oncological soft tissue margin over the primary site: either the distal or proximal humerus and the additional intraosseous lesion.

Surgical Anatomy

The entire humerus is covered by muscle that provides an anatomical barrier for tumour extension

- Brachialis muscle covers the anterior part of the distal humerus and protects the neurovascular bundle and biceps muscle
- Medial and lateral triceps originate at the posterior humerus and provide a good cuff of the muscle for a wide margin surgery
- All tendinous attachments and the common flexor and extensor origins of the forearm must be carefully evaluated for tumour extension.

W. F. N. B. W. Ismail (✉)
Prince Court Medical Center, Kuala Lumpur, Malaysia

Orthopaedic Oncology Reconstructive Unit, Universiti Sains Malaysia,
Kubang Kerian, Kelantan, Malaysia

A. Puri, W. F. N. B. W. Ismail (eds.), *Atlas of Orthopedic Oncology Volume 2*,
https://doi.org/10.1007/978-981-95-8962-3_13

Assessment

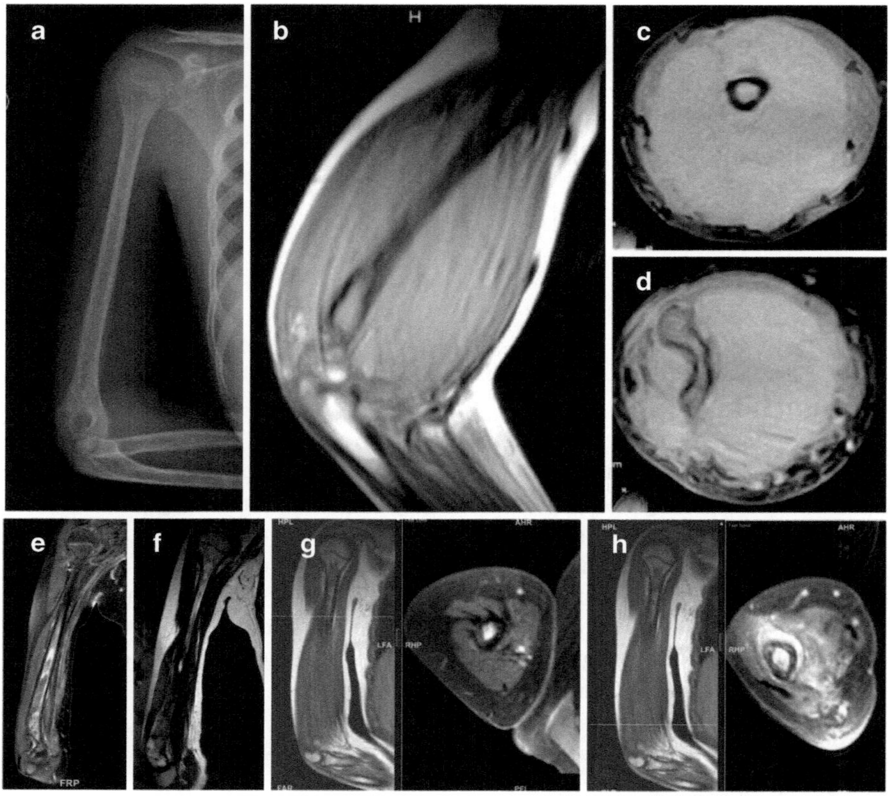

Ewing sarcoma of the distal humerus with intramedullary extension to just below the epiphyseal plate in the proximal humerus. The primary tumour responded well to chemotherapy; however, the brachialis muscle and medial triceps attached to the humerus showed gadolinium uptake and had to be removed together with the entire humerus for a wide oncological margin (Fig. 1a–h).

Surgical Steps (Fig. 1i–n)

The margin during resection of the entire humerus is based on tumour extension. Any remaining muscle that demonstrates residual gadolinium uptake will be removed with the entire humerus. The proximal or distal intramedullary extension is removed with a periosteum and soft tissue margin. Residual soft tissue is important for soft tissue reconstruction and stability and function of the shoulder and elbow.

- Exploration of the medial neurovascular structures—ulnar nerve is freed from the medial epicondyle.
- A lateral flap is created for exploration of the radial nerve between the brachioradialis and brachialis muscle.
- The entire biceps muscle is mobilised medially with intact perforator from the brachial artery for its vascularity.
- Brachialis covering the anterior part of the humerus is included in the margin.
- Cuff of the medial and lateral triceps is included as the posterior margin.

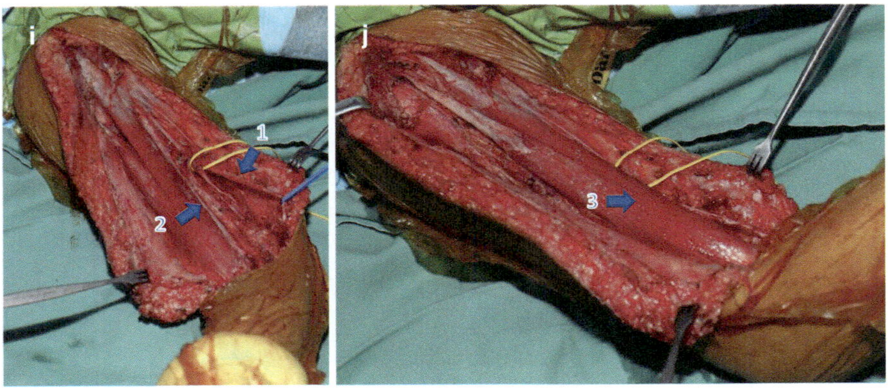

1. Mobilisation of ulnar nerve
2. Brachial artery and vein with median nerve
3. Biceps muscle

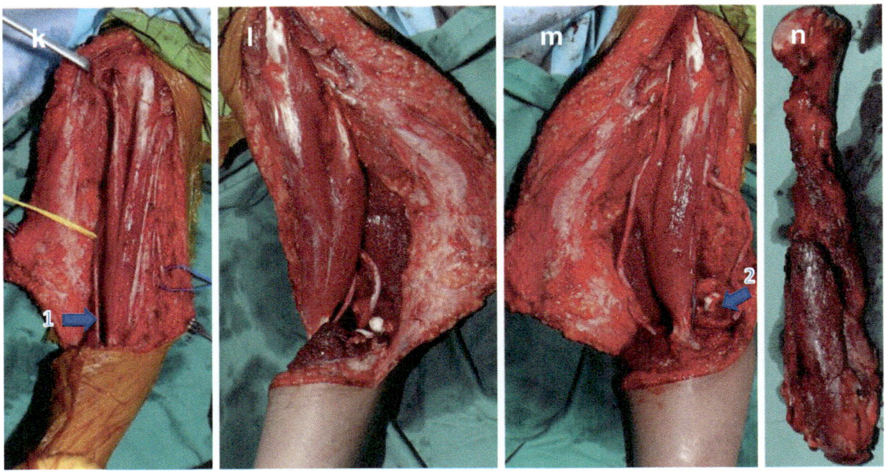

1. Mobilisation of radial nerve between brachialis and brachioradialis to the posterior compartment
2. Olecranon prepare for ulna stem total elbow replacement

Reconstruction

The elbow joint of total humerus endoprosthesis is reconstructed using a hinged joint and cemented ulna stem. The proximal humerus head is stabilised with remnants of the capsule and reinforced with a Dacron or Prolene graft. The rotator cuff tendon and proximal humerus muscle are reattached for some functional muscle activity (Fig. 1o–q).

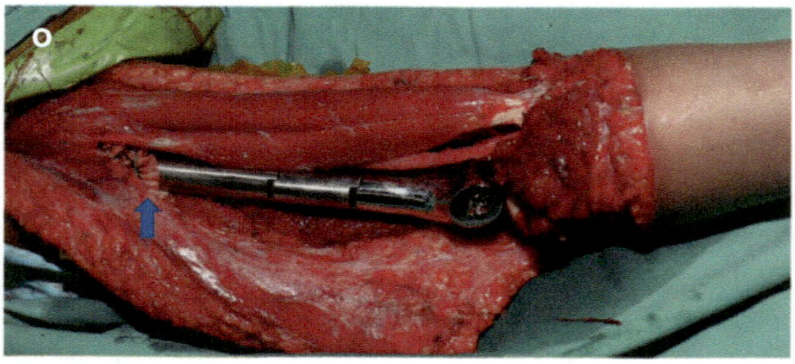

- Shoulder stability were reconstructed using PTFE graft or Trevira tube

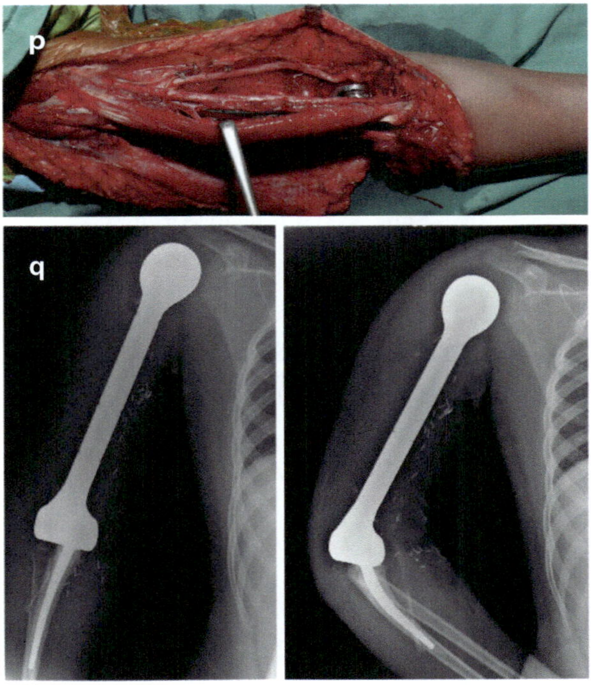

A total humerus replacement aims for painless and stable upper limb function to optimise elbow and hand function. The shoulder suspension permits minimal abduction and flexion. (Refer proximal humerus for shoulder stability reconstruction)

Allograft Total Elbow Prosthesis Reconstruction

Reconstruction with an allograft over the proximal humerus allows soft tissue reconstruction for attachment of the supraspinatus, infraspinatus, and subscapularis muscle for a stable shoulder and active abduction. Elbow reconstruction with total elbow replacement allows for a stable early functional elbow.

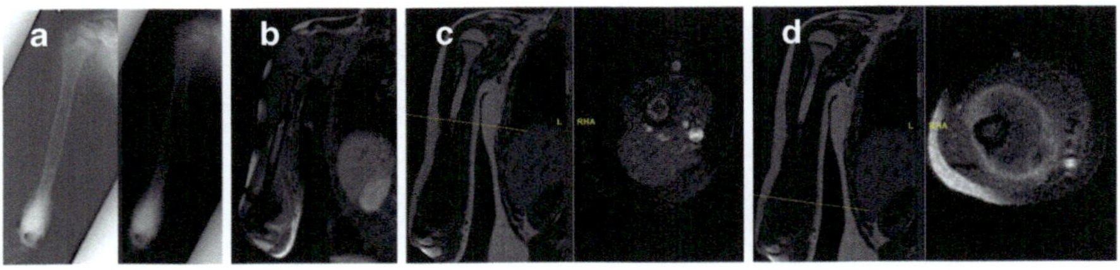

A case of distal humerus osteosarcoma with partial response to chemotherapy. The intramedullary involvement was near the epiphyseal plate (Fig. 2a–d). A total humerus resection was planned to achieve good oncological margins. The entire humerus was reconstructed with an allograft prosthesis composite (prosthesis for elbow reconstruction).

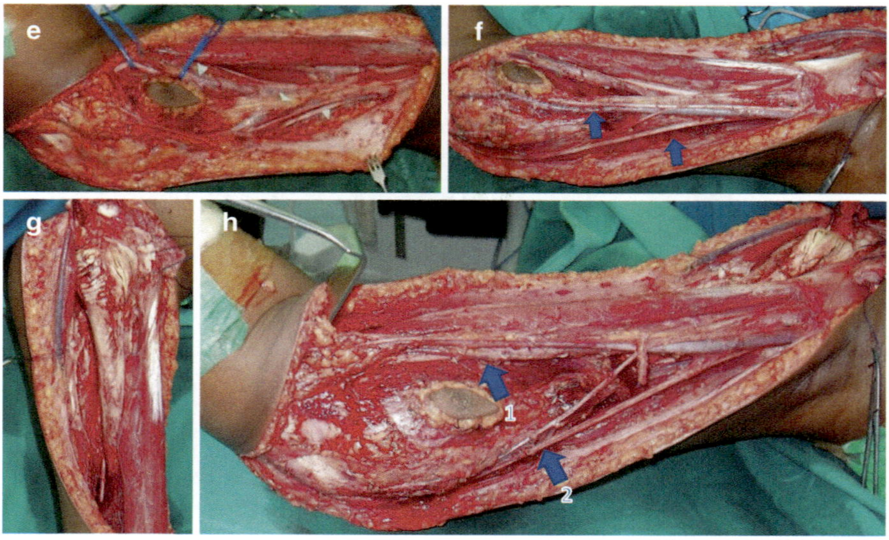

Following exploration of the medial neurovascular bundle, the entire brachialis muscle was included as surgical margin together with the medial triceps origin. The rotator cuff tendons were transacted near their attachment for final reconstruction with the remnant allograft tendon (Fig. 2e–h).

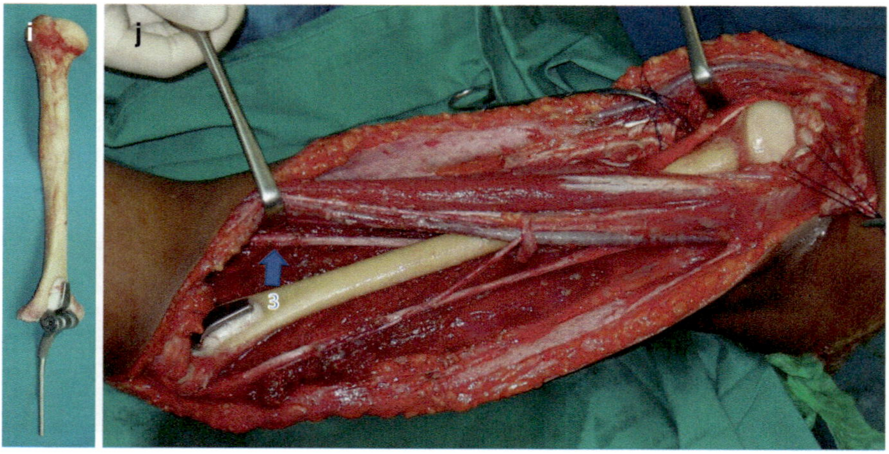

1. Brachial vessels and medial nerve
2. Ulnar nerve
3. Radial nerve

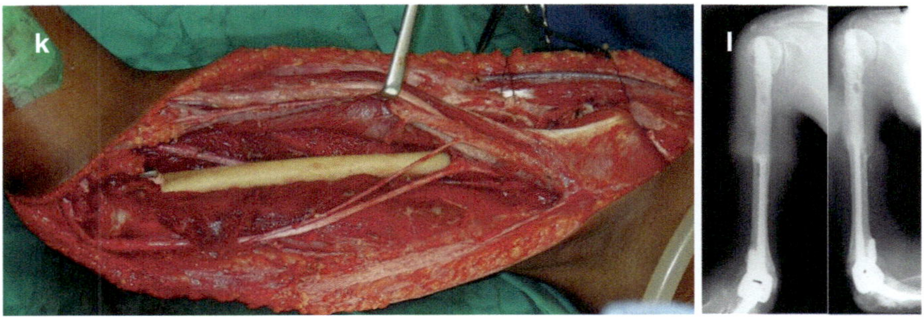

Allograft total elbow prosthesis reconstruction (Fig. 2i–l).

Suggested Reading

1. Kotwal S, Moon B, Lin P, Satcher R Jr, Lewis V. Total humeral endoprosthetic replacement following excision of malignant bone tumors. Sarcoma. 2016;2016:6318060.
2. Weber KL. Total humeral reconstruction. In: Master techniques in orthopaedic surgery orthopaedic oncology and complex reconstruction. Lippincott Williams & Wilkins, A Wolters Kluwer; 2011. p. 347–57.
3. Jeys LM, Morris GV, Kurisunkal V. Implant reconstruction of the humeral diaphysis: total humerus prosthesis. In: Orthopedic surgical oncology for bone tumors. Springer Nature Switzerland; 2022. p. 465–81.
4. Natarajan M, Sameer M, Kunal D, Balasubramanian N. Custom-made endoprosthetic total humerus reconstruction for musculoskeletal tumours. Int Orthop. 2012;36(1):125–9.
5. Puri A, Gulia A. The results of total humeral replacement following excision for primary bone tumour. J Bone Joint Surg Br. 2012;94(9):1277–81.
6. Wafa H, Reddy K, Grimer R, Abudu A, Jeys L, Carter S, Tillman R. Does total humeral endoprosthetic replacement provide reliable reconstruction with preservation of a useful extremity? Clin Orthop Relat Res. 2015;473(3):917–25.
7. Weber KL, Lin PP, Yasko AW. Complex segmental elbow reconstruction after tumor resection. Clin Orthop Relat Res. 2003;415:1–14.

Distal Humerus Resection

Wan Faisham Nu'man Bin Wan Ismail

Introduction

The distal humerus is a rare site for primary bone sarcoma. Limb salvage surgery with good oncological margins is possible, as the brachialis muscle acts as an anatomical barrier to the anterior part of the distal humerus and protects the major neurovascular structures. The ulnar nerve is in close proximity to the medial epicondyle and should be evaluated carefully for direct tumour infiltration. The modularity of distal humerus endoprosthesis reconstruction which provides a stable and functional elbow, results in good outcomes.

Surgical Anatomy

The distal humerus is covered by muscles that provide an anatomical barrier for tumour extension.

- Anterior—brachialis muscle attached to the midshaft of the humerus
- Posterior—medial triceps attached to the distal humerus above the olecranon fossae
- Medial and lateral—attachment of the common flexor and extensor of the forearm

The brachial vessels and median nerve cross the elbow and lie between the brachialis and biceps muscle and tendon. The radial nerve runs between the brachialis muscle and brachioradialis anteriorly and crosses posteriorly above the medial

W. F. N. B. W. Ismail (✉)
Prince Court Medical Center, Kuala Lumpur, Malaysia

Orthopaedic Oncology Reconstructive Unit, Universiti Sains Malaysia, Kubang Kerian, Kelantan, Malaysia

A. Puri, W. F. N. B. W. Ismail (eds.), *Atlas of Orthopedic Oncology Volume 2*,
https://doi.org/10.1007/978-981-95-8962-3_14

triceps. The ulnar nerve is very closely attached to the medial epicondyle and must be thoroughly assessed for infiltration.

Assessment

Anatomical boundaries around the distal humerus are an important part of assessment to achieve a wide surgical margin:

- Brachialis muscle infiltration, including the insertion to the ulna
- Origin of the medial triceps
- Origin of the common flexor and extensor forearm muscles
- Elbow and radio capitulum joint
- Ulnar nerve

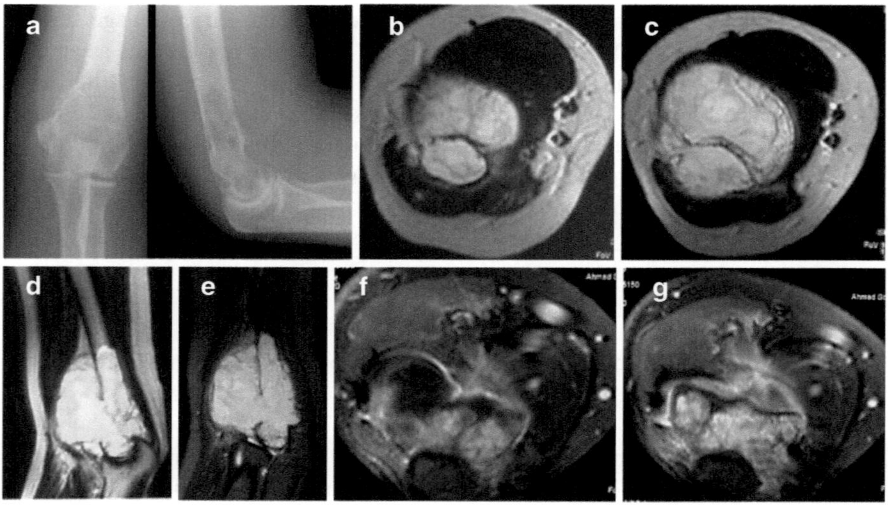

Chondromyxoid fibroma had occupied the entire distal humerus with anterior extension beneath the brachialis muscle. The brachial vessels and median nerve were spared, and the ulnar nerve was not closely attached to the tumour. The radio capitulum joint and ulna humeral joint were not involved (Fig. 1a–g).

Surgical Steps (Fig. 1h–q)

Distal humerus resection procedure:

- Exploration of the brachial artery and median nerve through a medial approach with a lateral incision curved at the cubital fossa.

- The entire bicep was elevated anteriorly from the brachialis muscle.
- The ulnar nerve was isolated and dissected free from the medial epicondyle and cubital tunnel.
- The radial nerve was explored after a lateral flap was created between the brachioradialis and brachial muscle and freed until it passed anteriorly to the lateral intermuscular septum.
- The medial common flexor and pronator teres origin were released from the distal medial epicondyle.
- The anterior elbow joint was opened after detaching the brachial insertion over the coronoid process. The medial collateral was transacted prior to the posterior arthrotomy. This procedure destabilised and subluxated the elbow.
- Proximal osteotomy allowed for manipulation of the lateral structures, facilitating release of the brachioradialis, extensor carpi radialis, and common extensor origin.

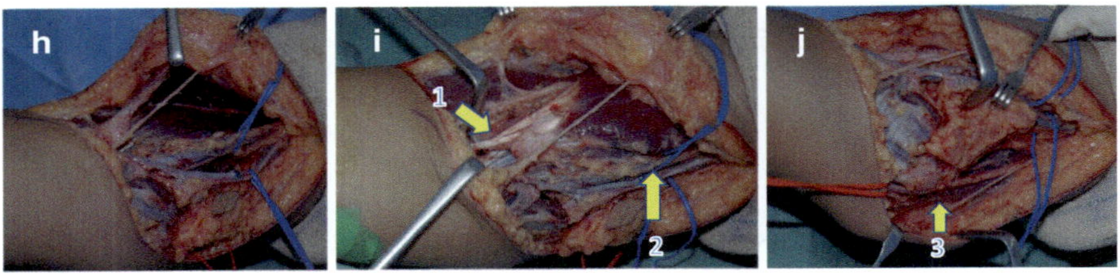

1. Biceps tendon
2. Brachial vessels
3. Mobilisation of the ulnar nerve below the medial epicondyle by detaching Osborne fascia

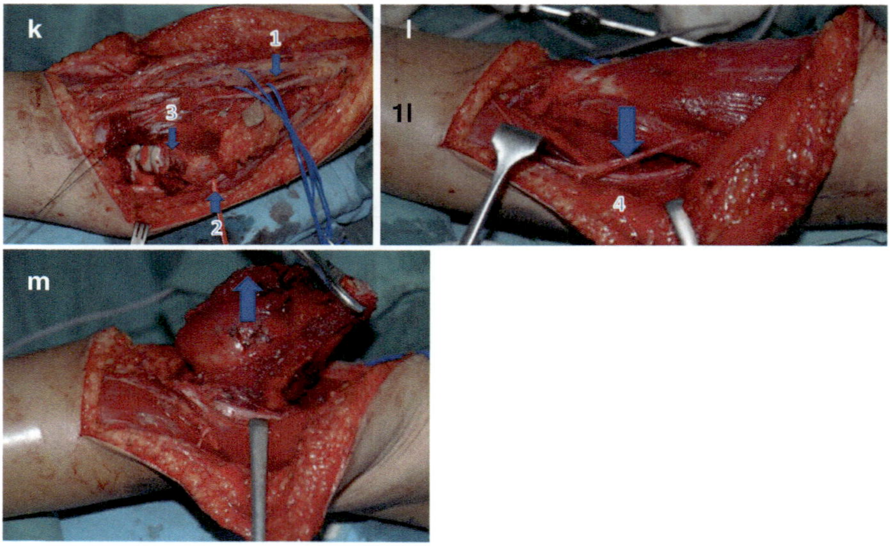

1. Brachial artery
2. Ulnar nerve
3. Brachialis muscle transected to expose the medial joint
4. Lateral exploration: radial nerve and cutaneous branch of musculocutaneous nerve

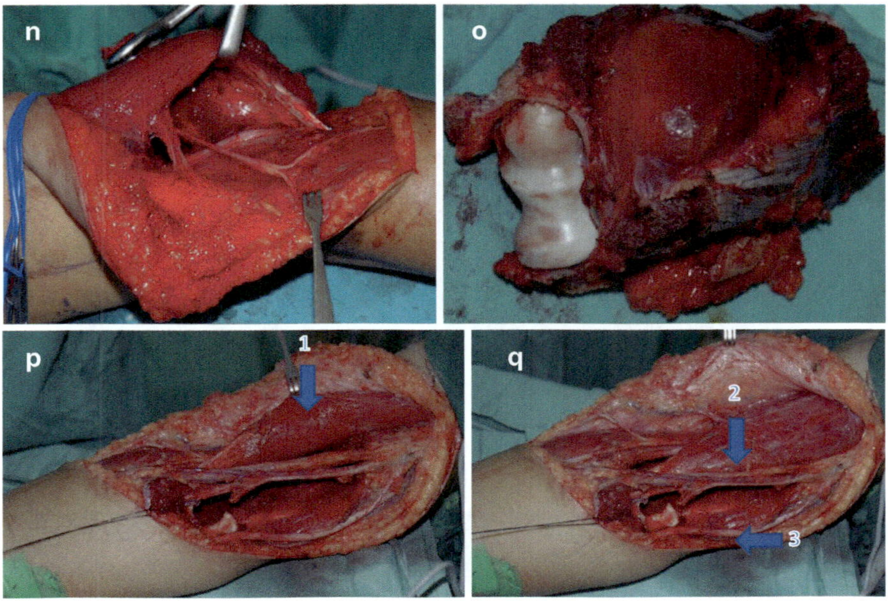

1. Biceps muscle
2. Brachial vessels with median nerve
3. Ulnar nerve

Options for distal humerus and elbow reconstruction:

- Distal humerus endoprosthesis
- Osteoarticular allograft
- Allograft prosthesis composites
- Recycled bone: extracorporeal radiation/cryotherapy with prosthesis

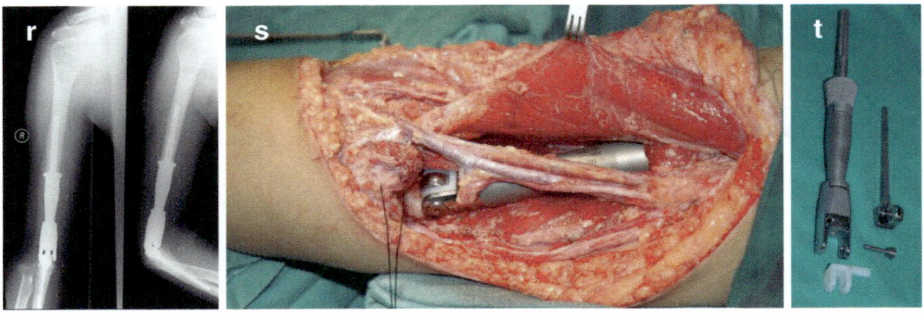

Distal humerus hinged endoprosthesis provides modularity for osseous defect reconstruction and provides immediate stability for rehabilitation and function (Fig. 1r–t).

Soft Tissue Sarcoma with Bone Involvement

A low-grade soft tissue sarcoma over the entire postero-medial distal humerus, which was closely attached to and infiltrated the bone (Fig. 2a–e).

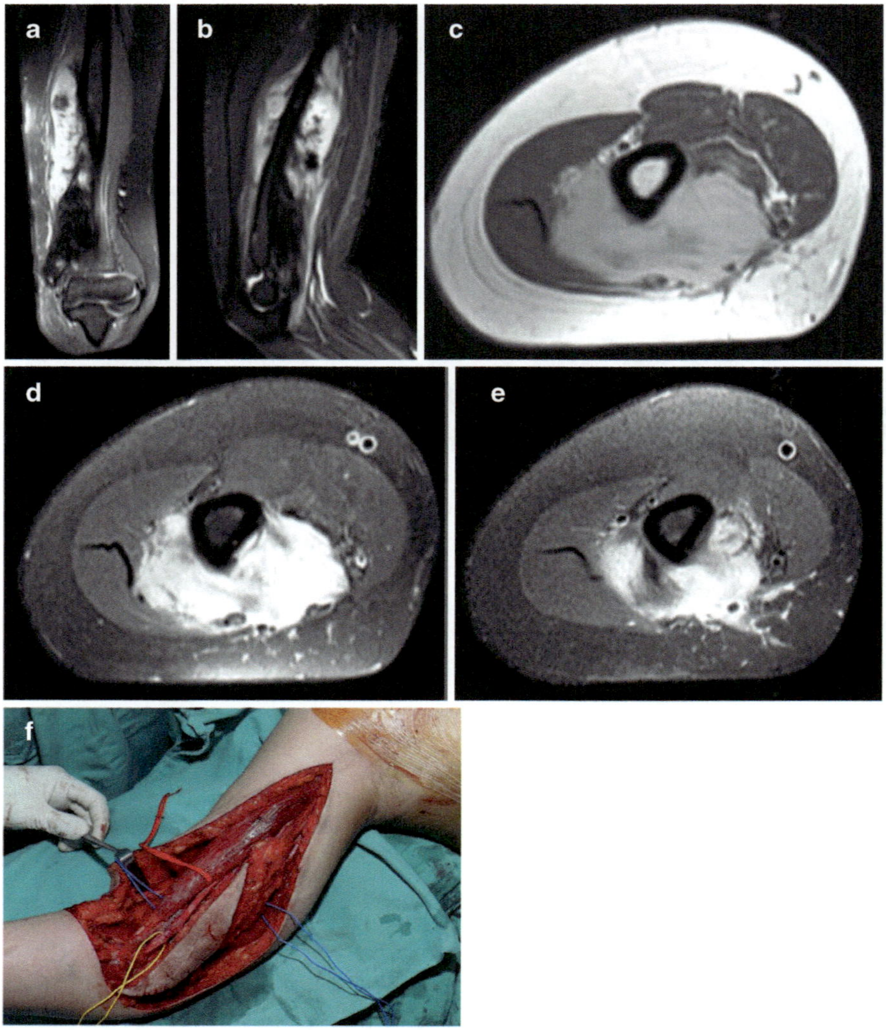

The surgical approach was designed for exploration of the medial neurovascular, including the ulnar and medial nerves. It crossed the elbow laterally for exploration of the radial nerve as well as exposed the entire common extensor origin. The common extensor and flexor origin had to be visualised to ensure adequate margins during detachment of the distal humerus (Fig. 2f–h).

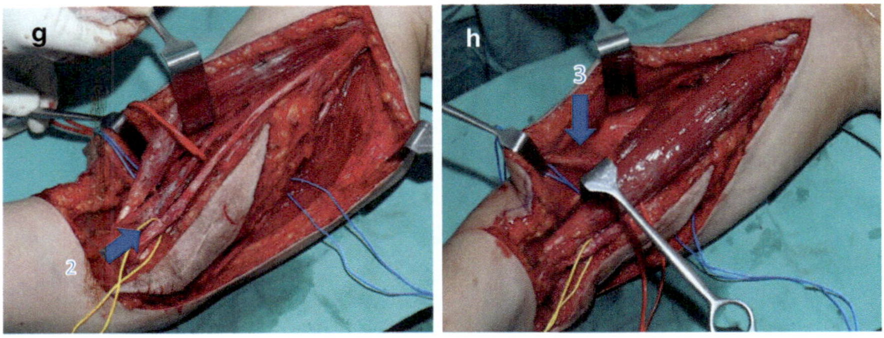

1. Mobilisation of biceps muscle and tendon from brachialis muscle
2. Median nerve and brachial vessels
3. Lateral exploration and identification of radial nerve

Common flexor origin was completely detached from medial epicondyle, the brachialis tendon was detached, and the entire anterior elbow capsule was opened permitting dislocation. Humerus osteotomy was performed, and the entire distal humerus was mobilised medially for proper visualisation of the lateral condyle and final delivery of the tumour (Fig. 2i–k).

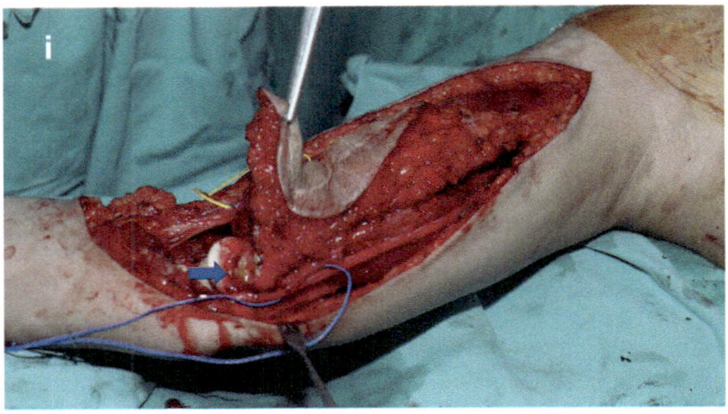

Arrows—common flexor origin, brachialis tendon, and medial collateral were detached from their origin to sublux the elbow joint.

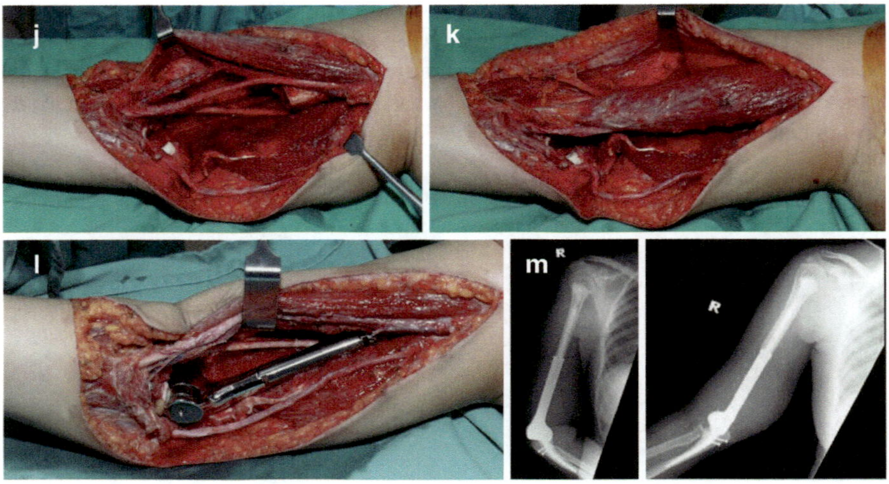

Distal humerus with total elbow prosthesis for reconstruction of bony defect (Fig. 2l, m).

Suggested Reading

1. Morrey BF, Sanchez-Sotelo J. Massive bone loss about the elbow. In: Master techniques in orthopaedic surgery orthopaedic oncology and complex reconstruction. Lippincott Williams & Wilkins, A Wolters Kluwer; 2011. p. 377–39.
2. Funovics PT, Schuh R, Adams SB Jr, Sabeti-Aschraf M, Dominkus M, Kotz RI. Modular prosthetic reconstruction of major bone defects of the distal end of the humerus. J Bone Joint Surg Am. 2011;93(11):1064–74.
3. Henrichs MP, Liem D, Gosheger G, Streitbuerger A, Nottrott M, Andreou D, Hardes J. Megaprosthesis replacement of the distal humerus: still a challenge in limb salvage. J Should Elbow Surg. 2019;28(5):908–14.
4. Weber KL. General considerations: elbow and wrist. In: Master techniques in orthopaedic surgery orthopaedic oncology and complex reconstruction. Lippincott Williams & Wilkins, A Wolters Kluwer; 2011. p. 371–7.
5. Funovics PT. Implant reconstruction of the distal humerus and elbow: modular prosthesis. In: Orthopaedic surgical oncology for bone tumors. Springer Nature Switzerland AG; 2022. p. 481–94.
6. Sarlikiotis T, Kaspiris A, Papagelopoulos PJ. Bone tumours around the elbow: a rare entity. EFORT Open Rev. 2019;4(4):133–42.
7. Schneider KN, Ellerbrock M, Gosheger G, Westphal LM, Deventer N, Klingebiel S, Rickert C, Theil C. Distal humeral replacement in patients with primary bone sarcoma: the functional outcome and return to sports. Cancers. 2023;15(13):3534.
8. Weber KL, Lin PP, Yasko AW. Complex segmental elbow reconstruction after tumour resection. Clin Orthop Relat Res. 2003;415:1–14.

Radial Neck-to-Humerus Trochlea Transposition

Ajay Puri, Rudra Pratap Singh, and Ashwin Prajapati

Introduction

Reconstruction after proximal ulna resection is challenging due to its complex bony anatomy, multiple musculoligamentous attachments, and subcutaneous location. With various biological and nonbiological options having their own limitations, transposition of the radial neck to the humerus trochlea can be a stable, mobile, and durable reconstruction option.

Surgical Anatomy

- Proximal ulna has two articulating facets, to articulate with the humerus trochlea and the radial head. These enable uniaxial hinge like flexion extension of the elbow and pronation-supination of the forearm, respectively.
- The attachments to the annular ligament, ulnar collateral ligament, and joint capsule act as static stabilisers of the elbow joint.
- Multiple muscular attachments like insertion of brachialis, triceps, anconeus and origin of supinator, flexor carpi ulnaris (FCU), pronator teres (ulnar head), and flexor digitorum superficialis (FDS) muscle need to be erased for while resecting the proximal ulna.
- Ulnar nerve traversing through the cubital tunnel on the posteromedial aspect can be close and requires meticulous dissection.
- Median nerve along with brachial vessel continuing as ulnar vessel lies anteriorly, just opposite to the posterior incision taken for proximal ulna resection.
- Due to its subcutaneous locations, raised fasciocutaneous flaps usually are thin and care needs to be taken to preserve their vascularity during dissection.

A. Puri (✉) · R. P. Singh · A. Prajapati
Department of Surgical Oncology, Tata Memorial Centre, Mumbai, India

A. Puri, W. F. N. B. W. Ismail (eds.), *Atlas of Orthopedic Oncology Volume 2*,
https://doi.org/10.1007/978-981-95-8962-3_15

Assessment

An MRI assessment of the elbow joint and proximal forearm includes the following:

- Intramedullary and intraarticular extent of the disease to plan oncologically safe resection
- Triceps tendon involvement
- Status of ulnar nerve, median nerve, and brachial vessels
- Biceps tenon, brachialis, anconaeus, and supinator involvement

Alternative options to reconstruction include a megaprosthesis, an osteoarticular allograft, or reimplantation of sterilised autograft.

Radius neck to humerus transposition offers a biological reconstructive option using native bone that provides long-term stability and durability while continuing to retain elbow function.

Surgical Steps

Position Lateral position with the arm resting on a bolster, tourniquet over the proximal arm, and the forearm draped and kept free.

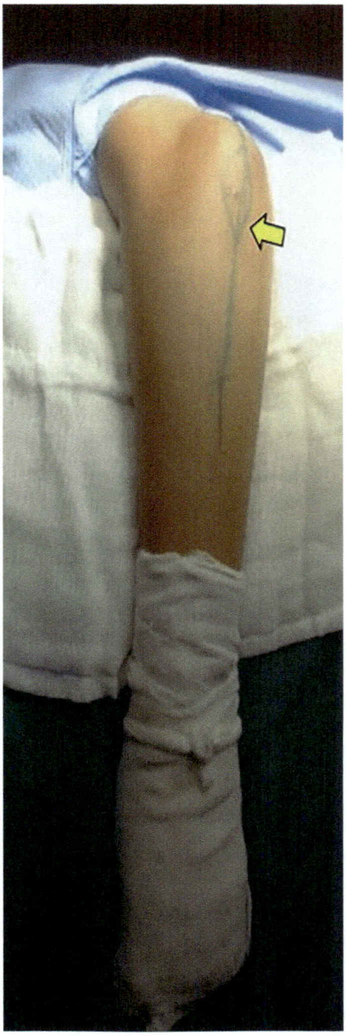

Resection Resection involves complete removal of the proximal ulna (osteoarticular) along with surrounding muscles for oncologic margins.

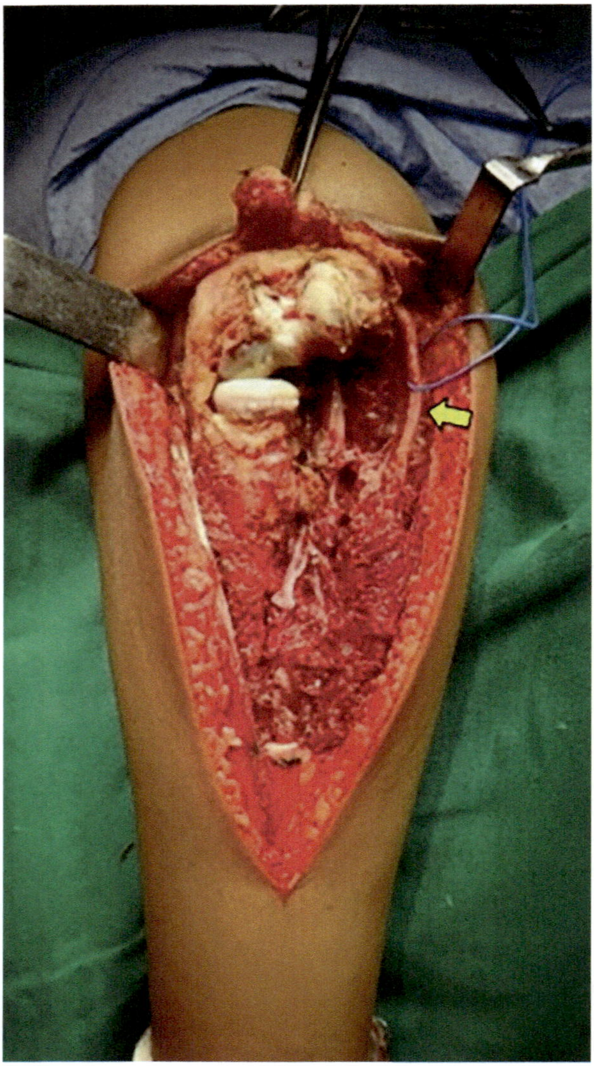

- A midline posterior vertical skin incision is taken starting from the distal arm, going over the subcutaneous border of the ulna, distal to the disease extent while islanding out the biopsy scar.
- Skin flaps are raised with adequate thickness without compromising margins.
- The ulnar nerve is identified posterior to the medial epicondyle of humerus and dissected off the tumour by releasing the cubital tunnel.
- After releasing the anconeus and supinator, triceps tendon is erased from olecranon preserving its length for subsequent reattachment to the radial head.
- Elbow joint capsule and collateral ligaments are released from their humeral attachment.

- Ulnar diaphyseal osteotomy is performed ensuring adequate oncological margin.
- Muscles originating from the proximal ulna (flexor digitorum superficialis, flexor digitorum profundus, abductor pollicis longus, pronator teres deep head) are sectioned at the level of the proposed osteotomy of ulna.
- Specimen can now be manipulated with a bone holding forceps applied at the distal end, provided the bone stock is good to cut the interosseous membrane and enter the volar compartment.
- Care is taken not to cut the biceps insertion on radial tuberosity.
- The annular ligament is cut close to the radius.
- Brachialis insertion is erased. Brachial, ulnar, radial vessels, and the median nerve lying anteriorly are dissected.
- Finally, the anterior capsular attachment is erased and specimen is delivered out.

Reconstruction

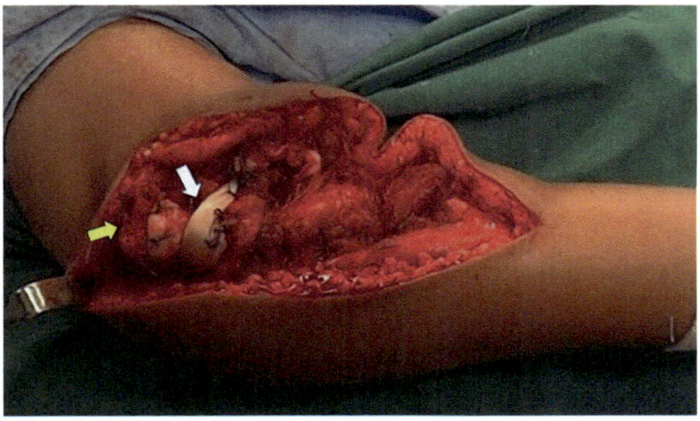

- Lateral collateral ligament, capsular and muscular attachments (except biceps tendon) are released from proximal radius, which allows its translocation in a medial, posterior and proximal direction.
- Care is taken not to erase the insertion of the biceps tendon which acts as a restraint to posterior subluxation of the radius.
- A tendon graft (allograft/semitendinosus autograft) is sutured to the soft tissue remnants on one humeral epicondyle with No 2 Ethibond Excel TM sutures (Nonabsorbable, braided, Polyester suture manufactured by Johnson & Johnson Ltd, Ethicon division, Chihuahua 32575 Mexico).
- A sling is created around the radial neck by winding the graft 360° around it, and under adequate tension, the tendon graft is secured to the soft tissue remnants on the opposite epicondyle with the elbow in 90-degree flexion and the forearm in neutral rotation.
- The tendon can be doubled (longitudinally folded on itself) if it is too thin, to increase the strength of the construct.
- After final positioning, the tendon graft should allow full supination, pronation, flexion, and extension of the elbow and limit medio-lateral and antero-posterior translation.

- The triceps tendon is attached to the radial head (remaining tendon graft can be used to increase its length if required) in 90-degree flexion.
- Suture anchors/cancellous screws with washers can be used to secure attachment of triceps tendon to the radial head.
- Haemostasis is achieved after deflation of the tourniquet and closure is accomplished over a negative suction drain.
- An above elbow plaster slab is applied in neutral position after adequate dressing.

Case Study: Radial Neck Humerus Trochlea Transposition—Reconstruction Using Autologous Semitendinosus Graft

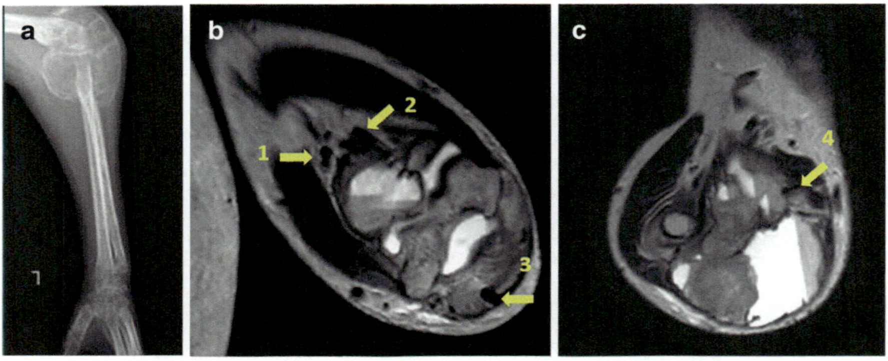

1. Brachial vessels
2. Median nerve
3. Ulnar nerve
4. Biceps tendon

Large osteosarcoma involving the proximal ulna is presented. Extraosseous component is abutting brachial vessels and median nerve anteriorly. Tumour is involving triceps insertion (Fig. 1a–c).

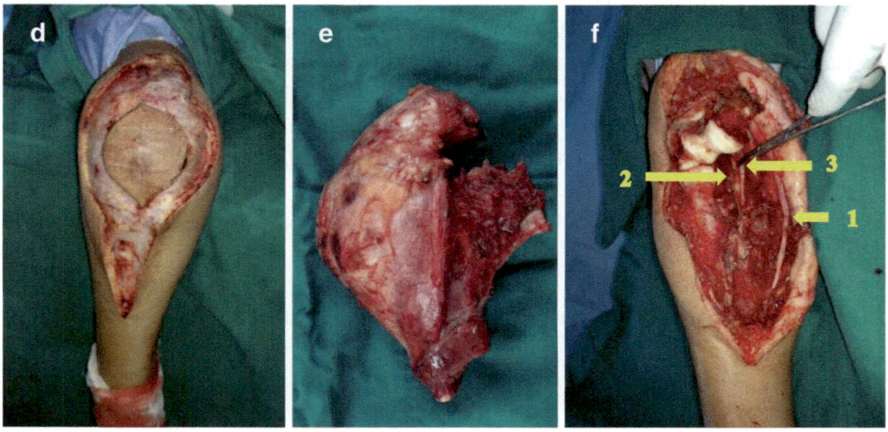

1. Ulnar nerve
2. Brachial vessels
3. Median nerve

A midline posterior incision is taken and skin flaps of adequate thickness raised islanding out the scar of open biopsy. Specimen is removed with adequate margins preserving the ulnar nerve, median nerve, and the brachial vessels (Fig. 1d–f).

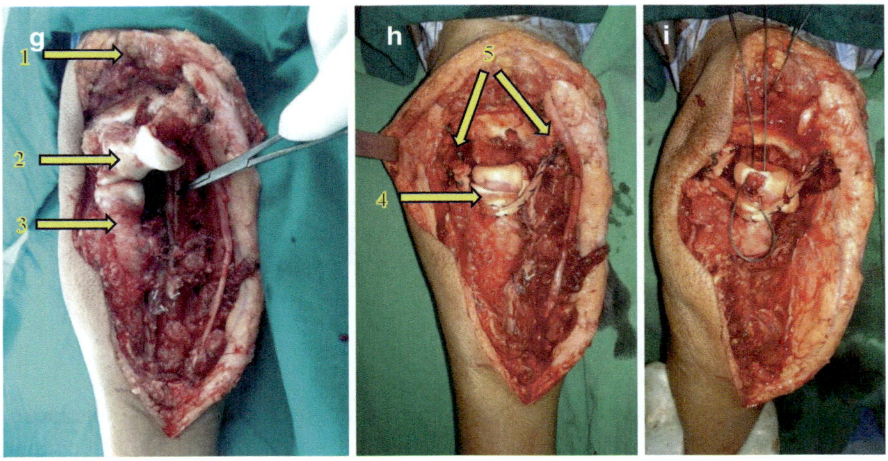

1. Triceps tendon
2. Trochlea
3. Radial neck
4. Semitendinosus graft sling
5. Humerus epicondyles

The proximal radius is mobilised medially and proximally such that radial head lies at the level of olecranon fossa. An autologous semitendinosus graft is harvested (or a tendon allograft) and used as a 360° sling around the radial neck for stability. Ends of this sling are attached to humeral epicondyles with nonabsorbable sutures maintaining neutral position at the elbow. Transosseous sutures are taken through radial head for the attachment of triceps tendon (Fig. 1g–i).

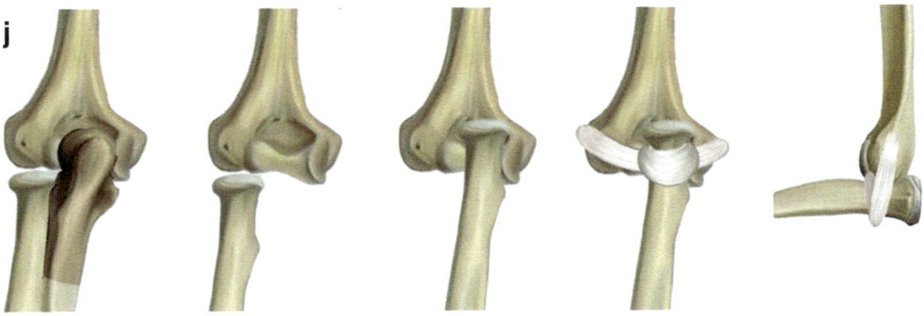

Figure 1j: Diagrammatic representation of radial neck transposition and tendon graft sling

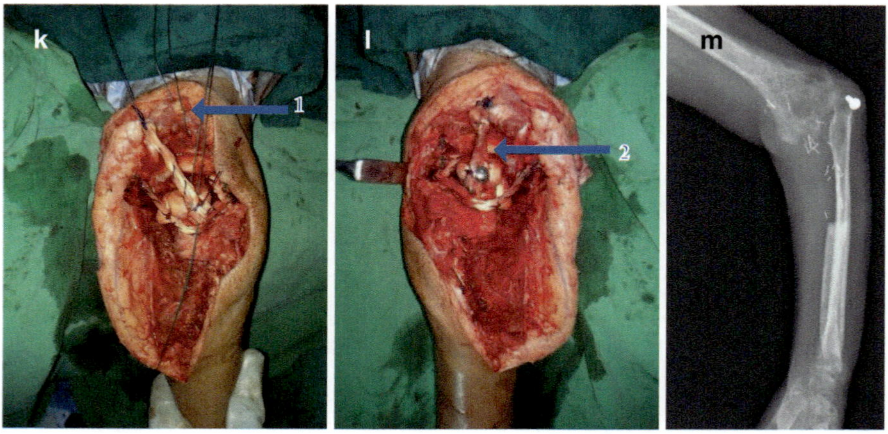

1. Triceps tendon
2. Semitendinosus graft

Since a part of triceps tendon was excised as margin, remaining semitendinosus graft was used to augment the length of the triceps tendon for a tension free repair at 90 degrees elbow flexion. Attachment of the semitendinosus graft on the radial head was reinforced with a cancellous screw and washer. Suture anchors can be used for securing the attachment of the triceps tendon on the radial head (Fig. 1k–m). After achieving haemostasis, the wound is closed in layers over a negative suction drain.

Rehabilitation

The forearm is immobilised in neutral position with the elbow in 90-degree flexion in an above elbow slab for 4 weeks. After 4 weeks, elbow and forearm movement are started using a hinged elbow brace that provides mediolateral stability. Assessment of stability during rehabilitation guides the timing for discontinuation of the hinged elbow brace, and it usually occurs around 10 weeks from surgery. Muscle strengthening exercises are continued, and 3 months after surgery, patients are allowed to use the limb for light household activities.

Right side is the operated limb—showing range of extension, supination, and flexion (Fig. 1n).

n

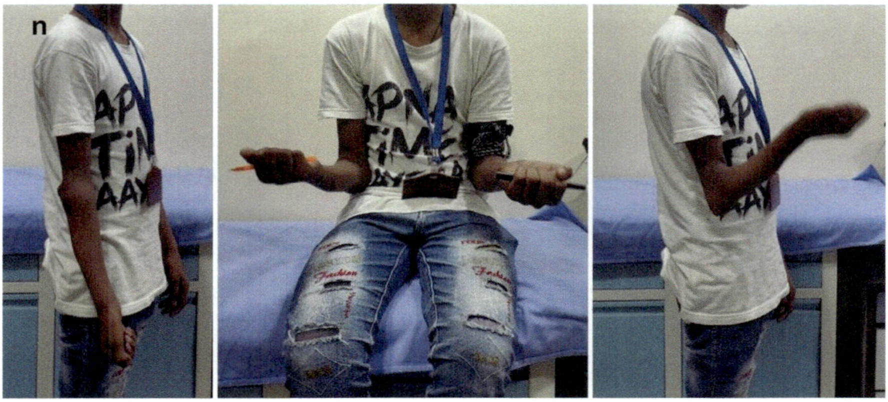

Suggested Reading

1. Rydholm A. Reconstruction after resection of the proximal ulna. Report of a case of chondrosarcoma. Acta Orthop Scand. 1987;58(6):671–2.
2. Duncan SFM, Athanasian EA, Healey JH. Radius neck-to-humerus trochlea transposition for elbow reconstruction after resection of the proximal ulna: report of 2 cases. J Hand Surg Am. 2008;33(8):1384–7.
3. Houdek MT, Gupta S, Griffin AM, Wunder JS, Ferguson PC. Radial neck-to-humerus transposition for elbow reconstruction following oncologic resection of the proximal ulna: a report of two cases. JBJS Case Connect. 2019;9(4):e0451.
4. Sułko J. Elbow reconstruction following an extensive resection of the proximal part of the ulna in a patient with Ewing sarcoma. JBJS Case Connect. 2013;3(4):e111.
5. Chen F, Xia J, Wei Y, Wang S, Wu J, Huang G, et al. Radius neck-to-humerus trochlea transposition elbow reconstruction after proximal ulnar metastatic tumor resection: case and literature review. Eur J Med Res. 2012;17(1):23.

Distal Radius Resection

Wan Faisham Nu'man Bin Wan Ismail and Ajay Puri

Introduction

Surgical resection of the distal radius tumour creates a bony defect and warrants reconstruction to achieve painless hand function. Achieving oncological margins to minimise risk of local recurrence while preserving good hand function are the main aims in this location with unique anatomical constraints, such as proximity to complex joints, limited surrounding soft tissue coverage and close relationship of important vessels, nerves, and tendons.

W. F. N. B. W. Ismail (✉)
Prince Court Medical Center, Kuala Lumpur, Malaysia

Orthopaedic Oncology Reconstructive Unit, Universiti Sains Malaysia, Kubang Kerian, Kelantan, Malaysia

A. Puri (✉)
Department of Surgical Oncology, Tata Memorial Centre, Mumbai, India

A. Puri, W. F. N. B. W. Ismail (eds.), *Atlas of Orthopedic Oncology Volume 2*,
https://doi.org/10.1007/978-981-95-8962-3_16

Surgical Anatomy

Distal radius is covered by pronator quadratus anteriorly and thick fibro-osseous structures posteriorly. However, there are a few potential areas for direct tumour infiltration. Anatomical correlation to the distal radius must be understood for surgical margin when the deep layer of anatomical boundaries is violated by large tumour or inappropriate biopsy.

- Carpal tunnel is formed by two layers: a deep carpal arch and superficial flexor retinaculum. The deep carpal arch forms a concave surface, which is converted into a tunnel by the overlying flexor retinaculum (transverse carpal ligament). It contains the median nerve and nine tendons: four tendons of the flexor digitorum superficialis, four tendons of the flexor digitorum profundus, and one tendon of the flexor pollicis longus.
- The space of Parona is a potential space in the distal forearm/volar wrist, deep in the flexor tendons. The space lies between the fascia of the pronator quadratus muscle and flexor digitorum profundus tendon sheath.
- Guyon's canal formed by the roof of the canal is created by the volar carpal ligament. The transverse carpal ligament forms the dorsal portion/floor of the canal. It contains the ulnar nerve and vessels and must be evaluated in large tumour with ulnar extension.
- Dorsal ligament and fibro-osseous tunnel form a part of the dorsal radiocarpal joint capsule and connects the dorsal radial rim with the lunate and triquetral bone. It is a broad and trapezoid like shaped ligament. It is connected to the extensor retinaculum, a fibrous, thickened band that holds the extensor tendons at the dorsum of the wrist.

The radial artery crosses the elbow distal to tendon of the biceps brachii muscle and travels along the medial aspect of the neck of the radius to the styloid process of the anterior surface of the radius. It is situated below the brachioradialis muscle lateral to the flexor carpi radialis. The radial artery is at risk in large tumour that can breach the deep anatomical boundaries covering the distal radius. At the wrist joint, the artery winds laterally around the wrist, passing through the anatomical snuff box and between the heads of the first dorsal interosseous muscle. It passes anteriorly between the heads of the adductor pollicis and becomes the deep palmar arch, which joins with the deep branch of the ulnar artery. The terminal branch must be mobilised prior to distal resection at the wrist joint or row carpectomy.

The ulnar artery lies medial to the flexor digitorum profundus, and distal to the flexor carpi ulnaris and flexor digitorum superficialis and finally enters Guyon's canal accompanied by the ulnar nerve. It is accompanied by two venae commitantes and overlapped in its middle third by the flexor carpi ulnaris. The ulnar nerve lies on the medial side of the lower two-thirds of the artery, and the palmar cutaneous branch of the nerve descends on the lower part of the vessel to the palm of the hand.

Anterior interosseous artery is a terminal branch of the ulnar artery. It pierces the interosseous membrane behind the pronator quadratus muscle. It must be ligated for distal radius resection and is a good recipient vessel for vascularised fibula graft.

The median nerve descends to the elbow in a superficial course. Initially, it is lateral to the brachial artery and eventually becomes medial. It passes between the deep and superficial heads of the pronator teres muscle and runs between the flexor digitorum profundus and flexor digitorum superficialis and enters the hand through the carpal tunnel. It is rarely involved in the tumour unless the Parona space is infiltrated or contaminated by procedures.

Assessment

Distal radius is covered by the pronator quadratus anteriorly and thick fibro-osseous structures posteriorly. However, there are few potential areas for direct tumour infiltration. Parona space is an extension from carpal tunnel containing the flexor tendon and median nerve boarder by flexor digitorum profundus and pronator quadratus. Pronator quadratus muscle is a good barrier for tumour extension to the Parona space.

- Wrist joint-wrist joint capsule, radio lunate, and radio scaphoid joint
- Distal radioulnar joint
- Attachment of the brachioradialis tendon
- For proximal tumour above the parona space
- Origin of the flexor pollicis longus, radialis longus, and brevis and flexor digitorum on the palmar aspect fibro-osseous tunnel, tendon of extensor compartment, and extensor muscle origin must be evaluated for direct infiltration and extension of the tumour

Anatomical boundaries around the distal radius for assessment to achieve wide resection include the following:

- Pronator quadratus
- Dorsal ligament and fibro-osseous tunnel
- Triangular fibrocartilage and distal radioulnar joint
- Wrist joint and capsule
- Parona space and its content
- Origin of the flexor pollicis longus/digitorum profundus
- Insertion of the brachioradialis

Simple Resection with Proximal Fibula Reconstruction

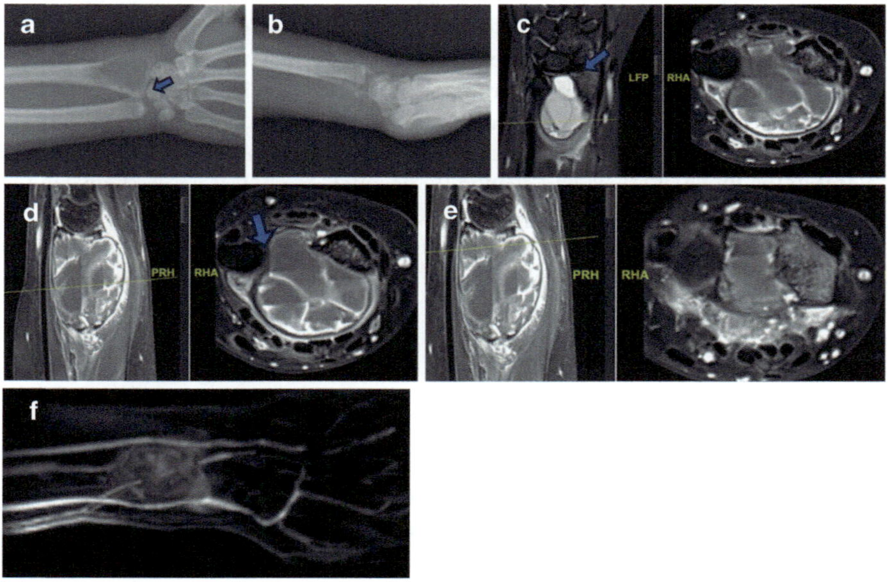

A case of distal radius giant cell tumour with infiltration to the pronator quadratus. However, the posterior fibro-osseous ligament was still intact with good margin. The distal radioulnar joint and wrist joint capsule were free without infiltration (Fig. 1a–f).

Surgical Steps (Fig. 1g–j)

The surgical margin is narrow in the distal radius due to close proximity with the fibro-osseous tunnel at the dorsal compartment. Pronator quadratus is a good anatomical barrier against tumour extension anteriorly. Thus, it protects against contamination of main flexor tendons and neuro-vascular bundles.

- A cuff of muscle must be removed together with tumour that breaks the anterior cortex and extends anteriorly.
- Dorsal fibro-osseous fascia strongly attached to the radius prevents tumour extension and infiltration of the extensors tendon and its pulley systems. It is a good anatomical barrier, and quality adequate margin can be achieved by elevating all extensor tendon from the fibro-osseous tunnel for function as well as good margin.

- Distal radioulnar joint can be potentially contaminated in aggressive tumour. Evaluation of the dorsal wrist ligament and ventral radio-lunate and radio-scaphoid ligament is important if we plan to use the ligament and capsule for wrist joint reconstruction with proximal fibula.

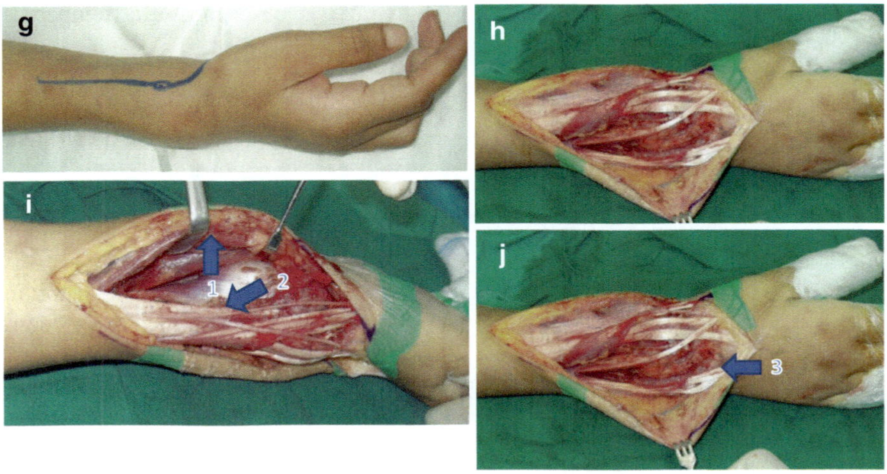

1. Radial vessels and entire flexor tendon mobilised from the pronator quadratus exposing the volar wrist joint
2. Superficial radial nerve
3. Extensor retinacula mobilised ulnarly exposing the extensor tendon

Option of Reconstruction

Resection arthroplasty: a non-vascularised or vascularised autogenous fibular graft and allograft replacement

- Proximal fibula graft has a near anatomical similarity in shape and size to the distal radius and is suitable for mobile reconstruction
- Custom prosthetic replacement
- ulnar translocation

Arthrodesis/wrist fusion (pan-carpal fusion)

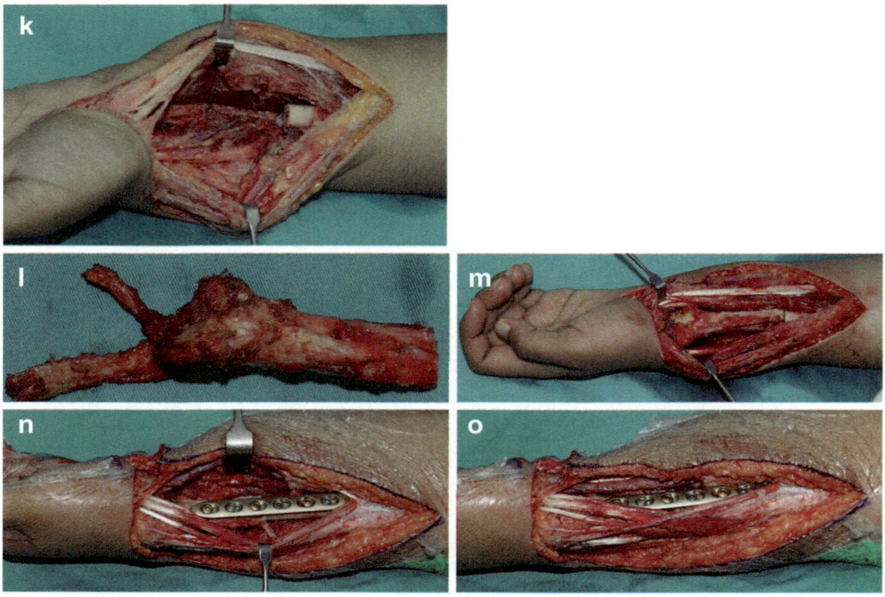

Biological reconstruction with autologous proximal fibula graft has advantages of anatomical congruency of the carpal joint, rapid incorporation, and minimal donor site morbidity. Reconstruction of the fibula-carpal joint by suturing the lateral collateral ligament and biceps femoris tendon of the fibula to the remaining capsule. Remaining capsule and ligament is sutured to the fibula head for wrist joint stability. The exposure for reconstruction and stability assessment is best done prior stabilisation with plate and screw (Fig. 1k–o).

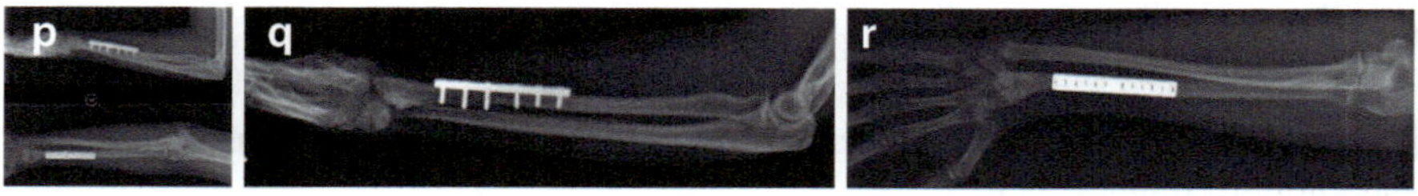

Wrist reconstruction developed a carpal subluxation after 8 years and disabling wrist pain. Degenerative arthritis between the head of the fibula and carpal bones occurs due to articular incongruity (Fig. 1p–r). No articular remodelling observed following this reconstruction, particularly in adults.

Major Resection with Vascularised Fibula Flap

Resection of the distal radius with extensive soft tissue extension and long segment of bone needs a vascularised bone to minimise wound complication and late resorption and fracture of the fibula graft. Radial vascular bundles can be explored as a donor vessel for vascularised fibula graft. Furthermore, it provides good soft tissue cover for mobile reconstruction and loose soft tissue for tendon gliding. Anterior interosseous vessel is also an option for vessel reconstruction.

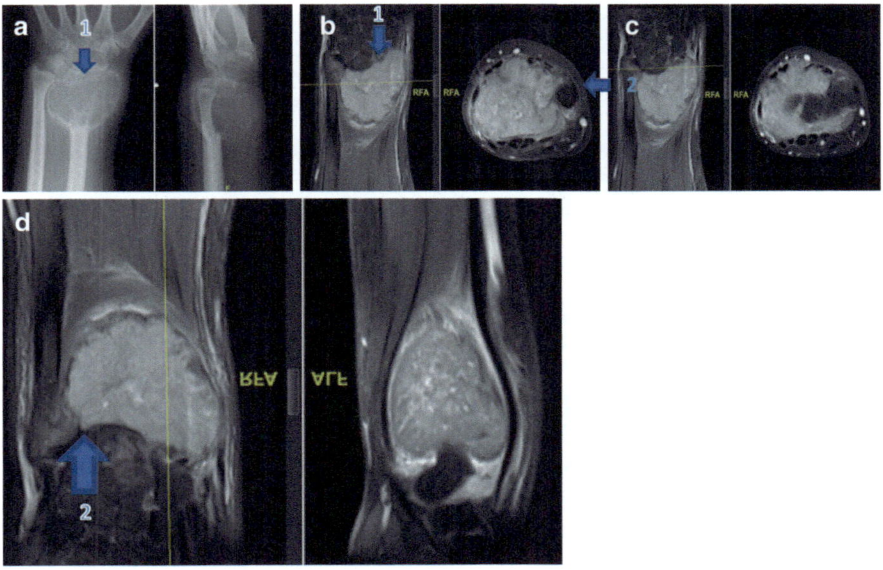

1. Wrist joint and proximal row of the carpus involved by the tumour
2. Distal radioulnar joint was involved

Distal radius giant cell tumour with wrist joint contamination and scaphoid involvement. The extra-osseous component involves the entire pronator quadratus to the ulna insertion and dorsal and volar ligament to the proximal row of carpus. The tumour involved the distal radioulnar joint and was abutting over the ulna (Fig. 2a–d).

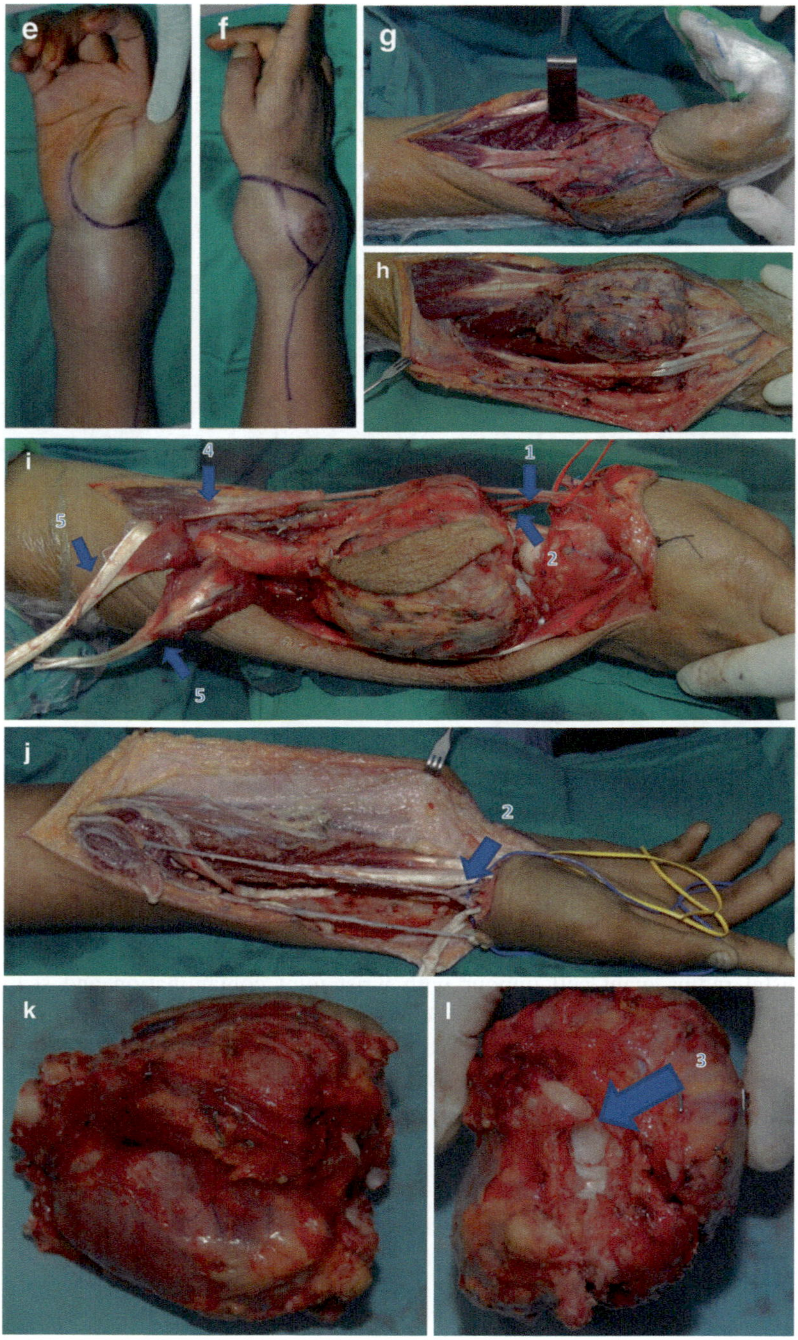
e
f
g
h
i
4
1
5
2
5
j
2
k
l
3

1. Superficial radial nerve
2. Mobilisation of the radial artery to its terminal branch to form palmar arch and dorsal interossei artery
3. Second row of the carpus

Large tumour that infiltrates to the carpus bone needs good exposure within the carpal tunnel by elevating the common flexors and median nerve. The dorsal tendon is elevated from the fibro-osseous tunnel and should be excised as margin. The radial artery that crosses the radial border to the dorsal compartment must be released and secured. Resection of the first row can be performed through the radial border by ulna deviation and subsequently dorsal and volar ligament excision by palmar and dorsiflexion of the wrist (Fig. 2e–l).

Extensor tendon can be sacrificed for better surgical margin and provided as tendon graft for function with remnants of tendon:

4. Brachioradialis
5. Flexor/extensor carpi radialis and ulnaris, which are not used once wrist joint fuse

The first-row carpus resection was done to improve the surgical margin in view of wrist joint contamination. The optimum hand function is expected with solid fusion. The fascia of the fasciocutaneous vascularised fibula was mobilised dorsally to improve gliding extensor function and minimise bowstringing of the tendons. Radioulnar joint stability also can be reconstructed in a similar manner.

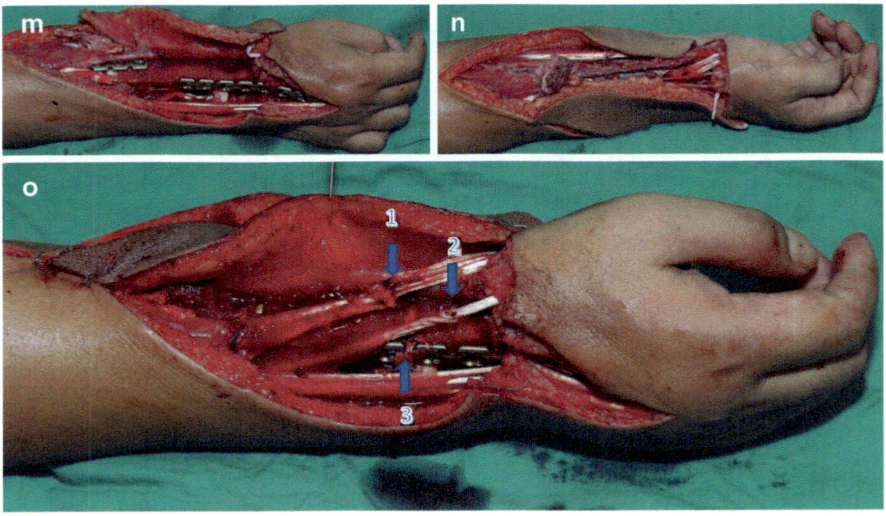

Reconstruction of:

1. Extensor pollicis longus
2. Abductor pollicis
3. Distal radioulnar joint

The finger cascade of the hand was maintained

Wrist flexors and extensors can be sacrificed in wrist fusion reconstruction. Part of the tendon can be used as a tendon graft for extensors of the finger in case the tendon is involved by the tumour. In proximal row resection of the carpus with distal radius, option of reconstruction is limited to wrist fusion with vascularised fibula graft. Distal ulna is not stable and must be stabilised with the fascia of the fibula graft. The cascade of the finger flexors was maintained with proper tension of the flexor and extensor tendons (Fig. 2m–q).

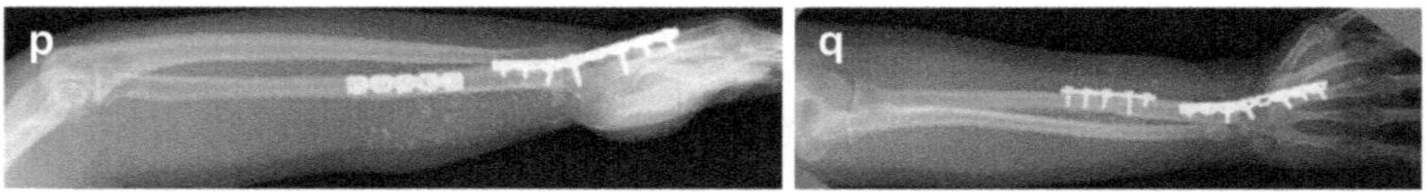

Resection of Both the Radius and Ulna

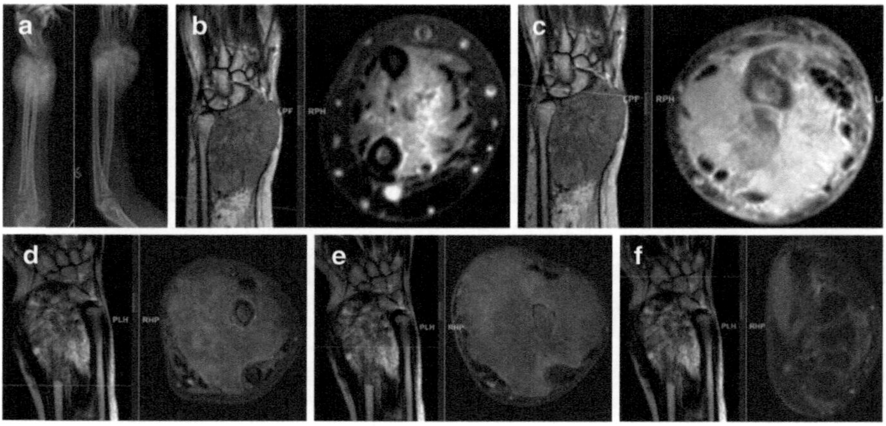

A case of osteosarcoma distal radius with good response to chemotherapy due to massive early soft tissue extension the soft tissue component entirely involving the volar and dorsal compartment and circumferentially abutting the ulna. The carpal tunnel and space of Parona are still preserved with patent ulna vessels. The medial and ulnar nerve still have a clear plane from the tumour margin. The distal radius osteosarcoma also shows extension to the proximal row of carpus and this needs to be resected together for oncological clearance (Fig. 3a–f).

Massive tissue involvement in malignant sarcoma needs more wider margins, especially the palmar compartment. Ulnar bone must be removed together with the radius as part of resection. Clinically, skin over the radial border was thin and tethered to the tumour and must be included as margin (Fig. 3g–k).

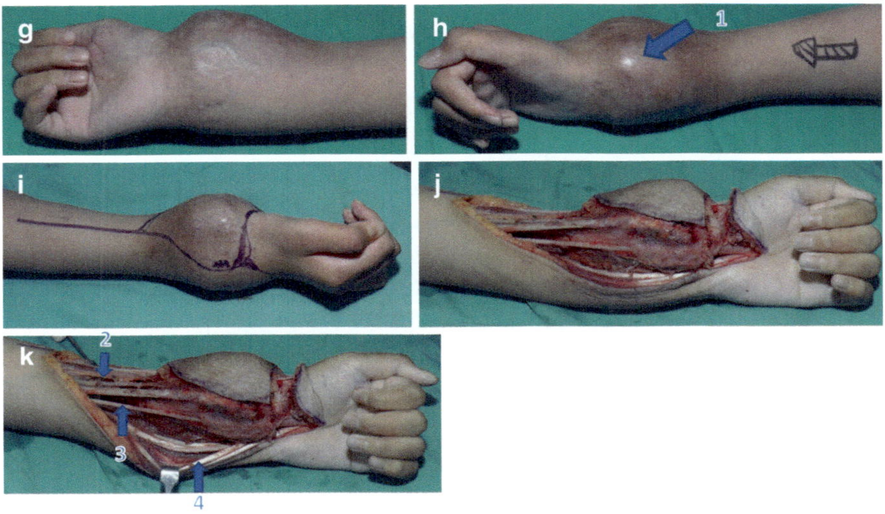

1. Skin involvement and biopsy tract as included in the resection margin
2. Radial vessels involved—included as margin and remnant vessels is a good recipient for vascularised fibula graft
3. Median nerve explored and freed from the tumour through epineural margin resection
4. Flexor digitorum superficialis muscle and tendon was mobilised, the flexor digitorum profundus and pollicis longus in the carpal tunnel were transected, leaving the muscle origin to be included as margin

Flexor digitorum profundus was attached to the tumour and its muscle origin must be included as part of margin. The remaining tendon was attached to the superficial tendons to achieve group flexion of the fingers. Flexor pollicis longus can be reconstructed to the remaining tendon of flexor carpi radials for thumb flexion. The ulna border was approach by elevating the lateral part of flexor superficialis and profundus together with ulna neurovascular structures (Fig. 3l, m).

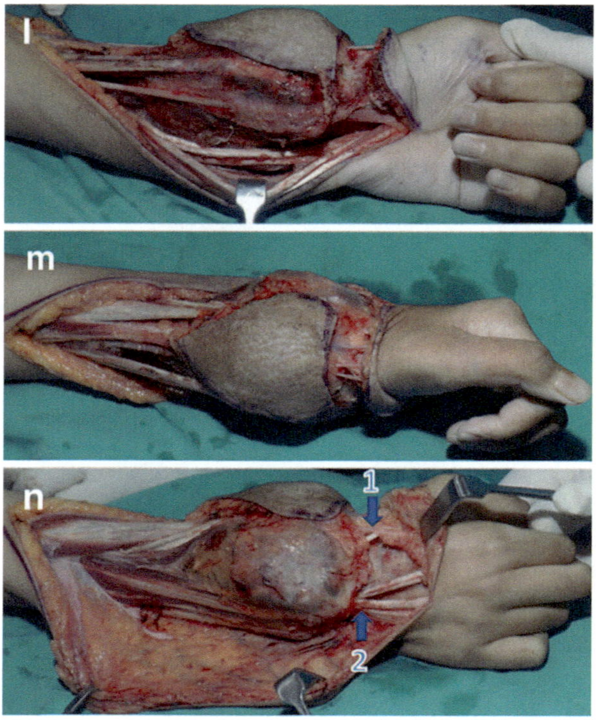

1. Extensor and abductor pollicis tendon trapped within the tumour
2. Extensor digitorum communis and digiti minimi were pushed ulnarly and not involved

Dorsally, the distal ulnar was freed by elevating the fascia with subcutaneous tissue. The extensor wrist retinaculum was mobilised to expose the entire fibro-osseous compartment. The tendon was mobilised from the tumour prior to resection and the involved tendon was resected segmentally (Fig. 3m–r).

- Resection of both the radius and ulna with cuff of tissue attached to both segment resected.

Multiple tendons were resected segmentally: flexor pollicis longus, flexor digitorum profundus, extensor pollicis longus, and abductor pollicis longus.

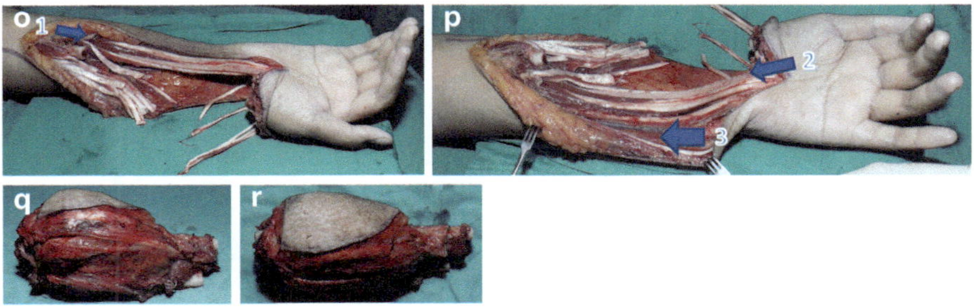

Reconstruction options

- Palmaris longus, flexor radialis longus, and extensor radialis can be used to reconstruct flexion, extension and abduction of the thumb.
- For resection of FDP—the remaining tendon is tagged to the FDS as it has similar function.

Vascularised graft is aligned to the ulna for better function of the elbow and centralised to the 2nd and 3rd metacarpal bone. In general, the fibular graft is best reconstructed to the ulna for centralisation of the wrist. However, if the remaining ulna bone is adequately long, radial reconstruction and wrist fusion is an option and the functional outcome is expected to be good (Fig. 3s–aa).

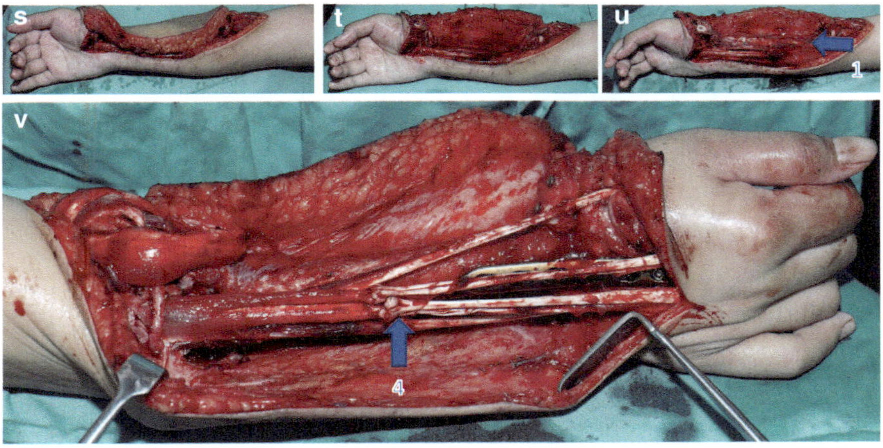

1. Remnant of the radial vessels used as recipient peroneal vessels of the fibular graft
2. Median nerve
3. Ulnar vessels and nerve
4. Reconstruction of the common extensor and extensor pollicis tendon

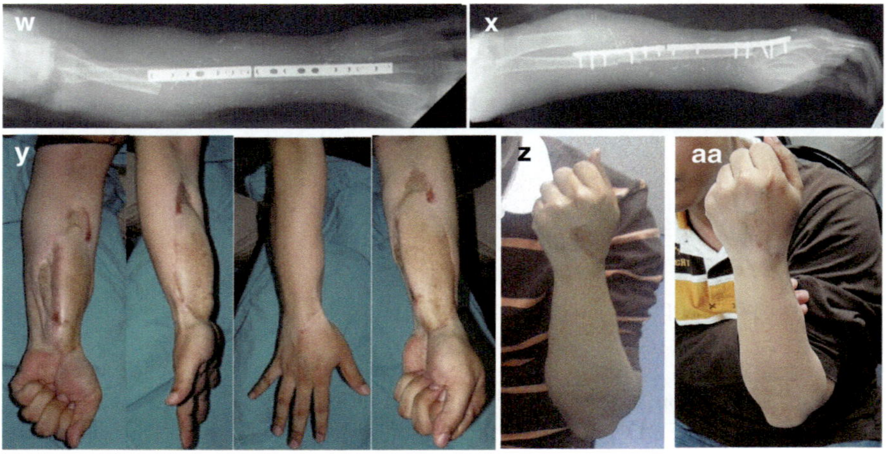

Reconstruction of Distal Radius with Long Segment Iliac Crest 'Deep Circumflex Iliac Artery-DCIA Flap'

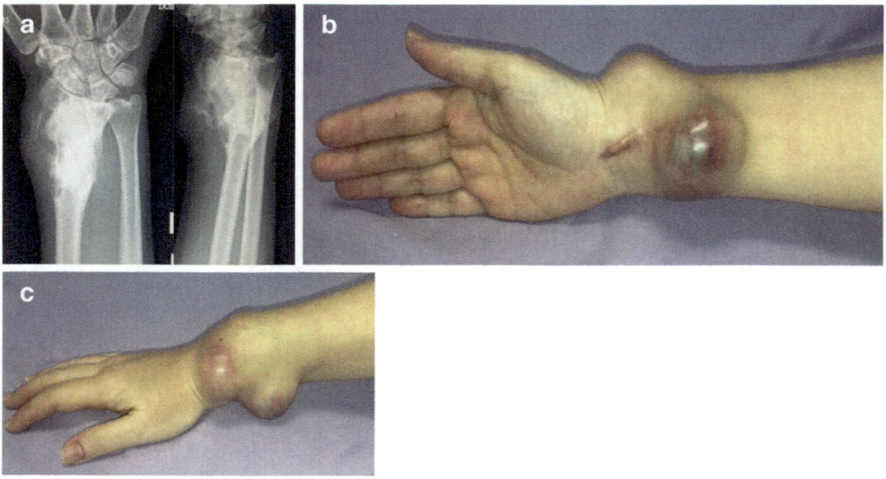

A case of recurrent giant cell tumour following extended curettage, note multiple area of contamination and tumour infiltration. Major parts of the skin were involved and must be removed as part of oncological margin (Fig. 4a–c).

Bilateral peroneal magna artery is a rare instance where vascularised fibula graft is contraindicated. DCIA provides osseous length with soft tissue. However, due to anatomical curvature of the iliac crest the positioning for reconstruction of the distal radius is a bit tricky (Fig. 4d–f).

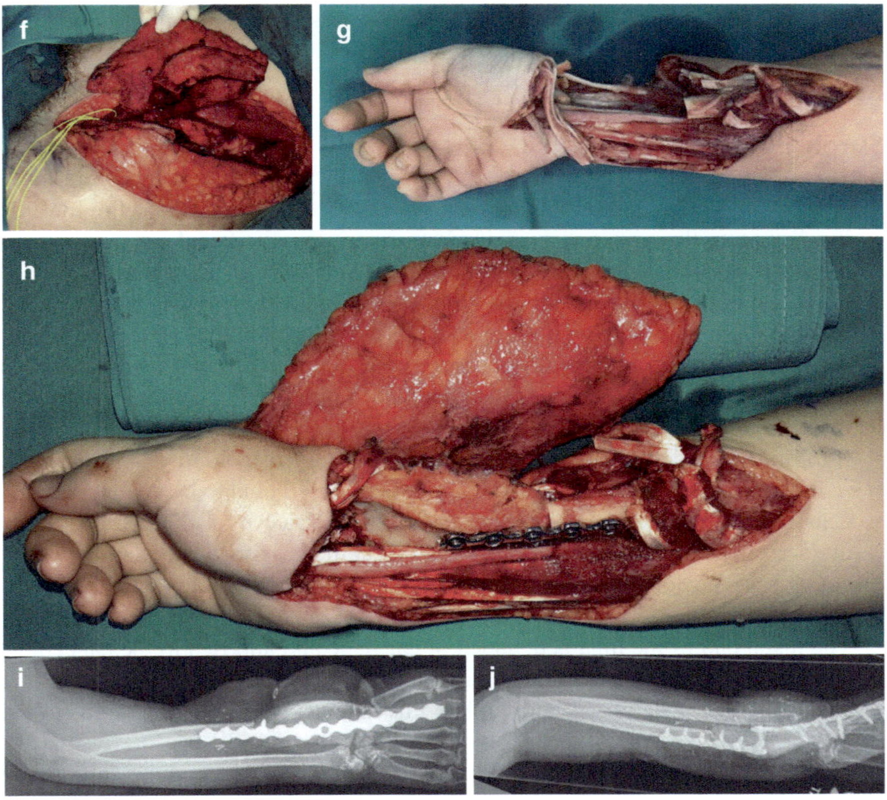

Long segment of the iliac crest is nonanatomical for reconstruction. However, curvature of the iliac crest can be positioned to maintain 30° dorsal angulations for wrist joint fusion (Fig. 4g–j). Care must be taken to maintain adequate radial length for good stability of the distal ulnar joint for rotational movement. Fasciocutaneous flap provides for soft tissue reconstruction, which is important for reconstruction of skin defect and gliding of repaired tendon in recurrent tumour.

Reconstruction with Ulna Transposition

Ajay Puri

Transposition of the ipsilateral ulna as a vascularised strut graft to bridge the defect after distal radius excision with wrist arthrodesis is yet another option for reconstruction.

Surgical Tips

- A single incision sited on the dorsolateral aspect of the radius curving towards the dorsum of the wrist (as opposed to two incisions, one dorsal and one ventral) provides adequate exposure to both dorsal and ventral surfaces of the tumour and enables safe resection while preserving neuro vascular structures and tendons.
- The ulna osteotomy is best done at a level 5 mm proximal to the proximal radial osteotomy. If the osteotomy is done more proximal, it is difficult to transpose the ulna (moving the osteotomised ulna distally in order to align it with the radius results in excessive soft tissue stripping).
- Prior to transposing the ulna the ulnar styloid is also osteotomised preserving it in its original position thus enabling the osteotomised ulna to be shifted radially.
- Care should be taken to ensure that the periosteal sleeve has been transversely divided circumferentially all around the ulna at the proximal osteotomy else you could have postoperative synostosis between the (neo) radius and the residual ulna.
- The distal end of the ulna is denuded of cartilage and apposed to the cancellous surfaces of the similarly denuded scaphoid and lunate.
- The construct is stabilised with a plate that extends from the host radius to the 2nd or 3rd metacarpal.
- Prior to fixing the plate check that the radius and the wrist are in the appropriate rotational alignment with respect to each other such that a complete range of prono supination is possible.

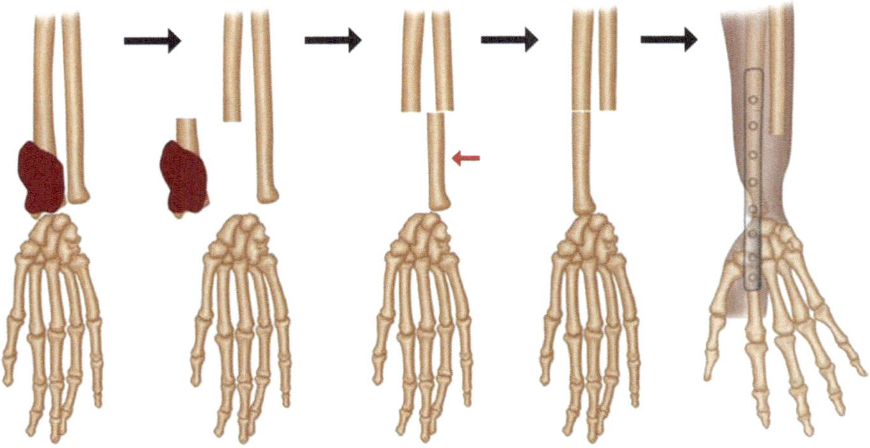

Schematic representation of proposed surgery

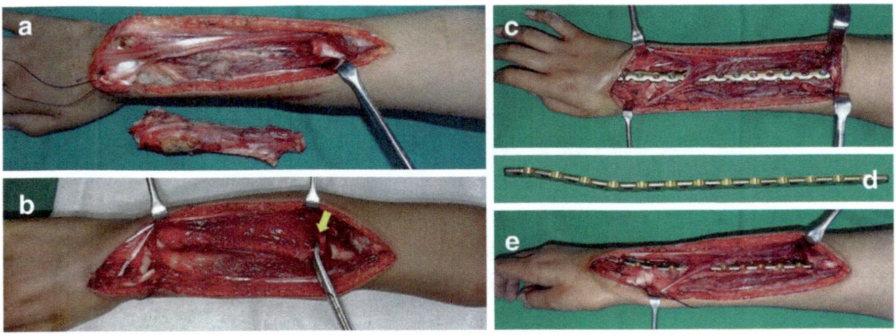

Distal radius tumour resected and osteotomised ulna [yellow arrow] being translocated to fill the radial defect and stabilised with an appropriately contoured plate (Fig. 5a–e).

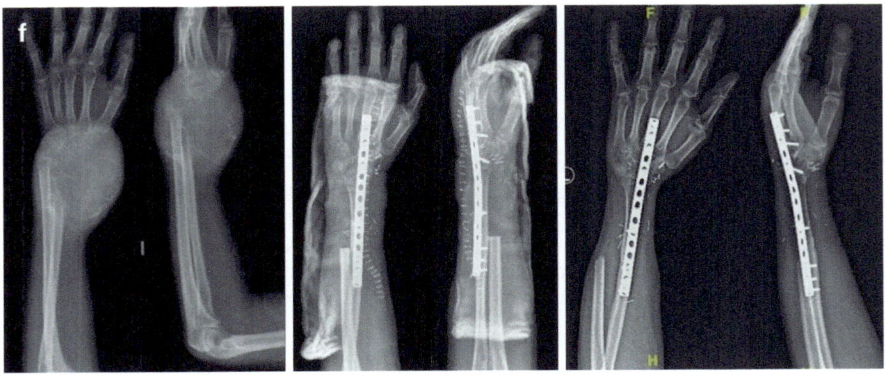

Case of giant cell tumour treated with excision and reconstructed with ulna transposition—initial X-ray, immediate postoperative X–ray, and 2-year follow-up X-ray (Fig. 5f).

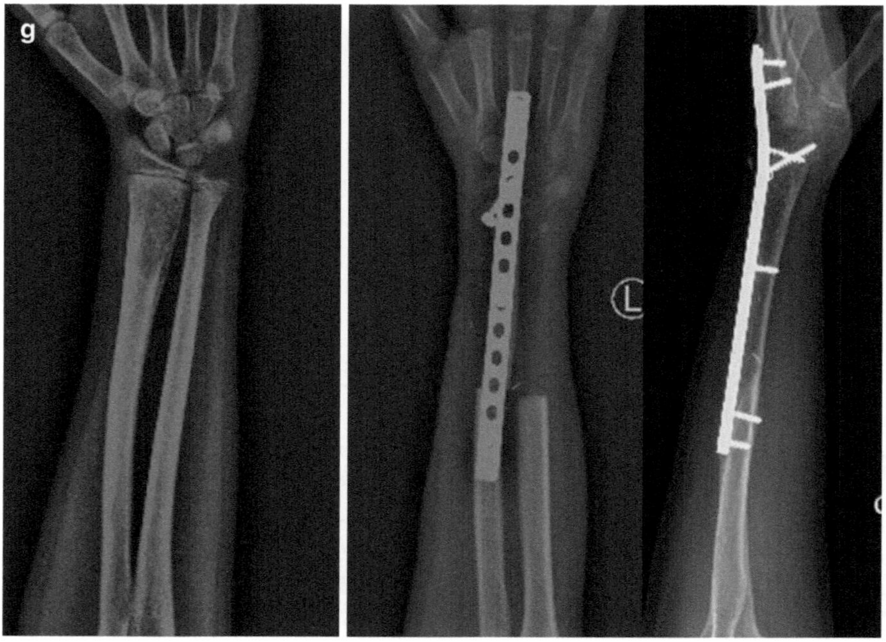

Case of Ewing sarcoma treated with excision and reconstructed with ulna transposition—initial X ray and 3-year follow-up X-ray (Fig. 5g)

Acknowledgements The author thanks Professor Wan Azman Wan Sulaiman, Professor Arman Zaharil Mat Saad, and Professor Ahmad Sukari Halim from the plastic reconstructive unit at Universiti Sains Malaysia and MSU Medical Centre, Management and Science University for their contributions and team member for managing the patients. All plastic reconstructive and microsurgery surgical procedures were performed by the team members. The author also thanks Professor Arman Zaharil Mat Saad, Nor Hazla Muhammad Haflah, Dr. Mohamed Hafizudin Abdullah Sani, and Dr. Levin Kesu Belani for their contributions on reconstruction DCIA flap of distal radius.

Suggested Reading

1. Puri A. Biological reconstruction of the forearm, wrist, and hand – II: transposition of the distal ulna. In: Orthopaedic surgical oncology for bone tumors. Springer Nature Switzerland; 2022. p. 503–13.
2. Choo CY, Mat-Saad AM, Wan-Azman WS, Wan Z, Nor-Azman MZ, Yahya S, Faisham WI. Functional outcome after treatment of aggressive tumours in the distal radius: comparison between reconstruction using proximal fibular graft and wrist fusion. Malay Orthopaed J. 2018;11(3):19–23.

3. Özger H, Alpan B, Tetik C. Biological reconstruction of the forearm, wrist, and hand – I: Free vascular fibula. In: Orthopaedic surgical oncology for bone tumors. Springer Nature Switzerland; 2022. p. 493–503.
4. Innocenti M, Delcroix L, Manfrini M, Ceruso M, Capanna R. Vascularized proximal fibular epiphyseal transfer for distal radial reconstruction. J Bone Joint Surg Am. 2004;86-A(7):1504–11.
5. Weber KL. General considerations: elbow and wrist. In: Master techniques in orthopaedic surgery orthopaedic oncology and complex reconstruction. Lippincott Williams & Wilkins, A Wolters Kluwer; 2011. p. 371–7.
6. Leung PC, Chan KT. Giant cell tumor of the distal end of the radius treated by the resection and free vascularized iliac crest graft. Clinical Orthop Rel Res. 1986;202:232–6.
7. Ayerza MA, Aponte-Tinao LA, Muscolo DL. Distal radius osteoarticular allograft. Orthopaedic oncology and complex reconstruction. Master technique in orthopaedic surgery. Walters Kluwer, Lippincott Willim & Wilkins.
8. Ayerza MA, Aponte-Tinao LA, Luis Muscolo D. Distal radius osteoarticular allograft master techniques in orthopaedic surgery orthopaedic oncology and complex reconstruction. Lippincott Williams & Wilkins, A Wolters Kluwer; 2011.
9. Puri A, Gulia A, Agarwal MG, Reddy K. Ulnar translocation after excision of a Campanacci grade – 3 giant-cell tumour of the distal radius: an effective method of reconstruction. J Bone Joint Surg Br. 2010;92(6):875–9.
10. Sadek AF, Halim AS, Faisham WI. Does distal radius reconstruction by free epiphyseal transfer lead to inferior radioulnar dissociation. Ann Clin Case Rep. 2016;1:1075.
11. Kumta Leung Ping Chung SM, Yip K, Kew J, Ponozzo K. Vascularized bone grafts in the treatment of juxta-articular giant-cell tumors of the bone. J Reconstruct Microsurg. 14(3):185–90.

GPSR Compliance

The European Union's (EU) General Product Safety Regulation (GPSR) is a set of rules that requires consumer products to be safe and our obligations to ensure this.

If you have any concerns about our products, you can contact us on ProductSafety@springernature.com

In case Publisher is established outside the EU, the EU authorized representative is:

Springer Nature Customer Service Center GmbH
Europaplatz 3
69115 Heidelberg, Germany

Batch number: 10726135

Printed by Printforce, the Netherlands